Recent Progress in the Treatment of Acute Lymphoblastic Leukemia

Guest Editors

WENDY STOCK, MD
MEIR WETZLER, MD

HEMATOLOGY/ONCOLOGY CLINICS OF NORTH AMERICA

www.hemonc.theclinics.com

October 2009 • Volume 23 • Number 5

SAUNDERS an imprint of ELSEVIER, Inc.

W.B. SAUNDERS COMPANY
A Division of Elsevier Inc.

1600 John F. Kennedy Blvd. ● Suite 1800 ● Philadelphia, PA 19103-2899

http://www.theclinics.com

HEMATOLOGY/ONCOLOGY CLINICS OF NORTH AMERICA Volume 23, Number 5
October 2009 ISSN 0889-8588, ISBN 13: 978-1-4377-1227-8, ISBN 10: 1-4377-1227-4

Editor: Kerry Holland

Hematology/Oncology Clinics (ISSN 0889-8588) is published bimonthly by Elsevier Inc., 360 Park Avenue South, New York, NY 10010-1710. Months of issue are February, April, June, August, October, and December. Application to mail at periodicals postage rates is pending at New York, NY and at additional mailing offices. Subscription prices are $283.00 per year (domestic individuals), $439.00 per year (domestic institutions), $141.00 per year (domestic students/residents), $321.00 per year (Canadian individuals), $537.00 per year (Canadian institutions) $382.00 per year (international individuals), $537.00 per year (international institutions), and $191.00 per year (international and Canadian students/residents). International air speed delivery is included in all *Clinics* subscription prices. All prices are subject to change without notice. **POSTMASTER:** Send address changes to *Hematology/Oncology Clinics of North America*, Elsevier Health Sciences Division, Subscription Customer Service, 3251 Riverport Lane, Maryland Heights, MO 63043. Customer Service (orders, claims, online, change of address): Elsevier Health Sciences Division, Subscription Customer Service, 3251 Riverport Lane, Maryland Heights, MO 63043. Tel: 1-800-654-2452 (U.S. and Canada); 314-447-8871(outside U.S. and Canada). Fax: 314-447-8029. E-mail: journalscustomerservice-usa@elsevier.com (for print support); journalsonlinesupport-usa@elsevier.com (for online support).

Reprints. For copies of 100 or more, of articles in this publication, please contact the Commercial Reprints Department, Elsevier Inc., 360 Park Avenue South, New York, New York 10010-1710; Tel.: 212-633-3813, Fax: 212-462-1935, E-mail: reprints@elsevier.com.

Hematology/Oncology Clinics of North America is covered in *MEDLINE/PubMed (Index Medicus), EMBASE/ Excerpta Medica, and BIOSIS.*

Printed and bound by CPI Group (UK) Ltd, Croydon, CR0 4YY

Transferred to Digital Print 2011

Contributors

GUEST EDITORS

MEIR WETZLER, MD, FACP
Professor of Medicine; and Chief, Leukemia Section, Roswell Park Cancer Institute,
Elm and Carlton Streets, Buffalo, New York

WENDY STOCK, MD
Professor of Medicine, University of Chicago Hospitals and Cancer Research Center,
Chicago, Illinois

AUTHORS

SYED A. ABUTALIB, MD
Section of Hematology and Oncology, Cancer Treatment Centers of America,
Zion, Illinois

PETER D. APLAN, MD
Genetics Branch, Center for Cancer Research, National Cancer Institute, Bethesda,
Maryland

DARIO CAMPANA, MD, PhD
Professor of Pediatrics, University of Tennessee Health Science Center; and Vice Chair for
Laboratory Research, Department of Oncology, and Member, Departments of Oncology
and Pathology, St. Jude Children's Research Hospital, Memphis, Tennessee

DANIEL J. DEANGELO, MD, PhD
Associate Professor of Medicine, Department of Medical Oncology, Dana-Farber Cancer
Institute, Harvard Medical School, Boston, Massachusetts

STEPHEN J. FORMAN, MD
Chair, Department of Hematology and Hematopoietic Cell Transplantation, City
of Hope National Medical Center; Director, Clinical Research, Department of Cancer
Immunotherapeutics and Tumor Immunology, City of Hope Comprehensive Cancer
Center, Duarte, California

DAVID P. HARPER, MD
Genetics Branch, Center for Cancer Research, National Cancer Institute; Department
of Pediatrics, Uniformed Services University of the Health Sciences, Bethesda, Maryland

LAURA A. JANZEN, PhD
Neuropsychologist, Department of Psychology, The Hospital for Sick Children, Toronto,
Ontario

SIMA JEHA, MD
Director, Leukemia/Lymphoma Developmental Therapeutics; and Member, Department
of Oncology, St. Jude Children's Research Hospital, Memphis, Tennessee

HAGOP M. KANTARJIAN, MD
Chairman; and Professor, Department of Leukemia, University of Texas M D Anderson
Cancer Center, Houston, Texas

PARTOW KEBRIAEI, MD
Assistant Professor, Department of Stem Cell Transplantation and Cellular Therapy,
The University of Texas M D Anderson Cancer Center, Houston, Texas

KRZYSZTOF MRÓZEK, MD, PhD
Division of Hematology and Oncology, Department of Internal Medicine, Comprehensive
Cancer Center, James Cancer Hospital, The Ohio State University, Columbus, Ohio

PAUL C. NATHAN, MD, MSc
Pediatric Hematologist/Oncologist, Division of Hematology/Oncology, Department of
Paediatrics, The Hospital for Sick Children; Assistant Professor of Pediatrics and Health
Policy, Management & Evaluation, The University of Toronto, Toronto, Ontario

SUSAN O'BRIEN, MD
Professor, Department of Leukemia, University of Texas M D Anderson Cancer Center,
Houston, Texas

ALBERT ORIOL, MD
Clinical Hematology Department, Institut Catala' d'Oncologia, Hospital Universitari
Germans Trias i Pujol, Badalona, Universitat Autonoma de Barcelona, Badalona, Spain

CHING-HON PUI, MD
Co-Leader, Hematological Malignancies Program; Fahad Nassar Al-Rashid Chair of
Leukemia Research Professor; and Chair, Department of Oncology, St. Jude Children's
Research Hospital, Memphis, Tennessee

FARHAD RAVANDI, MD
Associate Professor, Department of Leukemia, The University of Texas M D Anderson
Cancer Center, Houston, Texas

JOSEP-MARIA RIBERA, MD, PhD
Clinical Hematology Department, Institut Catala' d'Oncologia, Hospital Universitari
Germans Trias i Pujol, Badalona, Universitat Autonoma de Barcelona, Badalona

WENDY STOCK, MD
Professor of Medicine, University of Chicago Hospitals and Cancer Research Center,
Chicago, Illinois

DEBORAH A. THOMAS, MD
Associate Professor, Department of Leukemia, University of Texas M D Anderson Cancer
Center, Houston, Texas

KAREN WASILEWSKI-MASKER, MSc, MD
Pediatric Hematologist/Oncologist, Aflac Cancer Center and Blood Disorders Service,
Childhood Cancer Program; Assistant Professor of Pediatrics, Emory University School
of Medicine, Atlanta, Georgia

MEIR WETZLER, MD, FACP
Professor of Medicine; and Chief, Leukemia Section, Roswell Park Cancer Institute,
Buffalo, New York

Contents

Preface   **xi**

Meir Wetzler and Wendy Stock

Monoclonal AntibodyTherapy with Rituximab for Acute Lymphoblastic Leukemia   **949**

Deborah A. Thomas, Susan O'Brien, and Hagop M. Kantarjian

Significant advances have been achieved in the treatment of acute lymphoblastic leukemia (ALL) with the incorporation of targeted therapy agents. Targeting leukemia surface antigens with monoclonal antibodies is another promising strategy. This article comprehensively reviews available data regarding the use of rituximab for the treatment of Burkitt-type leukemia/lymphoma and CD20-positive precursor B-cell ALL. The incorporation of rituximab into frontline chemotherapy regimens for Burkitt-type leukemia/lymphoma appears to improve outcome. Preliminary data regarding the use of rituximab in frontline therapy for CD20- positive precursor B-cell ALL suggest its use may also be beneficial, particularly for the younger subsets.

Risk-adapted Treatment of Pediatric Acute Lymphoblastic Leukemia   **973**

Sima Jeha and Ching-Hon Pui

Optimal use of antileukemic agents and stringent application of risk-directed therapy in clinical trials have resulted in steady improvement in the outcome of children with acute lymphoblastic leukemia, with current cure rates exceeding 80% in developed countries. The intensity of treatment varies substantially among subsets of patients, as therapy is designed to reduce acute and long-term toxicity in low-risk groups while improving outcomes in poor risk groups by treatment intensification. Recent advances in genome-wide screening techniques, pharmacogenomic studies, and development of molecular therapeutics are ushering in an era of more refined personalized therapy.

Cytogenetics and Molecular Genetics of Acute Lymphoblastic Leukemia   **991**

Krzysztof Mrózek, David P. Harper, and Peter D. Aplan

Acute lymphoblastic leukemia (ALL) is a malignant disease that often features nonrandom numerical or structural chromosome aberrations that can be detected microscopically. The application of contemporary genome-wide molecular analyses is revealing additional genetic alterations that are not detectable cytogenetically. This article describes the cytogenetic methodology and summarizes major cytogenetic findings and their clinical relevance in ALL. The article provides a review of modern molecular techniques and their application in the research on the genetics and epigenetics of ALL.

Allogenic Hematopoietic Cell Transplantation for Acute Lymphoblastic Leukemia in Adults   1011

Stephen J. Forman

Acute lymphoblastic leukemia (ALL) is a hematologic malignancy of the bone marrow characterized by the rapid proliferation and subsequent accumulation of immature lymphocytes. ALL accounts for 20% of all acute leukemias that are seen in adults over the age of 20 years. In the past 2 decades, there has been substantial improvement in the understanding of the molecular biology of the disease and in the management of adult patients who have this disorder, including allogeneic transplantation This article reviews the biology of adult ALL, the relationship of specific disease characteristics to the natural history of the disease and the role of allogeneic hematopoietic cell transplantation in the management of adult patients with this disease.

Acute Lymphoblastic Leukemia in Adolescents and Young Adults   1033

Josep-Maria Ribera and Albert Oriol

Today, long-term survival is achieved in more than 80% of children 1 to 10 years old with acute lymphoblastic leukemia (ALL). However, cure rates for adults and adolescents and young adults (AYA) with ALL remain relatively low, at only 40% to 50%. Age is a continuous prognostic variable in ALL, with no single age at which prognosis deteriorates markedly. Within childhood ALL populations, older children have shown inferior outcomes, whereas younger adults have shown superior outcomes among adult ALL patients. The type of treatment (pediatric-based versus adult-based) for AYA has recently been a matter of debate. In this article the biology and treatment of ALL in AYA is reviewed.

Philadelphia Chromosome-Positive Acute Lymphoblastic Leukemia   1043

Farhad Ravandi and Partow Kebriaei

The Philadelphia (Ph) chromosome, a short chromosome 22, is the most frequent cytogenetic abnormality in adult patients with acute lymphoblastic leukemia (ALL). It occurs in approximately 20% to 30% of adults and in about 5% of children with this disease. The incidence rises with age and occurs in approximately 50% of patients older than 50 years. This article reviews the treatment regimens for Ph+ ALL, including imatinib and second generation tyrosine kinase inhibitors (TKIs). The introduction of effective TKIs in the treatment of Ph+ ALL has introduced several avenues of research in a disease that was hitherto difficult to treat.

Long-term Outcomes in Survivors of Childhood Acute Lymphoblastic Leukemia   1065

Paul C. Nathan, Karen Wasilewski-Masker, and Laura A. Janzen

Cure rates for childhood acute lymphoblastic leukemia (ALL) now exceed 80%. Consequently, there is a growing population of survivors of childhood ALL who are at risk for developing late sequelae of their cancer therapy. The risk of developing a late effect of therapy is particularly high in those survivors treated with cranial radiation or hematopoietic stem cell transplantation; however, most children who survive after treatment in the current era are expected to live normal lives with minimal or no long-term morbidity. In this article, the more common, serious late effects of ALL therapy are reviewed, the treatment exposures that predispose some survivors to their development are discussed, and the need for life-long risk-based medical care for all survivors of childhood ALL is emphasized.

Role of Minimal Residual Disease Monitoring in Adult and Pediatric Acute Lymphoblastic Leukemia
1083

Dario Campana

Assays that measure minimal residual disease (MRD) can determine the response to treatment in patients with acute lymphoblastic leukemia (ALL) much more precisely than morphologic screening of bone marrow smears. The clinical significance of MRD, detected by flow cytometry or polymerase chain reaction-based methods in childhood ALL, has been established. Hence, MRD is being used in several clinical trials to adjust treatment intensity. Similar findings have been gathered in adult patients with ALL, making MRD one of the most powerful and informative parameters to guide clinical management. This article discusses practical issues related to MRD methodologies and the evidence supporting the use of MRD for risk assignment in clinical trials.

Looking Toward the Future: Novel Strategies Based on Molecular Pathogenesis of Acute Lymphoblastic Leukemia
1099

Syed A. Abutalib, Meir Wetzler, and Wendy Stock

There has been exponential growth in our understanding of the pathobiology of acute lymphoblastic leukemia (ALL) leading to the discovery of new prognostic markers and potential new treatment strategies. The inferior treatment outcome observed in adults with ALL in comparison with children with ALL means that new therapeutic approaches are required, preferably based on novel molecular insights. In this concluding article, the important themes that have been discussed in earlier articles are reviewed. Looking toward the future, the authors highlight several of the new therapeutic agents and discuss some of the recently described molecular genetic aberrations that might serve as therapeutic targets for future drug development.

Nelarabine for the Treatment of Patients with Relapsed or Refractory T-cell Acute Lymphoblastic Leukemia or Lymphoblastic Lymphoma
1121

Daniel J. DeAngelo

Nelarabine (506U78) is a soluble prodrug of 9- Darabinofuranosylguanine (ara-G), a deoxyguanosine derivative. Nelarabine has significant activity in patients with T-cell acute lymphoblastic leukemia (T-ALL) and lymphoma (T-LBL). Principal toxicity is grade 3 or 4 neutropenia and thrombocytopenia. Neurologic toxicity with Guillain-Barré syndrome, depressed level of consciousness, and peripheral neuropathy are concerning side effects. Nelarabine is well tolerated and has significant antitumor activity in T-ALL and T-LBL. Nelarabine was approved by the Food and Drug Administration for patients with T-ALL/LBL who failed at least two prior regimens. Nelarabine is being explored in children and will be explored in the near future in adults with newly diagnosed T-ALL.

Recent Progress in the Treatment of Acute Lymphoblastic Leukemia: Clofarabine   **1137**

Sima Jeha

Significant progress in the treatment of acute lymphoblastic leukemia (ALL) has been achieved through more effective use of established drugs in risk-adapted treatment regimens. As we are reaching the limits of optimizing current treatment strategies, new therapeutic targets are being identified, and novel formulation of older drugs are being explored. Clofarabine is a novel purine analog approved in 2005 for treating children in second or greater ALL relapse. Ongoing trials are studying the benefits of clofarabine combinations in less heavily pretreated patients, and the use of different dose schedules in a variety of hematologic malignancies.

Index   **1145**

FORTHCOMING ISSUE

December 2009
Chronic Immune Thrombocytopenia
Howard Liebman, MD, *Guest Editor*

RECENT ISSUES

August 2009
Neoplastic Hematopathology
Randy D. Gascoyne, MD
Guest Editor

June 2009
Advances in Melanoma
David E. Fisher, MD, PhD,
Guest Editor

April 2009
Bone Marrow Failure Syndromes
Grover C. Bagby, MD and
Gabrielle Meyers, MD, *Guest Editors*

THE CLINICS ARE NOW AVAILABLE ONLINE!

Access your subscription at:
www.theclinics.com

Preface

Acute Lymphoblastic Leukemia – Quo Vadis?

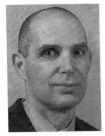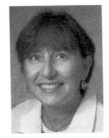

Meir Wetzler, MD, FACP   Wendy Stock, MD
Guest Editors

Acute lymphoblastic leukemia (ALL) is one of the most challenging malignant diseases in adults with respect to the intricacies of clinical presentation, diagnosis, and treatment. This preface previews the articles that follow, touching on current treatment strategies for ALL, presenting the controversies regarding the role of allogeneic stem cell and bone marrow transplantation (BMT) for ALL in first remission, and concluding with a look toward the future and a discussion concerning new data about the leukemia stem cells (LSCs) in this disease and how this knowledge will lead to new therapeutic strategies.

CURRENT ACUTE LYMPHOBLASTIC LEUKEMIA TREATMENT

Table 1 outlines the current treatment approaches for adults with ALL. Many of these approaches have been adapted from the successful treatment regimens developed for children with this disease. The article by Pui and colleagues, elsewhere in this issue reviews in detail the state-of-the-art treatment strategies for children with ALL. The survivorship in pediatric ALL now exceeds 80%. As a result, pediatricians are now turning more of their attention to concerns about sequelae of their treatment, as discussed in the article by Nathan and colleagues, elsewhere in this issue.

Overall, the outcome in adults with either B-cell or T-cell ALL with any of the approaches outlined in **Table 1** results in approximately 30% to 40% 5-year survival.[1] The main achievements in the last few years have been the inclusion of imatinib mesylate (Gleevec) and other tyrosine kinase inhibitors in Philadelphia-positive ALL (see article by Ravandi and colleagues, elsewhere in this issue), the approval of nelarabine (Arranon) for T-ALL (see article by DeAngelo and colleagues, elsewhere in this issue), the pediatric approach to treat ALL in adolescents and young adults (see article by Ribera and colleagues, elsewhere in this issue), and the inclusion of anti-CD20

Hematol Oncol Clin N Am 23 (2009) xi–xviii
doi:10.1016/j.hoc.2009.08.001
0889-8588/09/$ – see front matter

Table 1
Current and future adult ALL treatments

Characteristics	B	T	Ph +	Burkitt
Treatment	BFM-like regimen: Induction with VCR, PRED, daunorubicin, and L-ASP; Early intensification with CTX, ARA-C, 6-MP, VCR; Central nervous system prophylaxis with intrathecal MTX with either cranial irradiation or high-dose MTX and ARA-C; Late intensification with doxorubicin, VCR, DEXA, CTX, 6-TG and ARA-C; Maintenance with VCR, PRED, 6-MP and MTX to complete 24 months. Hyper-CVAD regimen: Alternating courses of CTX, VCR, doxorubicin and DEXA with MTX and high-dose ARA-C; Central nervous system prophylaxis includes intrathecal chemotherapy; Maintenance with VCR, PRED, 6-MP and MTX to complete 24 months.		Addition of imatinib to any of the approaches described for B-lineage diseases	CTX, VCR, doxorubicin, high-dose MTX and intrathecal therapy alternating with ifosfamide, VP-16, high-dose ARA-C, and intrathecal therapy
New aspects	Anti-CD20 Ab[a], different regimen for AYA[d]	Nelarabine[b], different regimen for AYA[d]	New TKIs[c]	Anti-CD20 Ab[a]

Abbreviations: Ab, antibody; ARA-C, cytosine arabinoside; AYA, adolescents and young adults; BFM, Berlin-Frankfurt-Münster; CTX, cyclophosphamide; CVAD, cyclophosphamide, vincristine, doxorubicin and dexamethasone; DEXA, dexamethasone; L-ASP, L-asparaginase; MTX, methotrexate; 6-MP, 6-mercaptopurine; PRED, prednisone; 6-TG, 6-thioguanine; TKI, tyrosine kinase inhibitors; VCR, vincristine; VP-16, etoposide.
[a] See article by Thomas and colleagues, elsewhere in this issue.
[b] See article by DeAngelo and colleagues, elsewhere in this issue.
[c] See article by Ravandi and colleagues, elsewhere in this issue.
[d] See article by Ribera and colleagues, elsewhere in this issue.
Data from Cavalli F, Hansen HH, Kaye SB, editors. The textbook of medical oncology. 4th edition. London: Informa Healthcare; 2009.

antibody into the ALL armamentarium (see article by Thomas and colleagues, elsewhere in this issue).

Two additional drugs are worth mentioning. One is pegylated asparaginase (Oncospar), which decreases the immunogenicity of the enzyme, thus reducing the risk of hypersensitivity reactions.[2] Another advantage of pegylated asparaginase is its long half-life. Its use in adult ALL has been lagging behind its use in pediatric ALL because of lack of pharmacokinetic and pharmacodynamic data in adults. However, two recent publications may change this trend. Specifically, the demonstration of the safety of intravenous pegylated asparaginase during remission induction in adult ALL with favorable pharmacodynamics and decreased hypersensitivity reactions[3] suggests that this route of administration will replace the intramuscular and subcutaneous routes. Furthermore, the findings that effective asparagine depletion with pegylated asparaginase resulted in improved outcome in adult ALL[4] suggest that monitoring for asparagine depletion will become part of the treatment approach in these patients.

The second drug worth noting is clofarabine (Clolar), a novel deoxyadenosine analog with clinical activity in refractory and relapsed pediatric ALL (see article by Jeha and colleagues, elsewhere in this issue). Its role in combination with other drugs in relapsed/refractory adult ALL is being investigated.[5,6] If efficacy of clofarabine combination therapy is identified in advanced stage ALL, it might be reasonable to explore the use of clofarabine as a front-line agent in adult ALL.

The concluding article by Abutalib and colleagues, elsewhere in this issue discusses other novel agents.

TO B(MT) OR NOT TO B(MT): A RISK-BASED DECISION

BMT is usually recommended to high-risk ALL patients in first remission and those in second and beyond remission. The recent Medical Research Council (MRC)/Eastern Cooperative Oncology Group (ECOG) trial[7] suggested a benefit for sibling donor transplantation in standard-risk ALL in first remission without any significant benefit for high-risk ALL. Others challenge this recommendation.[8] These data and the current controversies are reviewed elegantly in the article by Forman and colleagues, elsewhere in this issue and in the article by Ribera and colleagues, elsewhere in this issue. To understand the controversies about optimal treatment selection for adults with ALL reviewed in this issue, we highlight below some of the traditional and some of the newer biologic risk factors that prognosticate for treatment outcome in adult ALL.

The traditional ALL risk factors (high-risk factors denoted in parenthesis) are divided between the host and the disease.[9,10] The host-related factors include age (>60) and performance status (poor), while the disease-related factors include white blood cell count (>30 × 10^9/L for B-cell ALL and >100,000 × 10^9/L for T-cell ALL), mediastinal mass (present), immunophenotype (B-cell), karyotype (t[9;22], +8, t[4;11], −7 and hypodiploid karyotypes) and lactate dehydogenase (high level is associated with poor outcome and central nervous system disease). In addition, time to achieve complete remission (>4 weeks) is also recognized as a significant risk factor. Finally, the treatment team and the patient may also play a role in predicting outcome as it was recently implied that time to postremission treatment was an independent prognostic factor in adult ALL.[11] However, these traditional factors may not be sufficient to predict outcome of standard-risk ALL.

Recently, additional risk factors have been identified. The most important one on the host side is the presence of genetic variability in drug metabolism pathways.[12] Examples include 6-mercaptopurine, methotrexate, steroids, and asparaginase (see article by Abutalib and colleagues, elsewhere in this issue). On the disease side, novel molecular markers were identified that help determine outcome. In T-cell ALL, high expression of v-ets erythroblastosis virus E26 oncogene homolog (avian) (ERG); brain and acute leukemia, cytoplasmic (BAALC)[13]; and T-cell leukemia homeobox 3 (TLX3)[14] were associated with unfavorable outcome. In addition, expression of multi-drug resistance proteins in the leukemia blasts is associated with adverse outcome.[15] Finally, presence of minimal residual disease was shown to adversely affect outcome in both pediatric and adult studies (see article by Campana and colleagues, elsewhere in this issue). These risk factors, however, are currently only available through select and meticulously conducted clinical trials in academic centers. As we begin to study the impact of these factors in prospective trials, we will undoubtedly obtain critical insights that may help to guide the recommendation for a stem cell transplant in first remission.

ACUTE LYMPHOBLASTIC LEUKEMIA STEM CELLS

Hematopoiesis is the highly orchestrated process of blood cell production by which the billions of white blood cells, red blood cells, and platelets lost daily are replaced to maintain homeostasis.[16] Hematopoietic stem cells (HSCs) are the small population of long-lived, quiescent, undifferentiated, pluripotent cells characterized by a capacity of self-renewal, an exceptional proliferation potential, resistance to apoptosis, and the ability of multilineage differentiation into all types of blood cells mediated by the production of several lineage-committed progenitors.[16–20]

The central role of LSCs in the pathogenesis of leukemias has become well recognized over the last 2 decades. LSCs share many of the basic characteristics with normal HSCs, including quiescence, self-renewal, extensive proliferative capacity, and the ability to give rise to differentiated progeny in a hierarchical pattern.[21–27] Some scientists even view leukemia as a newly formed, abnormal hematopoietic tissue initiated by a few LSCs that undergo an aberrant and poorly regulated process of organogenesis analogous to that of normal HSCs.[28] The LSCs from different types of leukemias are likely to exhibit different biologic features, including survival and self-renewal pathways and immunophenotype.[29]

Many researchers believe that the persistence of LSCs, which are resistant to most of the traditional chemotherapeutic agents that kill the bulk of the leukemic cell populations, is a major cause of leukemia relapse after "successful" induction of remission. Subsequently, designing effective therapeutic modalities that specifically target the LSC is likely to reduce the incidence of relapse, and even possibly lead to cure. The main question that remains unanswered nowadays is: What are the LSCs in ALL?

Due to the clear limitations of conducting controlled experiments on humans, most of our current knowledge about human LSCs was obtained indirectly from in vitro studies, xenotransplantation of human cells into immunodeficient animals, and transplant experiments involving primates and other large animals.[16]

The hypothesis that a subset of leukemia cells has distinct stem cell properties implies that LSCs arise as an inherent property of tumor biology and development.[30,31] However, the bone marrow surroundings and the immune system offer support and are an intricate part of LSC survival and progression.[32] One current controversy in the LSC arena concerns the intrinsic characteristic of LSCs in the experimental setting of xenotransplantation, where appropriate microenvironment features are missing because of differences between humans and mice.[24] This may have significant adverse effects on leukemic initiating capacity when these human LSCs are transplanted into nonobese diabetic (NOD)/severe combined immune-deficient (SCID) mice.[33] Thus, LSCs that appeared to have failed transplantation may actually be fully leukemogenic in a microenvironmental setting with appropriate support.[34,35]

Initially, it was reported that immature ALL stem cells capable of long-term proliferation in vitro and in vivo are CD34(+)/CD10(−)/CD19(−).[36] Similar data were reported with Ph(+) ALL cells.[37] However, recent reports demonstrated that more mature [CD34(+)/CD19(+)] ALL cells can initiate leukemia by xenotransplantation.[38,39] These findings were associated with a switch to a more immune-deficient mouse strain, NOD/SCID/IL2rᵟnull.[40] This mouse has a mutation in the interleukin-2 receptor common gamma chain and is therefore devoid of not only T and B cells but also natural killer cells. Most recent twist to the theory of LSCs is the report that B precursor blasts in various stages of differentiation [CD34(+)/CD19(−), CD34(+)/CD19(+), CD34(−)/CD19(+)] displayed self-renewal capability, suggesting that leukemic lymphoid progenitors may not lose their self renewal capability with maturation[41] or are able to "move backward" in differentiation.

This recent finding brings in the potential malleability or plasticity of LSCs. The term *plasticity* refers to the ability of organ-specific stem cells to recover their ability to differentiate into cells of other lineages, either in vitro or after transplantation in vivo.[16,42,43] Here we use this term to describe the ability of more differentiated leukemic cells to reacquire the LSC characteristics. As a proof of concept, it was recently demonstrated that as few as 10 unselected ALL cells can initiate leukemia following xenotransplantation.[44]

These findings may explain the poor outcome in ALL since any remaining blasts can theoretically "dedifferentiate" and start a progeny after "successful" achievement of remission. If indeed these cells can also regain the other LSC characteristics, such as multidrug resistance and resistance to apoptosis, better treatments targeting these cells are needed.

HSCs reside in the bone marrow, close to the endosteal surfaces of the trabecular bone in what is commonly referred to as *the niche*.[45] A stem-cell niche can be defined as a structure in which HSCs are housed for an indefinite period of time and maintained by allowing progeny production through self-renewal in the absence of differentiation.[45–47] Several cell-surface receptors were implicated in controlling the localization of HSCs to the endosteal niche, among which is the chemokine receptor 4 (CXCR4). Its antagonist, AMD3100 (Mozobil) was recently approved as an HSC mobilizer before stem cell collection.[48]

Somewhat promising in this regard is the recent demonstration of dependency on the stromal-derived growth factor 1 (SDF-1α)/CXCR4 axis in Ph(+) ALL.[49] Specifically in this scenario, the Bcr-Abl kinase continued to be inhibited by imatinib, but the cells continued to proliferate in the presence of stromal support. The stromal effect did not require direct cell-cell contact and SDF-1α substituted for the presence of the stromal cells. These data imply that the stroma-selected imatinib-resistant Bcr-Abl cells were less dependent on the kinase activity; thus, interrupting the interaction between the lymphoblasts and the stroma may be of benefit in Ph(+) ALL and most probably also in Ph(−) ALL. Initial studies demonstrating a role for AMD3100 in pediatric ALL[50] offer promise for the future about our ability to mobilize the remaining lymphoblasts from their niche and eradicate them.

SUMMARY

This issue attempts to answer the question: *Quo vadis*? Where are we going with respect to ALL treatment in both children and adults? While health care teams caring for children now focus on tailoring their successful therapies to minimize long-term toxicities, those caring for adults are still working toward the goal of cure. The focus of therapy is increasingly based on the biologic characteristics of the patients. For one age group, adolescents and young adults, a pediatric approach seems warranted. However, this approach may be difficult to administer to older adults. This issue addresses current treatment strategies based on age and disease biology. The reader should be aware that the definition of "young" and "old" adults is in flux (ranging between 30 to 60 years old) and depends on the group (or the principal investigator) conducting the trial. The concluding article looks toward the future and reviews novel treatments that are moving into the clinic. Furthermore, we anticipate that that recent progress in our understanding LSC biology will shed light on the frequent relapses that occur after "successful" remission induction and will lead to therapeutic innovation and, ultimately, to the improved outcome of all patients with this challenging and heterogeneous disease.

ACKNOWLEDGEMENTS

The authors thank Dr. Hun J. Lee for his assistance preparing this preface.

Meir Wetzler, MD, FACP
Leukemia Section
Roswell Park Cancer Institute
Elm and Carlton Streets
Buffalo, NY 14263, USA

Wendy Stock, MD
University of Chicago Hospitals and Cancer Research Center
5841 S. Maryland Avenue
Chicago, IL 60637, USA

E-mail address:
meir.wetzler@roswellpark.org (M. Wetzler)

REFERENCES

1. Larson S, Stock W. Progress in the treatment of adults with acute lymphoblastic leukemia. Curr Opin Hematol 2008;15:400–7.
2. Zeidan A, Wang ES, Wetzler M. Pegasparaginase: where do we stand? Expert Opin Biol Ther 2009;9:111–9.
3. Douer D, Yampolsky H, Cohen LJ, et al. Pharmacodynamics and safety of intravenous pegaspargase during remission induction in adults aged 55 years or younger with newly diagnosed acute lymphoblastic leukemia. Blood 2007;109:2744–50.
4. Wetzler M, Sanford BL, Kurtzberg J, et al. Effective asparagine depletion with pegylated asparaginase results in improved outcomes in adult acute lymphoblastic leukemia: Cancer and Leukemia Group B Study 9511. Blood 2007;109:4164–7.
5. Faderl S, Gandhi V, O'Brien S, et al. Results of a phase 1-2 study of clofarabine in combination with cytarabine (ara-C) in relapsed and refractory acute leukemias. Blood 2005;105:940–7.
6. Karp JE, Ricklis RM, Balakrishnan K, et al. A phase 1 clinical-laboratory study of clofarabine followed by cyclophosphamide for adults with refractory acute leukemias. Blood 2007;110:1762–9.
7. Goldstone AH, Richards SM, Lazarus HM, et al. In adults with standard-risk acute lymphoblastic leukemia (ALL) the greatest benefit is achieved from a matched sibling allogeneic transplant in first complete remission (CR) and an autologous

transplant is less effective than conventional consolidation/maintenance chemo-therapy in All patients: final results of the international ALL trial (MRC UKALL XII/ ECOG E2993). Blood 2008;111:1827–33.

8. Larson RA. Allogeneic hematopoietic cell transplantation is not recommended for all adults with standard-risk acute lymphoblastic leukemia in first complete remission. Biol Blood Marrow Transplant 2008;15:11–6.

9. Hoelzer D, Thiel E, Loffler H, et al. Prognostic factors in a multicenter study for treatment of acute lymphoblastic leukemia in adults. Blood 1988;71:123–31.

10. Larson RA, Dodge RK, Burns CP, et al. A five-drug remission induction regimen with intensive consolidation for adults with acute lymphoblastic leukemia: cancer and leukemia group B study 8811. Blood 1995;85:2025–37.

11. Advani AS, Jin T, Ramsingh G, et al. Time to post-remission therapy is an independent prognostic factor in adults with acute lymphoblastic leukemia. Leuk Lymphoma 2008;49:1560–6.

12. Cheok MH, Pottier N, Kager L, et al. Pharmacogenetics in acute lymphoblastic leukemia. Semin Hematol 2009;46:39–51.

13. Baldus CD, Martus P, Burmeister T, et al. Low ERG and BAALC expression identifies a new subgroup of adult acute T-lymphoblastic leukemia with a highly favorable outcome. J Clin Oncol 2007;25:3739–45.

14. Ballerini P, Landman-Parker J, Cayuela JM, et al. Impact of genotype on survival of children with T-cell acute lymphoblastic leukemia treated according to the French protocol FRALLE-93: the effect of TLX3/HOX11L2 gene expression on outcome. Haematologica 2008;93:1658–65.

15. Swerts K, De Moerloose B, Dhooge C, et al. Prognostic significance of multidrug resistance-related proteins in childhood acute lymphoblastic leukaemia. Eur J Cancer 2006;42:295–309.

16. Smith C. Hematopoietic stem cells and hematopoiesis. Cancer Control 2003;10: 9–16.

17. Szilvassy SJ. The biology of hematopoietic stem cells. Arch Med Res 2003;34: 446–60.

18. Wang JC, Dick JE. Cancer stem cells: lessons from leukemia. Trends Cell Biol 2005;15:494–501.

19. Guo W, Lasky JL 3rd, Wu H. Cancer stem cells. Pediatr Res 2006;59:59R.

20. Huang X, Cho S, Spangrude GJ. Hematopoietic stem cells: generation and self-renewal. Cell Death Differ 2007;14:1851–9.

21. Terpstra W, Ploemacher RE, Prins A, et al. Fluorouracil selectively spares acute myeloid leukemia cells with long-term growth abilities in immunodeficient mice and in culture. Blood 1996;88:1944–50.

22. Guan Y, Gerhard B, Hogge DE. Detection, isolation, and stimulation of quiescent primitive leukemic progenitor cells from patients with acute myeloid leukemia (AML). Blood 2003;101:3142–9.

23. Guzman ML, Neering SJ, Upchurch D, et al. Nuclear factor-kappaB is constitutively activated in primitive human acute myelogenous leukemia cells. Blood 2001;98:2301–7.

24. Bonnet D, Dick JE. Human acute myeloid leukemia is organized as a hierarchy that originates from a primitive hematopoietic cell. Nat Med 1997;3:730–7.

25. Jordan CT. The leukemic stem cell. Best Pract Res Clin Haematol 2007;20:13–8.

26. Jordan CT. Unique molecular and cellular features of acute myelogenous leukemia stem cells. Leukemia 2002;16:559–62.

27. Jordan CT, Guzman ML. Mechanisms controlling pathogenesis and survival of leukemic stem cells. Oncogene 2004;23:7178–87.

28. Passegue E, Jamieson CH, Ailles LE, et al. Normal and leukemic hematopoiesis: are leukemias a stem cell disorder or a reacquisition of stem cell characteristics? Proc Natl Acad Sci U S A 2003;100(Suppl 1):11842–9.
29. Krause DS, Van Etten RA. Right on target: eradicating leukemic stem cells. Trends Mol Med 2007;13:470–81.
30. Dick JE. Stem cell concepts renew cancer research. Blood 2008;112:4793–807.
31. Bissell MJ, Labarge MA. Context, tissue plasticity, and cancer: are tumor stem cells also regulated by the microenvironment? Cancer Cell 2005;7:17–23.
32. Mantovani A. Cancer: Inflaming metastasis. Nature 2009;457:36–7.
33. Kelly PN, Dakic A, Adams JM, et al. Tumor growth need not be driven by rare cancer stem cells. Science 2007;317:337.
34. Hanahan D, Weinberg RA. The hallmarks of cancer. Cell 2000;100:57–70.
35. O'Brien CA, Pollett A, Gallinger S, et al. A human colon cancer cell capable of initiating tumour growth in immunodeficient mice. Nature 2007;445:106–10.
36. Cox CV, Evely RS, Oakhill A, et al. Characterization of acute lymphoblastic leukemia progenitor cells. Blood 2004;104:2919–25.
37. Cobaleda C, Gutierrez-Cianca N, Perez-Losada J, et al. A primitive hematopoietic cell is the target for the leukemic transformation in human philadelphia-positive acute lymphoblastic leukemia. Blood 2000;95:1007–13.
38. Castor A, Nilsson L, Astrand-Grundstrom I, et al. Distinct patterns of hematopoietic stem cell involvement in acute lymphoblastic leukemia. Nat Med 2005;11:630–7.
39. Hong D, Gupta R, Ancliff P, et al. Initiating and cancer-propagating cells in TEL-AML1-associated childhood leukemia. Science. 2008;319:336–9.
40. M Ito, Hiramatsu H, Kobayashi K,et al. NOD/SCID/gamma cnull mouse: an excellent recipient mouse model for engraftment of human cells. Blood 2002;100:3175–82.
41. le Viseur C, Hotfilder M, Bomken S, et al. In childhood acute lymphoblastic leukemia, blasts at different stages of immunophenotypic maturation have stem cell properties. Cancer Cell 2008;14:47–58.
42. Kondo M, Scherer DC, Miyamoto T, et al. Cell-fate conversion of lymphoid-committed progenitors by instructive actions of cytokines. Nature 2000;407:383–6.
43. Trounson A. Stem cells, plasticity and cancer - uncomfortable bed fellows. Development 2004;131:2763–8.
44. Morisot SWA, Bohana-Kashtan O, et al. Leukemia stem cell (LSC) are frequent in childhood precursor B acute lymphoblastic leukemia (ALL). Blood 2008;112.
45. Ohlstein B, Kai T, Decotto E, et al. The stem cell niche: theme and variations. Curr Opin Cell Biol 2004;16:693–6.
46. Spradling A, Drummond-Barbosa D, Kai T. Stem cells find their niche. Nature 2001;414:98–104.
47. Wilson A, Trumpp A. Bone-marrow haematopoietic-stem-cell niches. Nat Rev Immunol 2006;6:93–106.
48. Nervi B, Link DC, DiPersio JF. Cytokines and hematopoietic stem cell mobilization. J Cell Biochem 2006;99:690–705.
49. Mishra S, Zhang B, Cunnick JM, et al. Resistance to imatinib of bcr/abl p190 lymphoblastic leukemia cells. Cancer Res 2006;66:5387–93.
50. Juarez J, Dela Pena A, Baraz R, et al. CXCR4 antagonists mobilize childhood acute lymphoblastic leukemia cells into the peripheral blood and inhibit engraftment. Leukemia 2007;21:1249–57.

Monoclonal Antibody Therapy with Rituximab for Acute Lymphoblastic Leukemia

Deborah A. Thomas, MD*, Susan O'Brien, MD, Hagop M. Kantarjian, MD

KEYWORDS

- CD20 • Rituximab • Acute lymphoblastic leukemia
- Prognosis • Monoclonal antibody

Although a dramatic improvement in outcome was initially observed for adults with acute lymphoblastic leukemia (ALL) after incorporation of active chemotherapy agents, a period of stagnation ensued owing to limitations encountered with further dose intensification of standard chemotherapeutics. Significant advances have recently been achieved with the incorporation of targeted therapy agents such as tyrosine kinase inhibitors for Philadelphia (Ph)-positive ALL. Targeting leukemia surface antigens with monoclonal antibodies is another promising strategy. This article comprehensively reviews available data regarding the use of rituximab for the treatment of Burkitt-type leukemia/lymphoma and CD20-positive precursor B-cell ALL.

IMMUNOPHENOTYPIC CLASSIFICATION OF ACUTE LYMPHOBLASTIC LEUKEMIA

The prognostic relevance of immunologic subtypes of ALL relates to their association with particular cytogenetic and molecular aberrancies. For example, pro-B–cell ALL (universally CD10-, CD20-) is associated with the adverse karyotype of t(4:11), which involves the mixed lineage leukemia (MLL) proto-oncogene.[1] The subclassification of ALL by flow cytometric immunophenotyping not only characterizes the disease but also delineates potential therapeutic interventions by detecting surface antigens such as CD19, CD20, CD22, CD33, or CD52, which can be targeted by specific monoclonal antibodies (MoAbs).[2] The CD20 molecule in particular is a B-lineage specific antigen expressed on both normal and malignant cells during nearly all stages of

Department of Leukemia, University of Texas M D Anderson Cancer Center, 1515 Holcombe Blvd, Unit 428, Houston, TX 77030, USA
* Corresponding author.
E-mail address: debthomas@mdanderson.org (D.A. Thomas).

Hematol Oncol Clin N Am 23 (2009) 949–971
doi:10.1016/j.hoc.2009.07.005
0889-8588/09/$ – see front matter © 2009 Elsevier Inc. All rights reserved.

hemonc.theclinics.com

B-cell differentiation (except for hematopoeitic stem cells and plasma cells). Heterogeneity in the expression of CD20 among various B-cell malignancies has been well described.[3] For example, CD20 expression (defined as $\geq$20% of leukemia cells positive) ranges from 40% to 50% in precursor B-cell ALL compared with 80% to 90% in mature B-cell or Burkitt-type leukemia/lymphoma.

PROGNOSTIC SIGNIFICANCE OF CD20 EXPRESSION IN PRECURSOR B-CELL ACUTE LYMPHOBLASTIC LEUKEMIA

The CD20 molecule is a 33- to 37-kDa nonglycosylated hydrophobic transmembrane phosphoprotein that forms tetramers. The gene for CD20 has been mapped to chromosome 11 at position q12-13, centromeric to the Bcl-1 locus, which is involved in the translocation t(11;14)(q13;q32).[4] The CD20 antigen is not internalized or secreted on antibody binding, although circulating CD20 (bound to other proteins, cell membrane fragments, or large membrane complexes presumably after cells have undergone apoptosis) has been detected in the plasma of patients with B-cell malignancies.[5] CD20 functions as a calcium channel that ultimately influences cell cycle progression and differentiation via downstream signaling pathways. The modulations of surface CD20 and the resulting alterations in intracellular Ca^{2+} metabolism affect apoptosis pathways and levels of the proapoptotic proteins sarco/endoplasmic reticulum Ca(2+) (SERCA3) and Bax/Bak.[6] The constitutive activation of survival pathways involving nuclear factor-κB (NF-κB) and extracellular receptor kinase (ERK1/2) induced by CD20 results in the overexpression of the antiapoptotic protein Bcl-2 and associated Bcl-2 genes.[7] The hypothesis generated from these observations is that CD20 expression confers increased drug resistance through these mechanisms, resulting in the persistence of leukemia subclones that eventually resurge and lead to recurrence of the disease.

The prognostic relevance of CD20 expression in de novo childhood precursor B-cell ALL has been investigated, with conflicting results. CD20 expression was evaluated by the traditional arbitrary cut point of 20% and by mean fluorescence intensity (MFI) in 1231 children treated with risk-adapted Pediatric Oncology Group (POG) protocols.[8] Absolute CD20 expression and increasing MFI of CD20 were both independently associated with a significantly inferior event-free survival (EFS) irrespective of other known prognostic factors such as age and karyotypic aberrancies. Jeha and colleagues[9] retrospectively studied the influence of CD20 expression on outcome in 359 children with de novo precursor B-cell ALL treated on sequential St. Jude Total Therapy protocols. The overall incidence of CD20 expression was 48%, but decreased in frequency at the extremes of the age spectrum (younger than 1 year and older than 10 years). In contrast to the POG experience, CD20 expression was associated with a slightly more favorable prognosis (5-year EFS rate of 84% $\pm$ 2.9% vs 78% $\pm$ 3.1%, P = .08; 5-year overall survival [OS] rate of 88% $\pm$ 2.5% vs 83% $\pm$ 2.8%, P = .13). It was postulated that the disparate results could be accounted for by differences in the intensity of chemotherapy or the application of risk-adapted strategies between the POG and St. Jude chemotherapy regimens.

The significance of CD20 expression was then evaluated in 253 adolescents and adults with de novo precursor B-cell ALL treated in the pre-rituximab era with 1 of 2 sequential chemotherapy regimens of increasing intensity (VAD/CVAD [vincristine, doxorubicin, and dexamethasone/cyclophosphamide and VAD] or hyper-CVAD [fractionated cyclophosphamide, vincristine, doxorubicin, and dexamethasone alternating with high-dose methotrexate and cytarabine]).[10] Forty-seven percent of the cases were CD20-positive as defined by the traditional cut point of 20%. There were no significant associations between CD20 expression and the standard prognostic factors. Complete remission (CR) rates were similar within the regimens regardless of CD20 status (positive versus negative). However, CD20 expression was associated with a higher relapse rate (71% vs 53% for VAD/CVAD, $P = .08$; 61% vs 37% for hyper-CVAD, $P = .005$), lower 3-year CR duration (CRD) rates (22% vs 58% for hyper-CVAD, $P < .001$), and lower 3-year overall OS rates (27% vs 60% for hyper-CVAD, $P = .003$). The negative influence of CD20 expression on outcome appeared to be most pronounced in the younger subsets (eg, 3-year OS rates for hyper-CVAD if age 30 years or younger 35% vs 85%, $P = .009$; if age 31–59 years 28% vs 54%, $P = .04$). The elderly subgroup (age 60 years or older) did poorly irrespective of CD20 status; 3-year OS rates were 20% for hyper-CVAD.

In this study, multivariate analysis for EFS identified older age, leukocyte count $30 \times 10^9/L$ or more, presence of the Philadelphia chromosome, high systemic risk classification, and CD20 expression as independent adverse factors. Alternative cut points of CD20 expression such as 10% or 30% were also examined for prognostic relevance. The rate of CD20 expression increased from 47% to 67% with use of the 10% demarcation for CD20 positivity. The negative influence of CD20 expression on outcome (with to respect to CRD and OS) within each of the age subsets was nearly identical to that observed with the traditional cut point of 20% (**Fig. 1**). There was no correlation between increasing levels of CD20 expression and outcome; rather, the influence of CD20 expression appeared to be an "all or nothing phenomenon."[10]

Another retrospective analysis of CD20 expression in 143 adolescents and adults with de novo precursor B-cell ALL treated with the pediatric-inspired Group for Research in Adult Acute Lymphoblastic Leukemia (GRAALL)-2003 regimen identified a higher cumulative incidence of relapse (39% [95% confidence interval, 25–55] vs 20% [95% confidence interval, 13–31], $P = .02$) in the CD20-positive subset, although this did not translate into a difference in disease-free survival (DFS).[11,12] It also was noted that the negative prognostic influence of elevated leukocyte count or corticosteroid resistance on outcome was observed only in the CD20-positive subset, suggesting intrinsic resistance of the CD20-positive lymphoblasts to the dose intensification of alkylating agents applied in these scenarios.

UPREGULATION OF CD20 EXPRESSION IN PRECURSOR B-CELL ACUTE LYMPHOBLASTIC LEUKEMIA

The modulation of surface antigens on viable lymphoblasts during the induction phase of chemotherapy has been noted by several investigators. Serial analyses of surface leukemia antigen expression were performed on bone marrow (BM) samples collected from children with de novo precursor B-cell ALL during the induction phase of chemotherapy administered according to the Italian Association of Pediatric Hematology and Oncology/Berlin-Frankfurt-Munster (AIEOP-BFM) ALL 2000 protocol. The quantitative surface expressions of CD10 and CD34 were downmodulated, whereas the expressions of CD19, CD20, CD45RA, and CD11a were upregulated.[13] These findings were attributed to glucocorticoid effects because the modulations were detected as early as a few days after initiation of the prednisone phase of therapy.[14]

The modulation of CD20 on lymphoblasts in BM and peripheral blood (PB) samples was evaluated further during the induction phase of therapy (AIEOP-BFM ALL 2000 protocol) for 159 children with precursor B-cell ALL.[15] Expression of CD20 (using the traditional cut point of 20%) at diagnosis was noted in 46% and 51% of BM and PB samples, respectively. There was a good correlation in expression levels

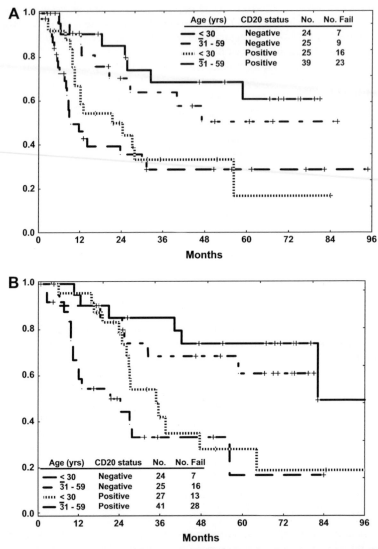

Fig. 1. Outcome for precursor B-cell ALL treated with hyper-CVAD in the pre-rituximab era by age category and CD20 status (positive or negative) using the 10% demarcation of expression. The 3-year rates for CRD (*A*) and OS (*B*) were nearly identical to those observed with the traditional cut point of 20% for CD20 expression.

between paired BM and PB samples, although significant variance (mean 13% ± 17%) was observed. There was no significant correlation between CD20 expression at diagnosis and age, BFM risk group, specific immunophenotype, or relapse. Subsequent specimens including PB samples collected on day 8 and BM samples collected on day 15 of the induction chemotherapy showed significantly increased levels of CD20 by expression and MFI. Of note, individual patient samples exhibited a significant increase in the proportion of CD20-positive lymphoblasts even if CD20 expression had been negative (by definition) at diagnosis, suggesting that therapy with anti-CD20 MoAbs may be applicable even in the CD20-negative subset. The one exception was the favorable category of TEL-AML1-rearranged cases in which the low baseline CD20 expression did not change significantly during induction chemotherapy. In contrast, samples from the high BFM risk group exhibited very high levels of CD20 expression (80% or more) at essentially all collection time points.

In this study, the upregulation of CD20 to a MFI of at least 50 (equivalent to CD20 expression of 80%) translated to a more efficient cytolysis of the lymphoblasts after in vitro exposure to rituximab.[15] In the cases positive for minimal residual disease (MRD, defined as $\geq 0.1\%$ lymphoblasts) at end-induction (day 33), CD20 expression at least 90% (or at least 80%) was observed in 52% (67%), as opposed to 5% (8%) at the time of diagnosis and 20% (25%) on day 15 of therapy. These findings certainly suggest that MoAb therapy directed against CD20 should be further investigated as a therapeutic intervention to eradicate residual disease.

Upregulation of surface CD20 expression via pharmacologic maneuvers may improve the efficacy of MoAb therapy. Venugopal and colleagues demonstrated an increase in surface CD20 expression on chronic lymphocytic leukemia (CLL) cells in vitro after exposure to the cytokines interleukin-4, granulocyte-macrophage colony-stimulating factor (GM-CSF), or tumor necrosis factor-α.[16] However, neither upregulation of CD20 nor an increase in the proportion of cells expressing CD20 was observed in patients with CLL who underwent PB sampling at various time points within a 24-hour span after a single dose of GM-CSF.[17] Despite these findings, GM-CSF has still been used as an adjunct to therapy with rituximab for CLL and indolent B-cell lymphomas, owing to its enhancement of antibody-dependent cellular cytotoxicity (ADCC) and augmentation of innate immunity against malignant cells.[18,19] Whether cytokines truly modulate CD20 expression remains to be elucidated. In vitro exposure of B-lineage non-Hodgkin lymphoma (NHL) cells to hypomethylating agents or bryostatin-1 (a modulator of the protein kinase C [PKC] pathway) has been shown to increase surface CD20 expression via processes detailed further in the section on mechanisms of resistance to rituximab.[20,21]

PRINCIPLES OF MONOCLONAL ANTIBODY THERAPY WITH RITUXIMAB

The activity of the chimeric MoAb rituximab (Rituxan, Genentech, South San Francisco, CA) is generally mediated by modulation of the CD20 receptor via induction of ADCC, complement-dependent cytotoxicity (CDCC), or direct apoptosis.[22] Rituximab is an IgG1 immunoglobulin that contains murine variable region sequences, and human constant κ and Fc region sequences. Rituximab recognizes a discontinuous epitope composed of the amino acids [170]ANPS[173] (alanine, asparagine, proline, serine) within the small extracellular domain of CD20.[23] Rituximab received approval by the Food and Drug Administration (FDA) in 1997 for the treatment of relapsed or refractory CD20-positive low-grade or follicular B-cell NHL based on its single-agent activity in the pivotal trials.[24-26] Rituximab was the first MoAb approved for the therapeutic treatment of malignancy.

Therapy with MoAbs directed against lymphoma or leukemia surface antigens is an attractive targeted treatment approach because it is subtype specific. When compared with chemotherapeutics, MoAbs generally effect cytolysis by different or complementary mechanisms, and therefore may have efficacy against malignant clones that are resistant to cytostatic drugs. The incorporation of MoAb into therapeutic regimens may therefore be particularly beneficial in instances whereby further intensification of chemotherapy is impossible, particularly when there is minimal overlapping toxicity. The clinical benefits of combining rituximab with CHOP (cyclo-phosphamide, doxorubicin, vincristine, and prednisone) chemotherapy for diffuse large B-cell lymphoma (DLBCL) were subsequently confirmed in randomized clinical trials; improvements in EFS and OS were evident not only in younger patients with good risk features but also in the elderly subsets.[27–29]

RITUXIMAB-BASED CHEMOIMMUNOTHERAPY FOR ADULT BURKITT-TYPE LEUKEMIA/LYMPHOMA

Burkitt-type lymphoma (BL) and mature B-cell ALL are composed of high-grade, rapidly proliferating, small noncleaved B lymphoid cells with a mature B-lineage immu-nophenotype characterized by expression of monotypic surface IgM, CD19, CD20, CD22, CD10, Bcl-6, and CD79a (negative for CD5, CD23, Bcl-2, and nuclear terminal deoxyribonucleotide transferase [TdT]). For mature B-cell ALL, the typical L3 morphology as per the French-American-British (FAB) classification and the presence of one of the characteristic translocations involving the proto-oncogene c-myc on band 8q24 [t8;14(q24;q32); t(2;8)(p12;q24); t(8;22)(q24;11)] have been hallmarks of the disease; an additional t(14;18)(q32;q21) may confer a worse prognosis owing to overexpression of the antiapoptotic protein bcl-2.[30,31] Prognosis has improved signif-icantly with use of short-term dose-intensive multiagent chemotherapy regimens, except for the elderly subgroup, which tends to be underrepresented in clinical trials (**Table 1**). The poor prognosis of older age (60 years or older) was initially reported on reviewing the outcome of mature B-cell ALL after chemotherapy as per the hyper-CVAD regimen.[35] A subsequent reanalysis of several multinational clinical trials of various chemotherapy regimens used for BL identified that 2-year OS rates were lower in most series for the subgroups aged 40 years or older.[45]

Significant activity of therapy with single-agent rituximab was initially observed in children with relapsed or refractory BL, or mature B-cell ALL.[46] Indeed, caspase-inde-pendent apoptosis has been reported in BL-derived cell lines after in vitro exposure to rituximab.[47] Rituximab has also been shown to sensitize B-lineage NHL cell lines to chemotherapeutic agents in vitro via selective downregulation of the antiapoptotic proteins Bcl-2 and Bcl-X_L.[48,49] Bcl-X_L protects cells from cytotoxicity, thus conferring a multidrug-resistant phenotype; downregulation of Bcl-X_L induced by rituximab could modulate this effect. Rituximab has therefore been incorporated into established regi-mens for Burkitt-type leukemia/lymphoma to exploit the universally high CD20 expres-sion and potential synergy with chemotherapeutic agents, particularly given the successes observed with chemoimmunotherapy approaches for DLBCL and other lymphoproliferative disorders. Given the relative rarity of these disease entities, these nonrandomized clinical trials have relied on historical comparisons for determination of clinical benefit.

As alluded to earlier, outcome for the elderly subset of de novo BL and mature B-cell ALL treated with the hyper-CVAD was particularly poor. The 3-year OS rates ranged from 17%–19% compared with 70%–77% for their younger counterparts, in part attributable to a higher induction mortality (10%) incurred from infections and to a higher incidence of disease recurrence (50%).[35,40] Further intensification of the chemotherapy was not deemed feasible. Standard-dose rituximab (375 mg/m^2) was therefore incorporated into the first 4 of 8 cycles of intensive chemotherapy (8 treatments given on days 1 and 11 of the hyper-CVAD cycles, days 1 and 8 of the high-dose methotrexate/cytarabine cycles).[40] No other modifications were made to the hyper-CVAD regimen except for use of a protective environment for the elderly patients during induction chemotherapy until neutrophil recovery greater than 500.

An analysis of 31 patients (29% age 60 years or older) treated with hyper-CVAD and rituximab demonstrated clinical benefit from the addition of rituximab, particularly for the elderly subset.[40] Although overall the CR rates were similar (86% vs 85%), the CRD, EFS, and OS rates for the entire group treated with the combination were 91%, 89%, and 89% compared with 66%, 52%, and 53% (P<.05 for all comparisons), respectively, for the historical cohort treated with hyper-CVAD alone (**Table 1**). The improvement in outcome was most apparent for the elderly subgroup, with respective rates of 100%, 89%, and 89% compared with 44%, 19%, and 19% for hyper-CVAD without rituximab, owing to amelioration of induction deaths and absence of disease recurrence. Multivariate analysis for DFS identified younger age and treatment with rituximab as independent factors predictive for favorable outcome.

A recent update of outcome with the hyper-CVAD and rituximab regimen inclusive of 49 patients with de novo BL or mature B-cell ALL continued to show apparent clinical benefit from the addition of rituximab, predominantly for the elderly subset (**Fig. 2**).[50] Of note, with long-term follow-up (median 46 months), 3 of 37 (8%) younger patients treated with chemoimmunotherapy subsequently developed secondary blood dyscrasias (acute myelogenous leukemia [AML] at 7 years, myelodysplastic syndrome at 3.5 years, AML with t(8;21) at 3 years) without recurrence of the Burkitt disease, suggesting that monitoring for late toxicities beyond 2 years after chemoimmunotherapy is warranted.

Elderly patients older than 55 years with BL and mature B-cell ALL also had a poor outcome with the former protocol B-NHL90 without rituximab. The CR rate in 45 patients was 71% with an OS rate of 39%.[33] In the ensuing chemoimmunotherapy regimen developed for BL, mature B-cell ALL, and DLBCL by the German Multicenter Study Group for Adult ALL (GMALL B-ALL/NHL 2002), 8 standard doses of rituximab were applied (1 dose before each of the 6 chemotherapy cycles and 2 doses for consolidation).[44] Other modifications to the former protocol B-NHL90 included the addition of cycles containing high-dose cytarabine (2 g/m^2) besides other drugs (cycle C). Patients younger than 55 years received six cycles (ABCABC) of therapy with 1.5 g/m^2 of intravenous methotrexate, whereas older patients underwent dose reduction of the methotrexate to 0.5 g/m^2 without cycle C (ABABAB). Outcome for the BL (n = 146, median age 36 years, 18% >55 years) and mature B-cell ALL (n = 84, median age 46, 41% >55 years) subgroups was recently reported.[43] The CR rate was 90% and 83% with induction death rates of 3% and 11%, respectively. The 3-year OS rates were influenced by age (younger versus older) within the subtypes: rates were 91% versus 84% for BL and 84% versus 39% for mature B-cell ALL, respectively. The worse outcome noted in the older patients with mature B-cell ALL was attributed to the high incidence of central nervous system (CNS) relapses, likely related to the predetermined dose reductions of systemic methotrexate and omission of the high-dose cytarabine chemotherapy cycles.

Standard-dose rituximab has been incorporated into other previously established regimens for BL such as dose-modified CODOX-M/IVAC (cyclophosphamide, vincristine, doxorubicin, and high-dose methotrexate alternating with ifosfamide, etoposide, and high-dose cytarabine) and dose-adjusted EPOCH (etoposide, prednisone, vincristine, cyclophosphamide, and doxorubicin), with encouraging preliminary results.[51,52] Several studies have recently shown that the use of rituximab and intensive chemotherapy for human immunodeficiency virus (HIV)-related BL is feasible and can result in outcomes similar to the HIV-negative population, particularly in the setting of effective highly active antiretroviral therapy (HAART).[42,51,53]

Table 1
Regimens for adult Burkitt-type leukemia/lymphoma

Study	Therapy	No.	Age (Years)		% CR	% Continuous CR (No. of Years)	% OS (No. of Years)
			Median	% ≥ 60 [% ≥ 55]			
No rituximab							
Hoelzer et al[32]	B-NHL83	24	33	0	63	50 (8)	49 (8)
	B-NHL86	35	36	10	74	71 (4)	51 (4)
Hoelzer et al[33]	B-NHL 90	45	–	[100]	71	–	39 (6)
Magrath et al[34]	89-C-41 (CODOX-M/IVAC)	20	25	0	89	89 (2)	74 (4)
Thomas et al[35]	Hyper-CVAD	26	58	46	81	61 (3)	49 (3)
	Age < 60 y	14	38	–	3	83 (3)	77 (3)
	Age ≥ 60 y	12	–	–	–	–	17 (3)
Rizzieri et al[36]	CALGB 9521 Cohort 1	52	44	19	79	66 (3)	54 (3)
	Cohort 2	40	50	23	68	67 (3)	50 (3)
Di Nicola et al[37]	CMVVP-16/Ara-C/CDDP	22	36	–	77	68 (2)	77 (2)
Lacasce et al[38]	Modified CODOX-M/IVAC	14	47	–	86	64 (2)	71 (2)
Divine et al[39]	LMB95	72	33	–	72	–	70 (2)
Thomas et al[40]	Hyper-CVAD	48	48	33	85	60 (3)	53 (3)
	Age <60 y	25	–	–	–	73 (3)	70 (3)
	Age ≥60 y	23	–	–	–	44 (3)	19 (3)
Mead et al[41]	Modified CODOX-M/IVAC	53	37	9	–	–	67 (2)

With rituximab

Study	Regimen/Subgroup						
Thomas et al[40]	Hyper-CVAD + rituximab	31	46	29	86	88 (3)	89 (3)
	Age < 60 y	22	–	–	–	88 (3)	90 (3)
	Age ≥ 60 y	9	–	–	–	100 (3)	89 (3)
Oriol et al[42]	PETHEMA[a]	17	36	0	88	93 (2)	82 (2)
Hoelzer[43]	GMALL B-ALL/NHL 2002	146	36	[18]	90		
	BL						
	Age < 55 y					–	91 (3)
	Age ≥ 55 y					–	84 (3)
	B-ALL	84	46	[44]	83		
	Age < 55 y					–	79 (3)
	Age ≥ 55 y					–	39 (3)

Note: –, not available or not reported.

Abbreviations: B-ALL, mature B-cell ALL; BL, Burkitt lymphoma; CALGB, Cancer and Leukemia Group B; CMVVP-16/Ara-C/CDDP, cyclophosphamide, doxorubicin, high-dose methotrexate, vincristine, etoposide, cytarabine, cisplatin; CODOX-M/IVAC, cyclophosphamide, vincristine, doxorubicin, high-dose methotrexate alternating with ifosfamide, etoposide, high-dose cytarabine; CR, complete remission; CVAD, fractionated cyclophosphamide, vincristine, doxorubicin, dexamethasone alternating with high-dose methotrexate and cytarabine; GMALL, German Multicenter Study Group for Adult ALL; hyper-LMB, Lymphoma Malignancy B; NHL, non-Hodgkin lymphoma; OS, overall survival; PETHEMA, Programa para el Estudio de la Terapéutica en Hemopatías Malignas.
[a] Adapted from GMALL B-ALL/NHL 2002.

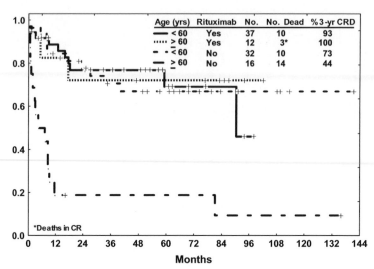

Fig. 2. Overall survival for de novo Burkitt leukemia/lymphoma by age and therapy (hyper-CVAD with or without rituximab). Late events in the younger group treated with hyper-CVAD and rituximab were related to secondary blood dyscrasias (refer to text).

RITUXIMAB-BASED CHEMOIMMUNOTHERAPY FOR ADULT PH-NEGATIVE PRECURSOR B-CELL ACUTE LYMPHOBLASTIC LEUKEMIA

Rituximab has also been incorporated into a modified hyper-CVAD regimen for adolescents and adults with de novo CD20-positive precursor B-cell ALL in a similar fashion to the regimen designed for BL or mature B-cell ALL. Comparative details of the modified hyper-CVAD chemoimmunotherapy regimens implemented since 1999 are provided in **Table 2**.[50,54] Since May 2000, 220 adolescents and adults with de novo ALL or lymphoblastic lymphoma were treated with the modified hyper-CVAD regimens, incorporating rituximab for the CD20-positive precursor B-cell subset (since October 2006 adolescents and young adults age 30 years or younger have been treated with an augmented BFM regimen without rituximab).[55] CD20 expression was noted in 53% of the 143 cases of precursor B-cell ALL. Overall CR rate was 94%, and was similar regardless of CD20 expression. In the CD20-positive subset, rituximab improved outcome compared with the historical experience with hyper-CVAD, with 3-year CRD rates (68% vs 28%, $P <$ .001) and OS rates (68% vs 35%, $P = $ .01) approaching those of the CD20-negative counterparts **(Fig. 3)**. In contrast to the experience with Burkitt-type leukemia/lymphoma, rituximab was not beneficial for the elderly group (age 60 years or older), with 3-year OS rates 48% versus 35%, P not significant.

In the elderly patients (>55 years) with CD20-positive precursor B-cell ALL treated according to the GMALL 2002 protocol, standard-dose rituximab was administered prior each cycle of dose-reduced chemotherapy and as consolidation for a total of 8 applications. In an interim analysis of 26 patients, the CR rate was 63% with a 1-year OS rate of 54%.[44] The younger patients with CD20-positive precursor B-cell ALL were treated per the GMALL 07/2003 protocol according to risk group. For the high-risk (HR) patients (leukocyte count >30 × 10^9/L or late achievement of CR), 3 standard doses of rituximab were administered immediately before each phase of induction (phase I, II), and the first consolidation chemotherapy cycle followed by allogeneic stem cell transplantation (SCT). The standard risk (SR) patients received 8

Table 2
Hyper-CVAD and modified hyper-CVAD chemoimmunotherapy regimens

	Modified Hyper-CVAD (± Rituximab)		Hyper-CVAD (1992–1999)
	Without Intensification (2001–Present)	With Intensification (2000–2001)	
Induction			
Hyper-CVAD (laminar air flow rooms if ≥60 y)	Y (Y)	Y (Y)	Y (N)
Consolidation			
Cycle 2 (intensification)			
Liposomal daunorubicin 150 mg/m² IV days 1–2; Cytarabine 3 g/m² IV every 12 h × 4 days 2–3; Prednisone 200 mg days 1–5	N	Y	N
Cycles 2, 4, 6, 8 or Cycles 3, 5, 7, 9			
Methotrexate 200 mg/m², then 800 mg/m² IV day 1; Cytarabine 3 g/m² IV every 12 h × 3 days 2–3; Solu-Medrol 50 mg IV every 12 h × 6 days 1–3	Y	Y	Y
Cycles 1, 3, 5, 7 or Cycles 1, 4, 6, 8			
Cyclophosphamide 300 mg/m² IV every 12 h × 6 days 1–3; Dexamethasone 40 mg days 1–4, 11–14; Doxorubicin 50 mg/m² CI IV day 4; Vincristine 2 mg IV days 1, 11	Y	Y	Y
Cycles 1–4			
IF CD20 ≥20%: 8 doses rituximab 375 mg/m²; Rituximab days 1, 11 (hyper-CVAD); Rituximab days 1, 8 (LDNR- or MTX-cytarabine)	Y	Y	N
CNS prophylaxis (No. intrathecals) Risk adapted (LDH >1400, S + G2M ≥14%)			
High	8	8	16
Indeterminate	8	8	8
Low	6	6	4
Maintenance			
POMP (6-mercaptopurine, VCR, methotrexate, prednisone)	Months 1–5, 8–17, 20–30	Months 1–5, 8–17, 20–30	Months 1–6, 8–10, 12–24
Intensification Hyper-CVAD; Rituximab 375 mg/m² days 1, 11 if CD20 ≥20%	Months 6, 18	Months 6, 18	N
Intensification Methotrexate 100 mg/m² IV day 1 weekly × 4; L-Asparaginase 20,000 units IV day 2 weekly × 4	Months 7, 19	Months 7, 19	Months 7, 11

Abbreviations: CI, continuous infusion; CNS, central nervous system; IV, intravenous; LDH, lactate dehydrogenase; LDNR, liposomal daunorubicin; MTX, methotrexate; VCR, vincristine.

applications of standard-dose rituximab before (day -1) the induction (phase I, II), reinduction, and 6 consolidation chemotherapy cycles. Preliminary results were reported for 185 patients with CD20-positive precursor B-cell ALL (133 SR, 52 HR); 117 (63%) received rituximab and were compared with the 70 patients who were treated with the same chemotherapy regimen before the incorporation of rituximab.[56] For SR patients, no difference in CR rate (94% vs 93%) was observed. However, the molecular CR rate (less than 10^{-4}) was superior with the rituximab therapy, 60% versus 19% at day 21 and 89% versus 57% at week 16. Improvement in the 3-year rates for CRD (64% vs 48%, $P = .009$) and for OS (75% vs 54%) were observed with the addition of rituximab. For HR pts, the 3-year rates for OS were 54% versus 32%. Allogeneic SCT was performed in 66% of the HR patients in first CR; OS was superior for the patients treated with rituximab (75% vs 40%) and was attributed to a reduction in the relapse rate. There was no difference in the incidence of deaths in first CR with the addition of rituximab (4% vs 3%).

The results of these 2 phase II nonrandomized clinical trials suggest that the addition of rituximab to established chemotherapy regimens for adolescents and adults with CD20-positive precursor B-cell ALL can improve outcome. Prospective clinical trials to further delineate the potential benefits of rituximab in a randomized fashion are either underway (randomization to rituximab versus no rituximab for CD20-positive precursor B-cell ALL) or planned (randomization of rituximab versus no rituximab for precursor B-cell ALL irrespective of CD20 expression). Based on preponderance of the data, the role of rituximab in the first-line treatment of adolescents and young adults with precursor B-cell ALL now treated with pediatric-based regimens should also be explored as a potential therapeutic intervention to eradicate MRD.

RITUXIMAB THERAPY IN PEDIATRIC BURKITT-TYPE LEUKEMIA/LYMPHOMA AND PRECURSOR B-CELL ACUTE LYMPHOBLASTIC LEUKEMIA

Until recently, there was a paucity of data regarding the use of rituximab for the treatment of BL or mature B-cell ALL in children and adolescents, despite extensive experience in the setting of posttransplant lymphoproliferative disease. Attias and Weitzman[57] reviewed the available literature up to the year 2007 and determined there was sufficient evidentiary support for the efficacy of rituximab as a single agent or in combination with chemotherapy, even in heavily pretreated patients. A subsequent clinical trial of rituximab combined with ifosfamide, carboplatin, and etoposide (RICE) for relapsed/refractory NHL or mature B-cell ALL was conducted by the Children's Oncology Group (COG ANHL0121).[58] The overall response rate was 64% in 14 patients with BL or mature B-cell ALL; there was no significant difference in toxicity profile compared with the historical experience with ICE. It was further postulated that the incorporation of rituximab into effective frontline chemotherapy could offset the negative prognostic influence of dose reductions (implemented for toxicities such as stomatitis, typhilitis, and infections) on EFS for children with de novo BL or mature B-ALL.[59] EFS was also inferior if features such as poor COP (cyclophosphamide, vincristine, and prednisone) response, combined BM/CNS disease, high tumor burden, or complex karyotype were present. Rituximab was therefore incorporated into French-American-British/Lymphoma Malignancy B (FAB/LMB) chemotherapy (4 doses in subpilot, 6 doses in pilot) for 48 children and adolescents with de novo intermediate risk advanced stage NHL (COG ANHL01P1), including 28 (59%) with BL. A preliminary report indicated an improvement in the 1-year EFS (96% vs 86%) compared with the historical experience with FAB/LMB96 without rituximab.[60] Randomized clinical trials are planned to confirm these findings.

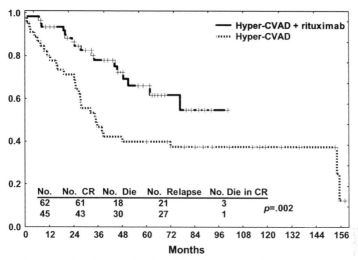

Fig. 3. Overall survival by therapy (modified hyper-CVAD with rituximab compared with hyper-CVAD alone) in the younger subsets (age less than 60 years) with de novo CD20-positive precursor B-cell ALL. No difference in survival was observed with rituximab for the elderly subset (not shown).

RITUXIMAB-BASED CHEMOIMMUNOTHERAPY WITH ALLOGENEIC STEM CELL TRANSPLANT FOR ACUTE LYMPHOBLASTIC LEUKEMIA

Investigators have reported an association between prior therapy with rituximab and a reduced incidence of acute and chronic graft-versus-host disease (aGVHD, cGVHD) after allogeneic SCT. Rituximab also has been efficacious as therapy for steroid-refractory GVHD, likely via depletion of donor and host antigen-presenting B cells that prime the T cells responsible for GVHD. In support of this hypothesis is the observation that infusion of a higher number of CD20-positive B cells from PB graft products correlated with a higher incidence of aGVHD.[61]

There are limited data regarding the use of rituximab for CD20-positive precursor B-cell ALL in the setting of allogeneic SCT. Kebriaei and colleagues[62] incorporated four weekly infusions of standard-dose rituximab (starting day −seven) into the standard preparative regimen of cyclophosphamide (Cy) and total body irradiation (TBI) for adolescents and adults with CD20-positive ALL. There was no delay in engraftment with the addition of rituximab. The cumulative incidence of aGVHD after matched sibling or matched unrelated donor SCT using the rituximab-based regimen was lower than that observed with the cohort of CD20-negative ALL patients treated over the same time period with the Cy/TBI regimen without rituximab (17% vs 39%, $P = .07$). Whether the addition of rituximab truly influenced outcomes such as survival and relapse-free survival could not be ascertained, because there were disparities with respect to the proportion of cases with B-lineage ALL (20% with T-lineage in the comparative group) and disease status at transplant (eg, in the rituximab group 74% were beyond first CR or had active disease whereas in the comparative group 54% were in first CR). Of note, the reduction in incidence of aGVHD with the use of rituximab did not seem to result in a significantly increased risk of relapse, as the direct antileukemic effects of rituximab likely offset any corresponding attenuation of graft-versus-leukemia (GVL) effect.

RITUXIMAB INTRATHECALLY FOR CENTRAL NERVOUS SYSTEM DISEASE IN ACUTE LYMPHOBLASTIC LEUKEMIA

Following systemic administration of rituximab, only 0.1% to 1.7% of the serum level was detectable in the cerebrospinal fluid (CSF), even in cases in which the blood-brain barrier was likely disrupted.[63,64] The CD20 antigen is not expressed by normal neurons or glial cells. Rituximab has been therefore been used intrathecally for the management of leptomeningeal infiltration in various lymphoproliferative disorders, including NHL.[65] There are limited data regarding the efficacy of this approach in CD20-positive ALL.[66] A small cohort of children and adolescents with CNS disease failing to respond triple intrathecal (IT) chemotherapy (methotrexate, cytarabine, hydrocortisone) underwent 4 weekly IT instillations of rituximab at a flat dose of 10 mg (in 6 mL of normal saline), followed by resumption of the triple IT therapy. All 7 patients cleared the CSF of malignant cells by the fourth dose of rituximab without significant toxicity. Although systemic relapses were noted in a few of the patients, the CNS was not a site of disease recurrence in any of the cases. The incorporation of rituximab concurrently with standard IT chemotherapy for de novo BL, mature B-cell ALL, or CD20-positive precursor B cell presenting with CNS involvement warrants further study in clinical trials.

EFFECTS OF RITUXIMAB ON DETECTION OF MINIMAL RESIDUAL DISEASE IN PRECURSOR B-CELL ACUTE LYMPHOBLASTIC LEUKEMIA

The use of multiparameter flow cytometry (MFC) for the detection and quantitation of MRD after induction and consolidation chemotherapy has been well established in childhood ALL.[67] The technique relies on aberrant leukemia-associated antigen expression patterns that allow discrimination from normal marrow precursor cells. The modulation of various surface leukemia antigens during induction chemotherapy (data from the AIEOP-BFM ALL 2000 protocol discussed earlier) did not compromise the ability to detect residual lymphoblasts.[13] In childhood ALL, the detection of MRD by MFC at levels 0.01% or greater at specific time points during chemotherapy has been associated with a higher propensity for disease recurrence. Risk-adapted therapeutic strategies have thus been implemented in these scenarios. Accurate assessments of MRD by MFC are therefore paramount.

Hematogones are normally occurring immature B-lineage cells that resemble malignant lymphoblasts morphologically and immunophenotypically. Hematogones may be particularly prominent in the regeneration phase following chemotherapy. The phenotypic stability and characteristic expression of antigens of these benign B-cell precursors has been well established.[68] In contrast, neoplastic lymphoblasts have aberrant antigen expression, maturational arrest, and immunophenotypic asynchrony (coexpression of early and late antigens). Despite these disparities, type 1 hematogones tend to have a similar phenotype to B lymphoblasts (CD34+ TdT+).

The use of MFC to detect MRD after induction and consolidation chemotherapy according to the modified hyper-CVAD regimen (with or without rituximab) for de novo CD20-positive precursor B-cell ALL (discussed earlier) was reviewed.[50] Rituximab appeared to induce a B-cell maturation arrest manifested by the detection of immature CD34+ TdT+ CD20− B cells in the marrow, potentially leading to a false positive diagnosis of MRD.[69] The use of additional markers such as CD38 (uniformly bright), CD58 (moderately positive), or CD9 (most cells positive) established a pattern of expression consistent with hematogones rather than residual ALL. The CD81 surface marker seems to be exceptionally discriminatory with respect to distinguishing residual precursor B-cell ALL (CD81 underexpressed) from hematogones (CD81 universally bright).[70] The effect of rituximab on the immunophenotype of marrow B-cell precursors could persist for as long as 6 months after completion of the immuno-therapy. These observations should be taken into consideration when performing MRD assays by MFC after rituximab-based chemoimmunotherapy.

TOXICITY OF RITUXIMAB

Rituximab is generally well tolerated, with the most common toxicity manifested by mild to moderate first-infusion reactions, although life-threatening anaphylaxis has been reported. In highly proliferative disease states such as Burkitt leukemia/lymphoma, the rapid cytolysis induced by rituximab may result in tumor lysis syndrome (TLS); the use of rasburicase for prophylaxis of TLS is considered manda-tory. Other potentially serious events associated with rituximab therapy have included reactivation of hepatitis B in chronic carriers leading to fulminant hepatic failure, severe mucocutaneous reactions, and progressive multifocal leukoencephalopathy (PML).[71] Prophylaxis of hepatitis B carriers with the antiviral agent lamivudine has been effective in preventing reactivation when commenced 1 week before initiation of rituximab and continued for at least 1 year after completion of therapy.[72] As a rare demyelinating infection of the CNS caused by the JC polyomavirus, PML is generally lethal, with a case-fatality ratio of 90%. A recent report summarized at least 50 cases, over a 10-year period following approval by the FDA, for which the develop-ment of PML was associated with rituximab (generally in the setting of prior or concur-rent immunosuppressive therapy).[73] Other rarely reported hematologic or immunologic events occurring subsequent to the completion of rituximab therapy include late onset neutropenia or transient hypogammaglobulinemia, neither usually associated with serious infections. Rituximab has rarely been linked to development of corticosteroid-responsive interstitial lung disease; it is an elusive diagnosis requiring exclusion of an underlying infectious etiology.

MECHANISMS OF RESISTANCE TO RITUXIMAB

Several potential mechanisms of resistance to rituximab have been characterized.[74] Development of rituximab-resistant B-lineage NHL cell lines (RRCL) has allowed the study of secondary or acquired resistance. The loss of protein expression, membrane exposure, or structural changes of CD20 can lead to primary resistance. Reduced expression of surface CD20 has been associated with hypermethylation of the transcription factor PU.1-encoding gene, which reputedly regulates CD20 expres-sion.[21] In vitro exposure to the hypomethylating agent 5-azacytidine restored CD20 mRNA expression of primary B-NHL cells.[20] Alterations of CD20 surface expression have been associated with increased histone acetylation, suggesting a possible role for histone deacetylase (HDAC) inhibitors.[6] Conformational changes of the CD20 protein that affect its affinity for rituximab have also been described.[6] The binding of rituximab to CD20 results in translocation and clustering of CD20 molecules into cholesterine-enriched lipid rafts. As inhibitors of cholesterol synthesis, statins have been shown to decrease rituximab-induced ADCC and CDCC.[75] The Fc region of rituximab is recognized by the complement component C1q, which activates the classic complement pathway and results in cytolysis via formation of the membrane attack complex (MAC). Specific Fc region or complement component polymorphisms, such as FgammaRIIIb (Val/Phe[158]), have been associated with reduced efficacy and increased propensity for disease recurrence after rituximab-based therapy.[76]

Within signaling platforms of the lipid rafts, CD20 is indirectly associated with the Src tyrosine kinases Lyn, Fyn, and Lck.[77] This process results in binding of downstream targets, triggering several intracellular signaling cascades, including NF-κB, phosphoinositide-3-kinase (PI3K)/Akt, p38 mitogen-activated kinases (MAPK), and ERK1/2.[7,49,78,79] Rituximab resistance has been associated with upregulation of these pro-proliferative signaling pathways. Resistance mechanisms also include upregulation of the antiapoptotic Bcl-2 protein family members Bcl-2, Bcl-X_L, and Mcl-1, as well as downregulation of proapoptotic Bak and Bax proteins.[80,81]

Pharmacologic targeting of NF-κB with bortezomib, histone deacetylase with vorinostat (SAHA), and Bcl-2 with the bcl-2 antisense oligonucleotide oblimersen may therefore restore sensitivity to rituximab. These agents interestingly have single-agent activity in a variety of lymphoproliferative disorders, and have been incorporated into chemoimmunotherapy regimens. Examples include bortezomib and hyper-CVAD with rituximab in de novo mantle cell lymphoma, and oblimersen with FCR (fludarabine, cyclophosphamide, and rituximab) in relapsed or refractory CLL.[82,83] Alterations of the PI3K/Akt pathway induced by inhibitors of the mammalian target of rapamycin (mTOR) (eg, temsirolimus and everolimus [RAD001]) appear to reverse resistance of lymphoblasts to anthracyclines and vinca alkaloids in vitro; combination therapy trials incorporating everolimus into hyper-CVAD and rituximab are planned.[84]

The downregulation of surface CD20 expression, increase in inhibitory complement-regulatory proteins CD55 and CD59, and upregulation of surface CD52 expression also seem to effect resistance to rituximab.[85] The CD52 antigen is a member of the glycosylphosphatidylinositol (GPI) anchored membrane glycoproteins, which seems to function in normal T-cell activation, release of cytokines, and signal transduction.[86] Targeting the CD52 antigen in vitro with alemtuzumab in RRCL induced significant cytolysis via CDCC, comparable with what has been observed with rituximab in sensitive cell lines.[85] Blocking the CD52 antigen using anti-CD52 F(ab')$_2$ fractions partially restored rituximab-associated CDCC, suggesting that CD52 may serve as an inhibitory protein.[85] An in vivo animal model of primary human ALL that coexpressed CD20 and CD52 was developed to assess response to rituximab, alemtuzumab, and the combination.[87] Whereas significant levels of residual ALL were identified in nearly all cases after administration of either MoAb singly, 90% achieved CR with the combination of rituximab and alemtuzumab. Faderl and colleagues[88] studied a regimen of 4 weekly standard doses of rituximab coadministered with alemtuzumab (7 full doses after 2 challenge doses) in relapsed or refractory CLL and other lymphoproliferative disorders, establishing the activity and tolerability of the regimen. The combination of rituximab with alemtuzumab could therefore be of further interest in the treatment of CD20-positive precursor B-cell ALL, based on the preclinical and clinical data.

It is notable that all of the mechanisms detailed here not only play a role in the primary or acquired resistance of lymphoblasts to rituximab but also in the sensitivity of the leukemia clones to chemotherapeutics. The countermeasures described that alter these pathways of leukemogenesis and resistance need to be studied further in the context of multitargeted chemoimmunotherapy.

NOVEL ANTI-CD20 MONOCLONAL ANTIBODIES

Ofatumumab (HuMax-CD20; GlaxoSmithKline, Collegeville, PA, and Genmab, Copenhagen, Denmark) is a second-generation fully human anti-CD20 IgG1 MoAb. This MoAb is directed at a unique small loop epitope of CD20 (different binding site than rituximab) with a longer release time from the target site and a superior CDCC effect compared with rituximab.[89] In vitro, ofatumumab exhibits its activity at a lower number of CD20 molecules per cell than rituximab, suggesting it would be more efficacious in diseases with inherently low CD20 expression, such as CLL.[90] Ofatumumab has indeed demonstrated promising clinical activity, with minimal infusional related toxicity in double refractory (fludarabine and alemtuzumab) or bulky fludarabine refractory CLL.[91] The use of ofatumumab in lieu of rituximab in frontline chemotherapy regimens for Burkitt-type leukemia/lymphoma and CD20-positive precursor B-cell ALL warrants investigation. Other candidate fully human anti-CD20 MoAbs undergoing development include veltuzumab (Immunomedics Inc., Morris Plains, NJ) in intravenous and subcutaneous formulations, and ocrelizumab (Biogen Idec Inc., Genentech Inc., Roche Holding AG, and Chugai Pharmaceuticals Co. Ltd).[92,93]

FUTURE DIRECTIONS

The incorporation of rituximab into frontline chemotherapy regimens for Burkitt-type leukemia/lymphoma seems to improve outcome. Preliminary data regarding the use of rituximab for CD20-positive precursor B-cell ALL suggest its use may also be beneficial, particularly for the younger subsets. Additional prospective studies are needed to confirm these findings and to determine the optimal use of rituximab in the treatment of CD20-positive (and possibly the CD20-negative subset based on upregulation of CD20 surface antigen expression) precursor B-cell ALL. To date, the development of these chemoimmunotherapy regimens has been entirely empirical. Future clinical trials should be guided by (1) levels of CD20 expression, (2) degree of CD20 modulation during induction chemotherapy, (3) presence or absence of circulating CD20 antigen, and (4) levels of rituximab. Unanswered questions include the potential benefits of early CD20 saturation (eg, more frequent or higher dosing of rituximab) versus administration solely to exploit chemosensitization (eg, standard dose concurrently with each cycle of chemotherapy). The incorporation of novel therapeutics that counter mechanisms of resistance to rituximab (eg, anti-Bcl-2 agents, mTOR inhibitors) may also improve the efficacy of chemoimmunotherapy by directly targeting the lymphoma or leukemia clone. The use of rituximab in combination with other MoAbs such as epratuzumab or alemtuzumab, for which safety and efficacy data exist, may also be beneficial for reasons detailed previously.[88,94,95] Although the preliminary data regarding the clinical activity of the novel anti-CD20 MoAbs seem promising, the improved efficacy alone is unlikely to ameliorate the need for multitargeted approaches required for a curative strategy in the treatment of adult ALL.

REFERENCES

1. Liedtke M, Cleary ML. Therapeutic targeting of MLL. Blood 2009;113:6061–8.
2. Craig FE, Foon KA. Flow cytometric immunophenotyping for hematologic neoplasms. Blood 2008;111:3941–67.
3. Ginaldi L, De Martinis M, Matutes E, et al. Levels of expression of CD19 and CD20 in chronic B cell leukaemias. J Clin Pathol 1998;51:364–9.
4. Riley JK, Sliwkowski MX. CD20: a gene in search of a function. Semin Oncol 2000; 27:17–24.
5. Manshouri T, Do KA, Wang X, et al. Circulating CD20 is detectable in the plasma of patients with chronic lymphocytic leukemia and is of prognostic significance. Blood 2003;101:2507–13.
6. Czuczman MS, Olejniczak S, Gowda A, et al. Acquirement of rituximab resistance in lymphoma cell lines is associated with both global CD20 gene and protein down-regulation regulated at the pretranscriptional and posttranscriptional levels. Clin Cancer Res 2008;14:1561–70.

7. Jazirehi AR, Vega MI, Bonavida B. Development of rituximab-resistant lymphoma clones with altered cell signaling and cross-resistance to chemotherapy. Cancer Res 2007;67:1270–81.

8. Borowitz MJ, Shuster J, Carroll AJ, et al. Prognostic significance of fluorescence intensity of surface marker expression in childhood B-precursor acute lymphoblastic leukemia. A Pediatric Oncology Group Study. Blood 1997;89:3960–6.

9. Jeha S, Behm F, Pei D, et al. Prognostic significance of CD20 expression in childhood B-cell precursor acute lymphoblastic leukemia. Blood 2006;108:3302–4.

10. Thomas DA, O'Brien S, Jorgensen JL, et al. Prognostic significance of CD20 expression in adults with de novo precursor B-lineage acute lymphoblastic leukemia. Blood 2009;113:6330–7.

11. Maury S, Huguet F, Pigneux A, et al. Prognostic significance of CD20 expression in adult B-cell precursor acute lymphoblastic leukemia [abstract 2829]. Blood 2007;110:832.

12. Huguet F, Leguay T, Raffoux E, et al. Pediatric-inspired therapy in adults with Philadelphia chromosome-negative acute lymphoblastic leukemia: the GRAALL-2003 study. J Clin Oncol 2009;27:911–8.

13. Gaipa G, Basso G, Maglia O, et al. Drug-induced immunophenotypic modulation in childhood ALL: implications for minimal residual disease detection. Leukemia 2005;19:49–56.

14. Gaipa G, Basso G, Aliprandi S, et al. Prednisone induces immunophenotypic modulation of CD10 and CD34 in nonapoptotic B-cell precursor acute lymphoblastic leukemia cells. Cytometry B Clin Cytom 2008;74:150–5.

15. Dworzak MN, Schumich A, Printz D, et al. CD20 up-regulation in pediatric B-cell precursor acute lymphoblastic leukemia during induction treatment: setting the stage for anti-CD20 directed immunotherapy. Blood 2008;112:3982–8.

16. Venugopal P, Sivaraman S, Huang XK, et al. Effects of cytokines on CD20 antigen expression on tumor cells from patients with chronic lymphocytic leukemia. Leuk Res 2000;24:411–5.

17. Yagci M, Akar I, Sucak GT, et al. GM-CSF does not increase CD20 antigen expression on chronic lymphocytic leukemia lymphocytes. Leuk Res 2005;29:735–8.

18. Schuster SJ, Venugopal P, Kern JC, et al. GM-CSF plus rituximab immunotherapy: translation of biologic mechanisms into therapy for indolent B-cell lymphomas. Leuk Lymphoma 2008;49:1681–92.

19. Ferrajoli A. Incorporating the use of GM-CSF in the treatment of chronic lymphocytic leukemia. Leuk Lymphoma 2009;50:514–6.

20. Hiraga J, Tomita A, Sugimoto T, et al. Down-regulation of CD20 expression in B-cell lymphoma cells after treatment with rituximab-containing combination chemotherapies: its prevalence and clinical significance. Blood 2009;113:4885–93.

21. Wojciechowski W, Li H, Marshall S, et al. Enhanced expression of CD20 in human tumor B cells is controlled through ERK-dependent mechanisms. J Immunol 2005;174:7859–68.

22. Maloney DG. Mechanism of action of rituximab. Anticancer Drugs 2001;12(Suppl 2):S1–4.

23. Binder M, Otto F, Mertelsmann R, et al. The epitope recognized by rituximab. Blood 2006;108:1975–8.

24. McLaughlin P, Grillo-Lopez AJ, Link BK, et al. Rituximab chimeric anti-CD20 monoclonal antibody therapy for relapsed indolent lymphoma: half of patients respond to a four-dose treatment program. J Clin Oncol 1998;16:2825–33.

25. Leget GA, Czuczman MS. Use of rituximab, the new FDA-approved antibody. Curr Opin Oncol 1998;10:548–51.
26. McLaughlin P, Hagemeister FB, Grillo-Lopez AJ. Rituximab in indolent lymphoma: the single-agent pivotal trial. Semin Oncol 1999;26:79–87.
27. Coiffier B, Lepage E, Briere J, et al. CHOP chemotherapy plus rituximab compared with CHOP alone in elderly patients with diffuse large-B-cell lymphoma. N Engl J Med 2002;346:235–42.
28. Feugier P, Van Hoof A, Sebban C, et al. Long-term results of the R-CHOP study in the treatment of elderly patients with diffuse large B-cell lymphoma: a study by the Groupe d'Etude des Lymphomes de l'Adulte. J Clin Oncol 2005;23:4117–26.
29. Pfreundschuh M, Trumper L, Osterborg A, et al. CHOP-like chemotherapy plus rituximab versus CHOP-like chemotherapy alone in young patients with good-prognosis diffuse large-B-cell lymphoma: a randomised controlled trial by the MabThera International Trial (MInT) Group. Lancet Oncol 2006;7:379–91.
30. Bennett JM, Catovsky D, Daniel MT, et al. Proposals for the classification of the acute leukaemias. French-American-British (FAB) co-operative group. Br J Haematol 1976;33:451–8.
31. D'Achille P, Seymour JF, Campbell LJ. Translocation (14;18)(q32;q21) in acute lymphoblastic leukemia: a study of 12 cases and review of the literature. Cancer Genet Cytogenet 2006;171:52–6.
32. Hoelzer D, Ludwig WD, Thiel E, et al. Improved outcome in adult B-cell acute lymphoblastic leukemia. Blood 1996;87:495–508.
33. Hoelzer D, Arnold R, Diedrich H. Successful treatment of Burkitt's NHL and other high-grade NHL according to protocol for mature B-ALL [abstract]. Blood 2002;100:159.
34. Magrath IT, Janus C, Edwards BK, et al. An effective therapy for both undifferentiated (including Burkitt's) lymphomas and lymphoblastic lymphomas in children and young adults. Blood 1984;63:1102–11.
35. Thomas DA, Cortes J, O'Brien S, et al. Hyper-CVAD program in Burkitt's-type adult acute lymphoblastic leukemia. J Clin Oncol 1999;17:2461–70.
36. Rizzieri DA, Johnson JL, Niedzwiecki D, et al. Intensive chemotherapy with and without cranial radiation for Burkitt leukemia and lymphoma: final results of Cancer and Leukemia Group B Study 9251. Cancer 2004;100:1438–48.
37. Di Nicola M, Carlo-Stella C, Mariotti J, et al. High response rate and manageable toxicity with an intensive, short-term chemotherapy programme for Burkitt's lymphoma in adults. Br J Haematol 2004;126:815–20.
38. Lacasce A, Howard O, Lib S, et al. Modified Magrath regimens for adults with Burkitt and Burkitt-like lymphomas: preserved efficacy with decreased toxicity. Leuk Lymphoma 2004;45:761–7.
39. Divine M, Casassus P, Koscielny S, et al. Burkitt lymphoma in adults: a prospective study of 72 patients treated with an adapted pediatric LMB protocol. Ann Oncol 2005;16:1928–35.
40. Thomas DA, Faderl S, O'Brien S, et al. Chemoimmunotherapy with hyper-CVAD plus rituximab for the treatment of adult Burkitt and Burkitt-type lymphoma or acute lymphoblastic leukemia. Cancer 2006;106:1569–80.
41. Mead GM, Barrans SL, Qian W, et al. A prospective clinicopathologic study of dose-modified CODOX-M/IVAC in patients with sporadic Burkitt lymphoma defined using cytogenetic and immunophenotypic criteria (MRC/NCRI LY10 trial). Blood 2008;112:2248–60.
42. Oriol A, Ribera JM, Bergua J, et al. High-dose chemotherapy and immunotherapy in adult Burkitt lymphoma: comparison of results in human immunodeficiency virus-infected and noninfected patients. Cancer 2008;113:117–25.

43. Hoelzer D. Recent results in the treatment of Burkitt lymphomas [abstract]. Ann Oncol 2008;19(Suppl 4):iv83.

44. Gokbuget N, Hoelzer D. Rituximab in the treatment of adult ALL. Ann Hematol 2006;85:117–9.

45. Kelly JL, Toothaker SR, Ciminello L, et al. Outcomes of patients with Burkitt lymphoma older than age 40 treated with intensive chemotherapeutic regimens. Clin Lymphoma Myeloma, in press.

46. de Vries MJ, Veerman AJ, Zwaan CM. Rituximab in three children with relapsed/ refractory B-cell acute lymphoblastic leukaemia/Burkitt non-Hodgkin's lymphoma. Br J Haematol 2004;125:414–5.

47. Daniels I, Abulayha AM, Thomson BJ, et al. Caspase-independent killing of Burkitt lymphoma cell lines by rituximab. Apoptosis 2006;11:1013–23.

48. Jazirehi AR, Gan XH, De Vos S, et al. Rituximab (anti-CD20) selectively modifies Bcl-xL and apoptosis protease activating factor-1 (Apaf-1) expression and sensitizes human non-Hodgkin's lymphoma B cell lines to paclitaxel-induced apoptosis. Mol Cancer Ther 2003;2:1183–93.

49. Jazirehi AR, Vega MI, Chatterjee D, et al. Inhibition of the Raf-MEK1/2-ERK1/2 signaling pathway, Bcl-xL down-regulation, and chemosensitization of non-Hodgkin's lymphoma B cells by Rituximab. Cancer Res 2004;64:7117–26.

50. Thomas DA, Kantarjian H, Faderl S, et al. Outcome after frontline therapy with the modified hyper-CVAD regimen with or without rituximab for de novo acute lymphoblastic leukemia (ALL) or lymphoblastic lymphoma (LL). [abstract 1931]. Blood 2008;112:674.

51. Abramson JS, Barnes JA, Toomey CE, et al. Rituximab added to CODOX-M/IVAC is highly effective in HIV-negative and HIV-positive Burkitt lymphoma. [abstract 3595]. Blood 2008;112:1229–30.

52. Dunleavy K, Little RF, Pittaluga S, et al. A prospective study of dose-adjusted (DA) EPOCH with rituximab in adults with newly diagnosed Burkitt lymphoma: a regimen with high efficacy and low toxicity. [abstract 009]. Ann Oncol 2008; 19(Suppl 4):iv83–4.

53. Cortes J, Thomas D, Rios A, et al. Hyperfractionated cyclophosphamide, vincristine, doxorubicin, and dexamethasone and highly active antiretroviral therapy for patients with acquired immunodeficiency syndrome-related Burkitt lymphoma/ leukemia. Cancer 2002;94:1492–9.

54. Thomas DA, O'Brien S, Cortes J, et al. Outcome with the hyper-CVAD regimens in lymphoblastic lymphoma. Blood 2004;104:1624–30.

55. Rytting M, Thomas D, Franklin A, et al. Young adults with acute lymphoblastic leukemia (ALL) treated with adapted augmented Berlin-Frankfurt-Munster (ABFM) therapy [abstract 3957]. Blood 2008;112.

56. Hoelzer D, Huettmann A, Kaul F, et al. Immunochemotherapy with rituximab in adult CD20 B-precursor ALL improves molecular CR rate and outcome in standard risk (SR) as well as in high risk (HR) patients with SCT. [abstract 481]. Haematologica 2009;94(Suppl 2).

57. Attias D, Weitzman S. The efficacy of rituximab in high-grade pediatric B-cell lymphoma/leukemia: a review of available evidence. Curr Opin Pediatr 2008; 20:17–22.

58. Griffin TC, Weitzman S, Weinstein H, et al. A study of rituximab and ifosfamide, carboplatin, and etoposide chemotherapy in children with recurrent/refractory B-cell (CD20+) non-Hodgkin lymphoma and mature B-cell acute lymphoblastic leukemia: a report from the Children's Oncology Group. Pediatr Blood Cancer 2009;52:177–81.

59. Cairo MS, Gerrard M, Sposto R, et al. Results of a randomized international study of high-risk central nervous system B non-Hodgkin lymphoma and B acute lymphoblastic leukemia in children and adolescents. Blood 2007;109: 2736–43.

60. Cairo MS, Lynch J, Harrison L, et al. Safety, efficacy, and rituximab levels following chemoimmunotherapy (rituximab + FAB chemotherapy) in children and adolescents with mature B-cell non-Hodgkin lymphoma (B-NHL): A Children's Oncology Group Report [abstract]. Blood 2008;112–310.

61. Iori AP, Torelli GF, De Propris MS, et al. B-cell concentration in the apheretic product predicts acute graft-versus-host disease and treatment-related mortality of allogeneic peripheral blood stem cell transplantation. Transplantation 2008;85: 386–90.

62. Kebriaei P, Saliba RM, Ma C, et al. Allogeneic hematopoietic stem cell transplantation after rituximab-containing myeloablative preparative regimen for acute lymphoblastic leukemia. Bone Marrow Transplant 2006;38:203–9.

63. Rubenstein JL, Combs D, Rosenberg J, et al. Rituximab therapy for CNS lymphomas: targeting the leptomeningeal compartment. Blood 2003;101:466–8.

64. Neuwelt EA, Specht HD, Hill SA. Permeability of human brain tumor to 99mTc-gluco-heptonate and 99mTc-albumin. Implications for monoclonal antibody therapy. J Neurosurg 1986;65:194–8.

65. Schulz H, Pels H, Schmidt-Wolf I, et al. Intraventricular treatment of relapsed central nervous system lymphoma with the anti-CD20 antibody rituximab. Haematologica 2004;89:753–4.

66. Jaime-Perez JC, Rodriguez-Romo LN, Gonzalez-Llano O, et al. Effectiveness of intrathecal rituximab in patients with acute lymphoblastic leukaemia relapsed to the CNS and resistant to conventional therapy. Br J Haematol 2009;144:794–5.

67. Campana D. Minimal residual disease in acute lymphoblastic leukemia. Semin Hematol 2009;46:100–6.

68. Kalff A, Juneja S. B-acute leukemic lymphoblasts versus hematogones: the wolf in sheep's clothing. Leuk Lymphoma 2009;50:523–4.

69. Siami K, Awagu S, Cooper DG, et al. Effects of rituximab on the immunophenotype of benign B-cell precursors: Implications for flow cytometric minimal residual disease detection in precursor B-acute lymphoblastic leukemia. Lab Invest 2006; 86(Suppl 1):246A–7A.

70. Muzzafar T, Medeiros J, Wang S, et al. Aberrant underexpression of CD81 in precursor B-cell acute lymphoblastic leukemia: utility in detection of minimal residual disease by flow cytometry. Amer J Clin Path, in press.

71. Ram R, Ben-Bassat I, Shpilberg O, et al. The late adverse events of rituximab therapy—rare but there! Leuk Lymphoma 2009;50:1083–95.

72. Lalazar G, Rund D, Shouval D. Screening, prevention and treatment of viral hepatitis B reactivation in patients with haematological malignancies. Br J Haematol 2007;136:699–712.

73. Carson KR, Evens AM, Richey EA, et al. Progressive multifocal leukoencephalopathy after rituximab therapy in HIV-negative patients: a report of 57 cases from the research on adverse drug events and reports project. Blood 2009;113: 4834–40.

74. Stolz C, Schuler M. Molecular mechanisms of resistance to rituximab and pharmacological strategies for its circumvention. Leuk Lymphoma 2009;50: 873–85.

75. Winiarska M, Bil J, Wilczek E, et al. Statins impair antitumor effects of rituximab by inducing conformational changes of CD20. PLoS Med 2008;5:e64.

76. Hatjiharissi E, Xu L, Santos DD, et al. Increased natural killer cell expression of CD16, augmented binding and ADCC activity to rituximab among individuals expressing the Fc{gamma}RIIIa-158 V/V and V/F polymorphism Blood 2007;110:2561–4.

77. Deans JP, Kalt L, Ledbetter JA, et al. Association of 75/80-kDa phosphoproteins and the tyrosine kinases Lyn, Fyn, and Lck with the B cell molecule CD20. Evidence against involvement of the cytoplasmic regions of CD20. J Biol Chem 1995;270:22632–8.

78. Suzuki E, Umezawa K, Bonavida B. Rituximab inhibits the constitutively activated PI3K-Akt pathway in B-NHL cell lines: involvement in chemosensitization to drug-induced apoptosis. Oncogene 2007;26:6184–93.

79. Vega MI, Huerta-Yepaz S, Garban H, et al. Rituximab inhibits p38 MAPK activity in 2F7 B NHL and decreases IL-10 transcription: pivotal role of p38 MAPK in drug resistance. Oncogene 2004;23:3530–40.

80. Stolz C, Hess G, Hahnel PS, et al. Targeting Bcl-2 family proteins modulates the sensitivity of B-cell lymphoma to rituximab-induced apoptosis. Blood 2008;112: 3312–21.

81. Olejniczak SH, Hernandez-Ilizaliturri FJ, Clements JL, et al. Acquired resistance to rituximab is associated with chemotherapy resistance resulting from decreased Bax and Bak expression. Clin Cancer Res 2008;14:1550–60.

82. Romaguera J, Fayad L, McLaughlin P, et al. Phase 1 trial of bortezomib in combination with rituximab-hyper-CVAD/methotrexate and cytarabine for untreated mantle cell lymphoma [abstract 3051]. Blood 2008;112:1049.

83. O'Brien S, Moore JO, Boyd TE, et al. Randomized phase III trial of fludarabine plus cyclophosphamide with or without oblimersen sodium (Bcl-2 antisense) in patients with relapsed or refractory chronic lymphocytic leukemia. J Clin Oncol 2007;25:1114–20.

84. Chanan-Khan A. Bcl-2 antisense therapy in hematologic malignancies. Curr Opin Oncol 2004;16:581–5.

85. Cruz RI, Hernandez-Ilizaliturri FJ, Olejniczak S, et al. CD52 over-expression affects rituximab-associated complement-mediated cytotoxicity but not antibody-dependent cellular cytotoxicity: preclinical evidence that targeting CD52 with alemtuzumab may reverse acquired resistance to rituximab in non-Hodgkin lymphoma. Leuk Lymphoma 2007;48:2424–36.

86. Ginaldi L, De Martinis M, Matutes E, et al. Levels of expression of CD52 in normal and leukemic B and T cells: correlation with in vivo therapeutic responses to Campath-1H. Leuk Res 1998;22:185–91.

87. Nijmeijer B, van Schie MLJ, Willemze R, et al. Rituximab and alemtuzumab in combination, but not alone, induce complete remissions in a preclinical animal model of primary human ALL: rationale for combination treatment [abstract 2833]. Blood 2007;112:833a–4.

88. Faderl S, Thomas DA, O'Brien S, et al. Experience with alemtuzumab plus rituximab in patients with relapsed and refractory lymphoid malignancies. Blood 2003;101:3413–5.

89. Castillo J, Milani C, Mendez-Allwood D. Ofatumumab, a second-generation anti-CD20 monoclonal antibody, for the treatment of lymphoproliferative and autoimmune disorders. Expert Opin Investig Drugs 2009;18:491–500.

90. Teeling JL, Mackus WJ, Wiegman LJ, et al. The biological activity of human CD20 monoclonal antibodies is linked to unique epitopes on CD20. J Immunol 2006; 177:362–71.

91. Osterborg A, Kipps TJ, Mayer J, et al. Ofatumumab (HuMax-CD20), a novel CD20 monoclonal antibody, is an active treatment for patients with CLL refractory

to both fludarabine and alemtuzumab or bulky fludarabine-refractory disease: Results from the planned interim analysis of an international pivotal trial [abstract 328]. Blood 2008;112:126–7.

92. Morschhauser F, Leonard JP, Fayad L, et al. Humanized anti-CD20 antibody, veltuzumab, in refractory/recurrent non-Hodgkin's lymphoma: phase I/II results. J Clin Oncol 2009;27:3346–53.

93. Hutas G. Ocrelizumab, a humanized monoclonal antibody against CD20 for inflammatory disorders and B-cell malignancies. Curr Opin Investig Drugs 2008;9:1206–15.

94. Leonard JP, Coleman M, Ketas J, et al. Combination antibody therapy with epratuzumab and rituximab in relapsed or refractory non-Hodgkin's lymphoma. J Clin Oncol 2005;23:5044–51.

95. Leonard JP, Schuster SJ, Emmanouilides C, et al. Durable complete responses from therapy with combined epratuzumab and rituximab: final results from an international multicenter, phase 2 study in recurrent, indolent, non-Hodgkin lymphoma. Cancer 2008;113:2714–23.

Risk-adapted Treatment of Pediatric Acute Lymphoblastic Leukemia

Sima Jeha, MD[a,b,]*, Ching-Hon Pui, MD[a,c]

KEYWORDS

- ALL treatment • Pediatric leukemia • ALL biology
- Risk-adapted therapy

Studies in pediatric acute lymphoblastic leukemia (ALL) have been a model for integration of basic and clinical research. As early as 1951, Burchenal and colleagues[1] noted that response of patients with ALL to antimetabolite therapy was less favorable when initial leukocyte count was high. Approximately 2 decades later, Aur and colleagues[2] first designed treatment specifically aimed at ALL at high risk of treatment failure. The 1980s and 1990s witnessed an extension of the observation of Burchenal and colleagues and the approach of Aur and colleagues as several groups adjusted therapy according to the risk of relapse, giving more drugs at higher dosage to patients with high leukocyte count and other features associated with treatment failure.[3] With improved understanding of the immunology and molecular pathways involved in ALL, current risk classification typically includes age, presenting leukocyte count, blast cell immunophenotype and genotype, and early treatment response (**Table 1**). Early response to therapy, as measured by minimal residual disease (MRD) evaluation, has played an increasing role in risk stratification of ALL. Adapting therapy according to the risk of relapse in individual patients is helping to improve the outcome of patients with high-risk leukemia while minimizing long-term sequelae and enhancing the quality of life in patients at low risk of relapse.[4]

This work was supported in part by a Cancer Center Support Grant (CA21765) from the National Cancer Institute and by the American Lebanese Syrian Associated Charities. Dr. Pui is an American Cancer Society Professor.

[a] Department of Oncology, St. Jude Children's Research Hospital, 262 Danny Thomas Place, Memphis, TN 38105, USA
[b] Leukemia/Lymphoma Developmental Therapeutics, Department of Oncology, St. Jude Children's Research Hospital, Memphis, TN, USA
[c] Hematological Malignancies Program, Department of Oncology, St. Jude Children's Research Hospital, Memphis, TN, USA
* Corresponding author. Department of Oncology, St. Jude Children's Research Hospital, 262 Danny Thomas Place, Memphis, TN 38105, USA.
E-mail address: sima.jeha@stjude.org (S. Jeha).

Hematol Oncol Clin N Am 23 (2009) 973–990
doi:10.1016/j.hoc.2009.07.009
0889-8588/09/$ – see front matter © 2009 Elsevier Inc. All rights reserved.

| Table 1 |
| Prognostic factors in childhood acute lymphoblastic leukemia |

Factor	Favorable	Intermediate	Unfavorable
Age (years)	1 to 9	$\geq 10^a$	<1 and *MLL*+
White blood cell count ($\times 10^9$/L)	<50	$\geq 50^a$	
Immunophenotype	Precursor B cell	T cell[a]	
Genetics	Hyperdiploidy >50 or DNA index >1.16 Trisomies 4,10, and 17 t(12;21)/*ETV6-CBFA2*	Diploid t(1;19)/*TCF3-PBX1*[a]	t(9;22)/*BCR-ABL1* t(4:11)/*MLL-AF4* Hypodiploid <44
CNS status	CNS1	CNS2[a] Traumatic with blasts	CNS3
MRD (end of induction)	<0.01%	0.01% to 0.99%	$\geq 1\%$

[a] These factors used to carry an unfavorable prognosis; however, outcome has improved with risk-directed contemporary therapy.

PROGNOSTIC FACTORS IN ACUTE LYMPHOBLASTIC LEUKEMIA TREATMENT

Optimal use of antileukemic agents and stringent application of risk-directed therapy in clinical trials have resulted in steady improvement in the outcome of children with ALL, with current cure rates exceeding 80% in developed countries. The intensity of treatment varies substantially among subsets of patients, as therapy is designed to reduce acute and long-term toxicity in low-risk groups while improving outcome in poor risk groups by treatment intensification. Recent advances in genome-wide screening techniques and pharmacogenomic studies and in the development of molecular therapeutics have ushered in an era of more refined personalized therapy. The intensity of contemporary ALL protocols is adjusted according to specific presenting clinical and biologic features and early treatment response (**Fig. 1**). These prognostic factors are often interrelated and largely dependent on the therapy administered.

Age and Leukocyte Count at Diagnosis

Many studies have established an inferior outcome of infants and adolescents with ALL compared with children of intermediate age and a poorer outcome associated with increasing leukocyte count.[3] The prognostic impact of age and, to a lesser extent, leukocyte count can be explained partly by their association with specific genetic abnormalities. For example, the overall favorable outcome of patients aged 1 to 9 years is associated with the preponderance of cases with hyperdiploidy and *ETV6-CBFA2* (also known as *TEL-AML1*) fusion, and the poor prognosis of infants is related to the preponderance of *MLL* rearrangement (70% to 80%) in this age group.[4,5] Philadelphia chromosome with *BCR-ABL1* fusion is more common in adolescents than in children of other age groups. Primary genetic features, however, do not entirely account for treatment outcome. Relapses are observed in up to 15% of patients with hyperdiploidy greater than 50 or *ETV6-CBFA2,* whereas a substantial proportion of patients with the t(9;22) and *BCR-ABL1* fusion who are 1 to 9 years old and have a low leukocyte count at diagnosis may be cured with intensive chemotherapy alone (pre-imatinib era).[6] Among patients with *MLL* rearrangement, infants and adults have a worse prognosis than children.[7–9]

St. Jude Total Therapy Study XVI: Risk Classification Schema

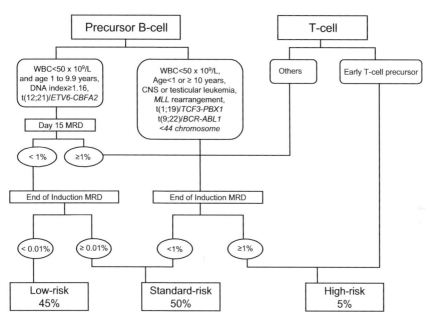

Fig. 1. Risk classification schema for patients with ALL treated in ongoing St. Jude Children's Research Hospital Total Study XVI.

Immunophenotype

Approximately 12% to 15% children with ALL have a T-cell immunophenotype (precursor T-cell ALL), and three fourths of these patients present at age older than 9 years or with elevated leukocyte count. Historically, the T-cell immunophenotype has been a marker of poorer prognosis in comparison to precursor B-cell ALL. Patients with precursor T-cell ALL are generally treated with intensive chemotherapy regardless of presenting age and leukocyte count. The introduction of intensive asparaginase and high-dose methotrexate treatment has significantly improved the outcome for patients with precursor T-cell ALL.[10–12] With the emergence of specific therapy,[13] there is an increasing tendency to assign patients with precursor T-cell ALL to a specific treatment protocol or strata. The US Children's Oncology Group has a separate trial for these children, which includes the purine nucleoside analog, nelarabine, for patients in intermediate and high-risk groups.

Although ALL can be further subclassified according to the recognized steps of normal maturation within the B lineage (pro-B, early pre-B, pre-B, transitional pre-B, and mature B) or T lineage (pre-T and mid and late thymocyte) pathways, the only distinctions used in treatment assignment in most studies are those between precursor T-cell, mature B-cell, and other B-lineage (precursor B-cell) immunophenotypes.[4] Recently, a distinct subset of T-cell ALL that retains stem cell-like features, termed early T-cell precursor ALL, was identified and associated with a dismal prognosis with conventional chemotherapy.[14]

Cytogenetics

Approximately 75% of childhood ALL cases can be classified into prognostically or therapeutically relevant subgroups based on the modal chromosome number (or DNA content measured by flow cytometry), specific chromosomal rearrangements, and molecular genetic changes.[15,16] Patients with precursor B-cell ALL and more than 50 chromosomes in blasts cells (or DNA index ≥1.16) have a good outcome, regardless of age and leukocyte count at presentation.[17,18] Hyperdiploidy (>50 chromosomes) is seen in approximately 25% of cases and its favorable prognosis may reflect an increased cellular accumulation of methotrexate and its polyglutamates, an increased sensitivity to antimetabolites and L-asparaginase, and a marked propensity of these cells to undergo apoptosis.[19–21] By contrast, hypodiploidy (<44) chromosomes is associated with an exceptionally poor prognosis.[22] More than 80% of patients with a favorable DNA index are 1 to 9 years old with low leukocyte count at presentation. Combined trisomy of chromosomes 4 and 10 was identified as an independent prognostic factor by the Pediatric Oncology Group.[23] Approximately 70% of patients with favorable DNA index have trisomy of chromosomes 4 and 10 compared with fewer than 5% of patients with unfavorable DNA index.

Approximately 20% to 25% of children with ALL present with the favorable t(12;21) translocation with *ETV6-CBFA2* fusion. The translocation t(9;22) (*BCR-ABL1*) is detected in approximately 2% to 4% of children with precursor B-cell ALL and the t(4;11) translocation with *MLL-AF4* fusion in 1% to 2% of children older than 12 months of age.[8,24–26] Patients with the unfavorable t(9;22) and t(4;11) translocations account for approximately 10% of patients older than 9 years at diagnosis and with high presenting leukocyte count. Approximately 3% of white and 12% of black children with ALL have the t(1;19)(*TCF3-PBX1*)[27]; one-half of these patients present with unfavorable age or high leukocyte count. Patients with the t(1;19) historically had a relatively poor outcome[28]; however, the outcome of patients with this genotype who are treated with contemporary intensive regimens is superior to that of other precursor B cases in pediatric and adult ALL.[29,30]

Molecular analyses can identify several submicroscopic genetic alterations, such as the *ETV6-RUNX1* fusion, intrachromosomal amplification of chromosome 21, deletions of tumor suppressor genes, and mutations of proto-oncogenes.[5,16,31,32] Fluorescence in situ hybridization and reverse transcriptase–polymerase chain reaction (RT-PCR) assays are used frequently to detect genetic rearrangements. More recently, the application of microarray-based genome-wide analysis of gene expression and DNA copy number, complemented by transcriptional profiling, resequencing, and epigenetic approaches, has identified specific genetic alterations with biologic and therapeutic implications.[33–35] Most notable is the identification of a subgroup of very high-risk precursor B-cell ALL with genetic profile similar to that of cases with *BCR-ABL1* fusion, characterized by deletion of *IKZF1*, encoding the transcription factor Ikaros, reviewed elsewhere in this issue.[33–35]

Early Response to Therapy

The degree of reduction of the leukemic cell clone early during remission induction therapy has greater prognostic strength than any other individual biologic or host-related feature, as it encompasses leukemic cell genetics, host pharmacokinetics and pharmacogenomics, the host microenvironment of leukemic cells, compliance with treatment, and treatment efficacy.[36] Assessing MRD by flow-cytometric detection of aberrant immunophenotypes or by PCR analysis of clonal antigen-receptor gene rearrangements provides a level of sensitivity and specificity that cannot be attained by traditional morphologic assessment, reviewed elsewhere in this issue. There is strong concordance between the assessment of MRD by flow cytometry and by PCR methods. More than 95% of patients can be followed by flow cytometry, which is a simple and rapid method.[36] PCR method could be reserved for the few patients whose leukemic cells lack a suitable immunophenotype.

TREATMENT

Childhood ALL cases are divided into three risk groups: low, intermediate, and high (also referred to as standard, high, and very high).[37] The Children's Oncology Group has used a four-category system that recognizes patients with a very low probability of relapse. Infants are often considered a special subgroup of ALL that requires different treatment.[38] Current treatment regimens consist of three main phases: remission induction, intensification/consolidation with reinduction segments, and prolonged continuation/maintenance phase. Central nervous system (CNS)-directed therapy starts early and overlaps other treatments. These regimens vary in intensity according to risk groups and are increasingly addressing the therapeutic needs of clinically and biologically distinct patient subgroups (including infant, *BCR-ABL1* positive, and T-cell ALL). Identification of new genetic and epigenetic alterations almost certainly will lead to the development of more specific targeted treatment.

Remission Induction

The induction regimen is typically administered over a 4- to 6-week period and includes a glucocorticoid (prednisone, prednisolone, or dexamethasone), vincristine, and asparaginase. Patients with intermediate- or high-risk ALL also receive an anthracycline.[4] The biologically equivalent doses of dexamethasone and prednisone are not certain and the optimal dose and schedule also remain to be determined.[39–41] Similarly, a role for pharmacogenomics in predicting glucocorticoid resistance may assist in treatment decisions.[1] Most regimens currently use prednisone during induction and reserve dexamethasone for postremission therapy, although some investigators advocate the use of dexamethasone during remission induction therapy.

As with glucocorticoids, the pharmacodynamics of asparaginase differ by formulation. Three forms are available: one derived from *Erwinia chrysanthemi*, another prepared from *Escherichia coli*, and a third made of a polyethylene glycol form of the *E coli* product (pegaspargase).[42] The amount of asparagine depletion, which reflects the dose intensity and duration of asparaginase treatment, is more important than the type of asparaginase used for leukemia control. The dose schedule of the three preparations is based on their half-lives. Pegaspargase, which has the longest half-life, usually is administered at 2500 IU/m² every other week for 1 to 2 doses in cases of newly diagnosed ALL. By contrast, the *Erwinia* preparation, which has the shortest half-life, is administered at 20,000 IU/m² 2 to 3 times per week for 6 to 12 doses. The doses of *E coli* L-asparaginase range from 6000 to 10,000 IU/m², administered every 2 to 3 days for 6 to 12 doses. Different preparations of the *E coli* enzyme also seem to have different pharmacologic and pharmacokinetic properties.[43] These differences mandate dosage adjustment to avoid lack of efficacy or excessive toxicity.[44,45] Because of lower immunogenicity and less frequent administration,[46,47] pegaspargase is replacing the native product as the first-line treatment for children and is also increasingly used in adult ALL trials.[48,49] Compared with *E coli* asparaginase, *Erwinia* asparaginase was associated with inferior antileukemic response but few toxic effects in some randomized trials, a finding now attributed to use of inadequate doses of the *Erwinia* drug.[50,51] Among various anthracyclines (daunorubicin, doxorubicin, and mitoxantrone) used, none has proved superior; however, daunorubicin is used most commonly.

Several studies have suggested that intensive therapy is unnecessary for children with standard-risk ALL, provided patients receive postinduction intensification therapy.[52] High-risk patients might benefit from intensifying induction therapy, which could potentially result in a faster and more robust reduction of the leukemic cell burden. This strategy, however, can lead to increased early morbidity and mortality.[53] Conceivably, intensified remission induction with targeted agents that have no overlapping toxicities (for example, monoclonal antibodies, or tyrosine kinase inhibitors for BCR-ABL1–positive ALL) can also improve treatment outcome.

The rapidity of response to induction therapy, as measured by clearance of peripheral and bone marrow blasts, is a predictor of outcome.[4,36,54] Approximately 98% of children attain complete morphologic remission (ie, <5% blasts in bone marrow) at the end of remission induction. These patients have various degrees of residual leukemia, and some can still have as many as 10 billion leukemic cells.[55] Because the extent of residual disease is well correlated with long-term outcome,[36] the concept of a "molecular" or "immunologic" remission, defined as leukemic involvement of less than 0.01% of nucleated marrow cells,[56] is beginning to supplant the traditional perception of remission, which is based solely on morphologic criteria. The authors and other investigators have found that patients with 1% blasts identified by MRD studies at end of induction had an outcome as poor as those with induction failure.[56]

Intensification (Consolidation) and Reinduction

This regimen starts when normal hematopoiesis is restored and is tailored to the leukemia subtype and risk group. This phase of therapy has improved outcome, even for patients with low-risk ALL.[57] The necessity of intensification in childhood ALL is not disputed; however, there is no consensus about the best regimen and duration of treatment. More commonly used regimens for childhood ALL include high-dose methotrexate with or without mercaptopurine;[58] high-dose L-asparaginase given for an extended period;[47,59] or a combination of dexamethasone, vincristine, L-asparaginase, and doxorubicin, followed by thioguanine, cytarabine, and cyclophosphamide.[11,60] Patients with ETV6-RUNX1 have an especially good outcome in clinical trials featuring intensive postremission treatment with glucocorticoids, vincristine, and asparaginase.[61,62] Adding doxorubicin to asparaginase favorably influenced the outcome of high-risk patients, in particular those with T-cell disease.[12,47]

Improved outcome was also reported for patients receiving early intensification treatment with intermediate-dose or high-dose methotrexate.[11,63–66] The optimal dose of methotrexate depends on the leukemic cell genotype and phenotype and host pharmacogenetic and pharmacokinetic parameters. Methotrexate at 2.5 g/m^2 is adequate for most patients with standard-risk ALL, but a higher dose (5 g/m^2) seems to improve outcome of those with T-cell or high-risk precursor B-cell ALL.[54,67] This observation is consistent with the finding that T-lineage blast cells accumulate methotrexate polyglutamates (active metabolites of the parent compound) less avidly than do precursor B-cell blasts[19]; therefore, higher serum levels of the drug are needed for an adequate therapeutic effect.[68] The fact that hyperdiploid ALL blast cells accumulate increased amount of methotrexate polyglutamate could partially explain the excellent outcome of children with this genotype treated on low-intensity antimetabolites-based regimens.[54,69,70] The conventional dose of methotrexate (1 g/m^2) may be too low for many patients with precursor B-cell ALL.[58] To this end, the authors' study showed that among precursor B-cell ALL, blasts with ETV6-RUNX1 or TCF3-PBX1 gene fusion accumulate significantly lower methotrexate polyglutamates compared with those with hyperdiploidy or other genetic abnormalities.[71] This finding suggested that patients with *ETV6-RUNX1* or *TCF3-PBX1* gene fusion benefit from a higher dose of methotrexate.

Because methotrexate is an antifolate, children with variant alleles in enzymes within the folate pathway (eg, 5,10-methylenetetrahydrofolate reductase and thymidylate synthase) are at a higher risk for relapse.[2,3] These findings suggest new approaches to predict and potentially overcome methotrexate resistance.

Reinduction therapy, pioneered by the Berlin-Frankfurt-Munster (BFM) consortium, consists of drugs similar to those used in remission induction therapy and is usually administered after 3 months of a less-intensive, interim maintenance chemotherapy.[11,54] The Children's Cancer Group confirmed the efficacy of delayed reinduction therapy in low-risk cases[72] and showed that a second reinduction at week 32 of treatment further improved outcome in patients with intermediate-risk disease.[73] An augmented intensification regimen consisting of the administration of additional doses of vincristine and asparaginase during delayed intensification periods of myelosuppression, and sequential escalating-dose parental methotrexate followed by asparaginase (Capizzi methotrexate regimen), improved the outcome of high-risk patients whose disease had responded slowly to initial multiagent induction therapy.[59] Additional pulses of vincristine and prednisone after one reinduction treatment did not improve outcome.[4] These data suggest that the benefit of double-delayed intensification (ie, two reinductions) resulted from the increased dose intensity of other agents, such as asparaginase or anthracycline, or the timing or scheduling of the intensification regimen.[73]

Continuation (Maintenance)

Excluding cases of mature B-cell leukemia, continuation therapy with 2 to 2.5 years of low-intensity metronomic chemotherapy is an integral part of ALL regimens. Attempts to shorten the duration of continuation treatment have led to inferior outcome in childhood and adult ALL.[74–76] Although it seems that two thirds of childhood cases could be cured with only 12 months of treatment,[77] it remains unclear which subgroups of childhood ALL can be cured with abbreviated therapy. In a meta-analysis of 42 trials, a third year of continuation therapy reduced the likelihood of relapse, but no advantage to prolonging treatment beyond 3 years was observed.[78] Early studies have demonstrated that the third year of continuation therapy benefits boys but not girls[79,80]; hence, most studies discontinue all therapy for girls after 2 to 2.5 years of treatment. It is uncertain whether or not improved contemporary treatment will reduce the need for a prolonged continuation.

Weekly low-dose methotrexate and daily mercaptopurine form the backbone of most continuation regimens. Adjusting chemotherapy doses to maintain neutrophil counts between 0.5 and 1.5 × 10^9/L and accumulation of higher intracellular concentrations of the active metabolites of methotrexate and mercaptopurine are associated with improved clinical outcome.[81–84] Overzealous use of mercaptopurine, to the extent that neutropenia necessitates chemotherapy interruption, reduces overall dose intensity and is counterproductive.[85] It is recommended to give mercaptopurine at bedtime to patients with an empty stomach[86] and to avoid concomitant intake of milk or milk products containing xanthine oxidase, which can degrade the drug.[87] Antimetabolite treatment should not be withheld because of isolated increased levels of liver enzymes, because such liver function abnormalities are tolerable and reversible.[88]

One in 300 patients inherits two nonfunctional variant alleles of the gene encoding thiopurine *S*-methyltransferase, the enzyme that inactivates mercaptopurine. In these patients, mercaptopurine should be given in much smaller doses (eg, 10-fold reduction) to avoid potentially fatal hematologic side effects.[89] Approximately 10%

of patients are heterozygous for the enzyme deficiency and have intermediate levels of thiopurine methyltransferase.[90] This subgroup can be treated safely with only moderate reductions in mercaptopurine dosage and seems to have better clinical outcomes than do patients with the homozygous wild-type phenotype. Patients with this enzyme deficiency are at risk for chemotherapy-related leukemia and radiation-related brain tumor.[91,92] Whether or not reducing the mercaptopurine dosage reduces the risk of therapy-related leukemia in these patients is unknown. This underscores the importance of understanding the inherited differences in drug metabolism and disposition resulting from genetic polymorphisms.[5,93,94] Thioguanine is more potent than mercaptopurine in model systems and leads to higher concentrations of thioguanine nucleotides in cells and cytotoxic concentrations in cerebrospinal fluid.[95] In randomized trials comparing the effectiveness of these two drugs, thioguanine, given at a daily dose of 40 mg/m^2 or more, produced superior antileukemic responses to mercaptopurine but was associated with profound thrombocytopenia, an increased risk of death, and unacceptable rate of hepatic veno-occlusive disease.[96,97] Although the lower activity of thiopurine methyltransferase was associated with the development of veno-occlusive disease, this measure could not reliably identify patients at risk.[98] Therefore, mercaptopurine remains the drug of choice for prolonged administration. Thioguanine could still be tested, however, in short-term courses during the intensification or continuation phase of therapy.

Regular pulses of vincristine and a glucocorticoid during the antimetabolite-based continuation regimens have been widely adopted.[78] The benefit of these pulses in the context of cotemporary therapy is not established. In a randomized trial featuring intensive reinduction, the addition of six pulses of vincristine and dexamethasone during early continuation treatment failed to improve outcome of children with intermediate-risk ALL.[99]

Central Nervous System–Directed Therapy

The CNS is a common sanctuary for leukemic cells. Presenting features associated with an increased risk of CNS relapse in ALL include a T-cell immunophenotype; hyperleukocytosis; the presence of t(9;22), t(4;11), or t(1;19); and CNS involvement.[29,100] Children or adolescents with T-cell ALL and a presenting leukocyte count of more than 100×10^9/L have a high risk of CNS and bone marrow relapse if CNS-directed treatment is suboptimal.[101]

The presence of any amount of blasts in the CSF at diagnosis,[102] including a traumatic lumbar puncture with leukemia blasts into the CSF[103–105] has been associated with a poor treatment outcome. Based on these observations, the authors proposed a new classification of CNS status: CNS1, no detectable blast cells in CSF; CNS2, fewer than five leukocytes per μL with detectable blast cells in a cytocentrifuged preparation of CSF; CNS3, the presence of overt CNS leukemia, as previously defined by the Rome workshop ($\geq$5 leukocytes per μL with identifiable blast cells or the presence of cranial-nerve palsies); and traumatic lumbar puncture with blasts.[100] The use of more effective systemic and CNS-directed treatment in contemporary trials has greatly reduced or eliminated the prognostic effect of a CNS2 status. In contrast, a traumatic lumbar puncture with blasts continues to predict a poor outcome.[103–105] In the authors' view, a CNS2 status or traumatic lumbar puncture with blasts warrants intensification of CNS-directed treatment to reduce the risk of relapse in these patients. To avoid traumatic lumbar punctures, especially at diagnosis when most patients have abundant circulating leukemia blasts, the procedure should be performed by an experienced clinician while a patient is under general anesthesia or deep sedation. The authors[100] also correct thrombocytopenia before the diagnostic lumbar puncture and then immediately give intrathecal treatment. Platelet transfusion is seldom necessary after the start of remission induction that includes a glucocorticoid and asparaginase, because most patients are in a hypercoagulable state and at low risk of bleeding despite thrombocytopenia.[106] Intrathecal medication given in a large volume (6 mL or more) attains a better distribution in the CNS than if given in a small volume. After the procedure, patients should remain in the prone position for at least 30 minutes. This position is shown to increase the intraventricular amount of medication in a nonhuman primate model.[107] Triple intrathecal therapy with methotrexate, cytarabine, and hydrocortisone is more effective than intrathecal methotrexate in preventing CNS relapse.[108] Systemic treatment, including high-dose methotrexate, and dexamethasone, and optimal intrathecal therapy, is important to control CNS leukemia.[100]

Cranial irradiation is an effective form of CNS-directed treatment, but its effectiveness is offset by substantial rates of secondary neoplasms (CNS tumors and carcinomas within the radiation port), multiple endocrinopathies, growth impairment, neurocognitive dysfunction, and neurotoxic effects.[109–111] Most contemporary pediatric ALL protocols limit the use of prophylactic cranial irradiation (12–18 Gy) to 2% to 20% of patients at especially high risk of CNS relapse[100] and do not specify cranial irradiation for infants or very young children, irrespective of their presenting features.[38,112] A recent study at St. Jude Children's Research Hospital tested the feasibility of total omission of prophylactic cranial irradiation in the context of risk-adapted intrathecal and systemic chemotherapy.[113] The 5-year survival rate for the 498 patients enrolled was 93.5% and the cumulative risk of an isolated CNS relapse rate was only 2.7%, a promising result suggesting that prophylactic cranial irradiation can be safely omitted in all patients in the context of the effective intrathecal and systemic chemotherapy. Although intensive intrathecal treatment can abolish the adverse prognostic effect of some risk factors, it is not without potential adverse effects, including postdural puncture headache, CNS hemorrhage, leukoencephalopathy, chemical meningitis, and neuropsychological and spinal-cord dysfunction.[114,115] Consequently, additional studies to determine the optimal number of doses for each group of patients are still needed in the context of the contemporary effective systemic chemotherapy regimen, which can improve the control of CNS leukemia.[100]

STEM CELL TRANSPLANTATION

Assessing the benefits of stem cell transplantation in first ALL remission is difficult due to the small numbers of patients studied and differences in selection criteria. Some studies suggest that allogeneic transplantation benefits certain high-risk patients, such as those with Philadelphia chromosome–positive ALL.[6] With recent improvement of chemotherapy and the addition of tyrosine kinase inhibitors, however, there is no apparent advantage in terms of early treatment outcome with the use of transplantation in children with Philadelphia chromosome–positive ALL.[116] Allogeneic transplantation does not seem to improve the outcome of children or infants with the t(4;11).[8,38] Because of their unfavorable prognosis, patients with a poor initial response to induction therapy commonly undergo allogeneic stem cell transplantation during the first remission. Studies to establish the efficacy of this intervention are also lacking, however. In an early BFM study, allogeneic transplantation with matched related or unrelated donor improved outcome of high-risk T-cell ALL cases.[117] In a subsequent study, however, intensive blocks of chemotherapy alone seemed to have improved the outcome for this group of patients.[118] Thus, the indications for allogeneic transplantation in first remission should be re-evaluated as chemotherapy and transplantation continue to improve.

TARGETED THERAPY

Addition of a tyrosine kinase inhibitor has greatly improved the remission induction rate and the duration of disease-free survival of patients with Philadelphia chromosome–positive ALL.[116,119–122] A second generation of more potent tyrosine kinase inhibitors has been developed to partly address the problem with resistance to imatinib.[123] It remains to be determined whether or not success in targeting BCR-ABL1 with tyrosine kinase inhibitors will translate into other successful molecular therapeutics targeted at other pathways, including NOTCH and FLT3 inhibitors. CD20 expression is associated with an inferior outcome in adult ALL[124] but not childhood ALL.[125] Pilot trials using anti-CD20 antibody have yielded some promising results in adults with CD20-positive precursor B-cell ALL.[126] An ongoing Children's Oncology Group study has demonstrated the feasibility of combining anti-CD22 epratuzumab with a standard chemotherapy backbone.[127] In a preliminary analysis, the rates of complete remission and clearance of minimal residual disease appeared favorable in comparison to historical experience with chemotherapy alone.[127] The cytotoxicity of monoclonal antibodies can be dramatically increased by linkage to toxic moieties including chemotherapeutic agents, bacterial and plant toxins, and radionuclides. Bacterial and plant toxins are highly potent and active in minute quantities and not susceptible to the multiple drug resistance gene (MDR)-mediated mechanism of resistance to chemotherapy.[128] Recombinant anti-CD22 immunotoxins are demonstrating promising activity in early clinical trials. Several other immunologic and molecular targets are under development. The novel mechanism of action along with the nonoverlapping toxicities will allow integration of the most promising targeting therapies into future personalized ALL therapy.

SUMMARY

Systematic enrollment of children and adolescents with ALL into well-designed clinical trials has allowed the establishment of prognostic parameters, leading to the design of risk-directed therapy. This has significantly contributed to the reduction of disease recurrence and improved quality of life of the patients by reducing acute and late side effects. Recent advances lead to departing from the use of traditional clinical risk stratification and instead using knowledge and insights about the biology and pharmacology to select treatment. As the limits of optimizing the use of standard therapy are reached, novel therapeutic approaches are designed according to the genetic constitution of the host and the leukemic cells. The design of future trials will be challenging but rewarding. As the focus increases on ever-smaller subsets of ALL, collaborations at the national and international levels are needed.

REFERENCES

1. Burchenal JH, Karnofsky DA, Kingsley-Pillers EM, et al. The effects of the folic acid antagonists and 2,6-diaminopurine on neoplastic disease, with special reference to acute leukemia. Cancer 1951;4(3):549–69.
2. Aur RJ, Simone JV, Pratt CB. Successful remission induction in children with acute lymphocytic leukemia at high risk for treatment failure. Cancer 1971; 27(6):1332–6.

3. Smith M, Arthur D, Camitta B, et al. Uniform approach to risk classification and treatment assignment for children with acute lymphoblastic leukemia. J Clin Oncol 1996;14(1):18–24.
4. Pui CH, Evans WE. Treatment of acute lymphoblastic leukemia. N Engl J Med 2006;354(2):166–78.
5. Pui CH, Relling MV, Downing JR. Acute lymphoblastic leukemia. N Engl J Med 2004;350(15):1535–48.
6. Arico M, Valsecchi MG, Camitta B, et al. Outcome of treatment in children with Philadelphia chromosome-positive acute lymphoblastic leukemia. N Engl J Med 2000;342(14):998–1006.
7. Mancini M, Scappaticci D, Cimino G, et al. A comprehensive genetic classification of adult acute lymphoblastic leukemia (ALL): analysis of the GIMEMA 0496 protocol. Blood 2005;105(9):3434–41.
8. Pui CH, Gaynon PS, Boyett JM, et al. Outcome of treatment in childhood acute lymphoblastic leukaemia with rearrangements of the 11q23 chromosomal region. Lancet 2002;359(9321):1909–15.
9. Gleissner B, Goekbuget N, Rieder H, et al. CD 10-negative pre-B acute lymphoblastic leukemia (ALL): a distinct high-risk subgroup of adult ALL associated with a high frequency of MLL aberrations. Results of the German Multicenter Trials for Adult ALL (GMALL). Blood 2005;106(13):4054–6.
10. Amylon MD, Shuster J, Pullen J, et al. Intensive high-dose asparaginase consolidation improves survival for pediatric patients with T cell acute lymphoblastic leukemia and advanced stage lymphoblastic lymphoma: a Pediatric Oncology Group study. Leukemia 1999;13(3):335–42.
11. Schrappe M, Reiter A, Ludwig WD, et al. Improved outcome in childhood acute lymphoblastic leukemia despite reduced use of anthracyclines and cranial radiotherapy: results of trial ALL-BFM 90. German-Austrian-Swiss ALL-BFM Study Group. Blood 2000;95(11):3310–22.
12. Goldberg JM, Silverman LB, Levy DE, et al. Childhood T-cell acute lymphoblastic leukemia: the Dana-Farber Cancer Institute acute lymphoblastic leukemia consortium experience. J Clin Oncol 2003;21(19):3616–22.
13. Ravandi F, Gandhi V. Novel purine nucleoside analogues for T-cell-lineage acute lymphoblastic leukaemia and lymphoma. Expert Opin Investig Drugs 2006;15(12):1601–13.
14. Coustan-Smith E, Mullighan CG, Onciu M, et al. Early T-cell precursor leukaemia: a subtype of very high-risk acute lymphoblastic leukaemia. Lancet Oncol 2009;10(2):147–56.
15. Pui CH, Robison LL, Look AT. Acute lymphoblastic leukaemia. Lancet 2008;371(9617):1030–43.
16. Meijerink JP, den Boer ML, Pieters R. New genetic abnormalities and treatment response in acute lymphoblastic leukemia. Semin Hematol 2009;46(1):16–23.
17. Look AT, Roberson PK, Williams DL, et al. Prognostic importance of blast cell DNA content in childhood acute lymphoblastic leukemia. Blood 1985;65(5):1079–86.
18. Trueworthy R, Shuster J, Look T, et al. Ploidy of lymphoblasts is the strongest predictor of treatment outcome in B-progenitor cell acute lymphoblastic leukemia of childhood: a Pediatric Oncology Group study. J Clin Oncol 1992;10(4):606–13.
19. Synold TW, Relling MV, Boyett JM, et al. Blast cell methotrexate-polyglutamate accumulation in vivo differs by lineage, ploidy, and methotrexate dose in acute lymphoblastic leukemia. J Clin Invest 1994;94(5):1996–2001.

20. Kaspers GJ, Smets LA, Pieters R, et al. Favorable prognosis of hyperdiploid common acute lymphoblastic leukemia may be explained by sensitivity to anti-metabolites and other drugs: results of an in vitro study. Blood 1995;85(3): 751–6.

21. Ito C, Kumagai M, Manabe A, et al. Hyperdiploid acute lymphoblastic leukemia with 51 to 65 chromosomes: a distinct biological entity with a marked propensity to undergo apoptosis. Blood 1999;93(1):315–20.

22. Nachman JB, Heerema NA, Sather H, et al. Outcome of treatment in children with hypodiploid acute lymphoblastic leukemia. Blood 2007;110(4):1112–5.

23. Harris MB, Shuster JJ, Carroll A, et al. Trisomy of leukemic cell chromosomes 4 and 10 identifies children with B-progenitor cell acute lymphoblastic leukemia with a very low risk of treatment failure: a Pediatric Oncology Group study. Blood 1992;79(12):3316–24.

24. Raimondi SC. Current status of cytogenetic research in childhood acute lympho-blastic leukemia. Blood 1993;81(9):2237–51.

25. Crist W, Carroll A, Shuster J, et al. Philadelphia chromosome positive childhood acute lymphoblastic leukemia: clinical and cytogenetic characteristics and treatment outcome. A Pediatric Oncology Group study. Blood 1990;76(3): 489–94.

26. Fletcher JA, Lynch EA, Kimball VM, et al. Translocation (9;22) is associated with extremely poor prognosis in intensively treated children with acute lympho-blastic leukemia. Blood 1991;77(3):435–9.

27. Pui CH, Sandlund JT, Pei D, et al. Results of therapy for acute lymphoblastic leukemia in black and white children. JAMA 2003;290(15):2001–7.

28. Raimondi SC, Behm FG, Roberson PK, et al. Cytogenetics of pre-B-cell acute lymphoblastic leukemia with emphasis on prognostic implications of the t(1;19). J Clin Oncol 1990;8(8):1380–8.

29. Jeha S, Pei D, Raimondi SC, et al. Increased risk for CNS relapse in pre-B cell leukemia with the t(1;19)/TCF3-PBX1. Leukemia 2009 [Epub ahead of print].

30. Garg R, Kantarjian H, Thomas D, et al. Adults with acute lymphoblastic leukemia and translocation (1;19) abnormality have a favorable outcome with hyperfrac-tionated cyclophosphamide, vincristine, doxorubicin, and dexamethasone alter-nating with methotrexate and high-dose cytarabine chemotherapy. Cancer 2009;115(10):2147–54.

31. Moorman AV, Richards SM, Robinson HM, et al. Prognosis of children with acute lymphoblastic leukemia (ALL) and intrachromosomal amplification of chromo-some 21 (iAMP21). Blood 2007;109(6):2327–30.

32. Paulsson K, Horvat A, Strombeck B, et al. Mutations of FLT3, NRAS, KRAS, and PTPN11 are frequent and possibly mutually exclusive in high hyperdiploid childhood acute lymphoblastic leukemia. Genes Chromosomes Cancer 2008;47(1):26–33.

33. Mullighan CG, Su X, Zhang J, et al. Deletion of IKZF1 and prognosis in acute lymphoblastic leukemia. N Engl J Med 2009;360(5):470–80.

34. den Boer ML, van SM, De Menezes RX, et al. A subtype of childhood acute lymphoblastic leukaemia with poor treatment outcome: a genome-wide classifi-cation study. Lancet Oncol 2009;10(2):125–34.

35. Mullighan CG, Miller CB, Radtke I, et al. BCR-ABL1 lymphoblastic leukaemia is characterized by the deletion of Ikaros. Nature 2008;453(7191):110–4.

36. Campana D. Minimal residual disease in acute lymphoblastic leukemia. Semin Hematol 2009;46(1):100–6.

37. Pui CH, Campana D, Evans WE. Childhood acute lymphoblastic leukaemia–current status and future perspectives. Lancet Oncol 2001;2(10):597–607.

38. Pieters R, Schrappe M, De Lorenzo P, et al. A treatment protocol for infants younger than 1 year with acute lymphoblastic leukaemia (Interfant-99): an observational study and a multicentre randomised trial. Lancet 2007;370(9583): 240–50.
39. Bostrom BC, Sensel MR, Sather HN, et al. Dexamethasone versus prednisone and daily oral versus weekly intravenous mercaptopurine for patients with standard-risk acute lymphoblastic leukemia: a report from the Children's Cancer Group. Blood 2003;101(10):3809–17.
40. Mitchell CD, Richards SM, Kinsey SE, et al. Benefit of dexamethasone compared with prednisolone for childhood acute lymphoblastic leukaemia: results of the UK Medical Research Council ALL97 randomized trial. Br J Haematol 2005;129(6):734–45.
41. Igarashi S, Manabe A, Ohara A, et al. No advantage of dexamethasone over prednisolone for the outcome of standard- and intermediate-risk childhood acute lymphoblastic leukemia in the Tokyo Children's Cancer Study Group L95-14 protocol. J Clin Oncol 2005;23(27):6489–98.
42. Asselin BL, Whitin JC, Coppola DJ, et al. Comparative pharmacokinetic studies of three asparaginase preparations. J Clin Oncol 1993;11(9):1780–6.
43. Vieira Pinheiro JP, Wenner K, Escherich G, et al. Serum asparaginase activities and asparagine concentrations in the cerebrospinal fluid after a single infusion of 2,500 IU/m(2) PEG asparaginase in children with ALL treated according to protocol COALL-06-97. Pediatr Blood Cancer 2006;46(1):18–25.
44. Liang DC, Hung IJ, Yang CP, et al. Unexpected mortality from the use of E. coli L-asparaginase during remission induction therapy for childhood acute lymphoblastic leukemia: a report from the Taiwan Pediatric Oncology Group. Leukemia 1999;13(2):155–60.
45. Ahlke E, Nowak-Gottl U, Schulze-Westhoff P, et al. Dose reduction of asparaginase under pharmacokinetic and pharmacodynamic control during induction therapy in children with acute lymphoblastic leukaemia. Br J Haematol 1997; 96(4):675–81.
46. Hak LJ, Relling MV, Cheng C, et al. Asparaginase pharmacodynamics differ by formulation among children with newly diagnosed acute lymphoblastic leukemia. Leukemia 2004;18(6):1072–7.
47. Silverman LB, Gelber RD, Dalton VK, et al. Improved outcome for children with acute lymphoblastic leukemia: results of Dana-Farber Consortium Protocol 91-01. Blood 2001;97(5):1211–8.
48. Douer D, Yampolsky H, Cohen LJ, et al. Pharmacodynamics and safety of intravenous pegaspargase during remission induction in adults aged 55 years or younger with newly diagnosed acute lymphoblastic leukemia. Blood 2007; 109(7):2744–50.
49. Wetzler M, Sanford BL, Kurtzberg J, et al. Effective asparagine depletion with pegylated asparaginase results in improved outcomes in adult acute lymphoblastic leukemia: Cancer and Leukemia Group B Study 9511. Blood 2007; 109(10):4164–7.
50. Moghrabi A, Levy DE, Asselin B, et al. Results of the Dana-Farber Cancer Institute ALL Consortium Protocol 95-01 for children with acute lymphoblastic leukemia. Blood 2007;109(3):896–904.
51. Duval M, Suciu S, Ferster A, et al. Comparison of Escherichia coli-asparaginase with Erwinia-asparaginase in the treatment of childhood lymphoid malignancies: results of a randomized European Organisation for Research and Treatment of Cancer-Children's Leukemia Group phase 3 trial. Blood 2002;99(8):2734–9.

52. Harms DO, Janka-Schaub GE. Co-operative study group for childhood acute lymphoblastic leukemia (COALL): long-term follow-up of trials 82, 85, 89 and 92. Leukemia 2000;14(12):2234–9.

53. Hurwitz CA, Silverman LB, Schorin MA, et al. Substituting dexamethasone for prednisone complicates remission induction in children with acute lymphoblastic leukemia. Cancer 2000;88(8):1964–9.

54. Schrappe M, Reiter A, Zimmermann M, et al. Long-term results of four consecutive trials in childhood ALL performed by the ALL-BFM study group from 1981 to 1995. Berlin-Frankfurt-Munster. Leukemia 2000;14(12):2205–22.

55. Borowitz MJ, Devidas M, Hunger SP, et al. Clinical significance of minimal residual disease in childhood acute lymphoblastic leukemia and its relationship to other prognostic factors: a Children's Oncology Group study. Blood 2008; 111(12):5477–85.

56. Pui CH, Campana D. New definition of remission in childhood acute lymphoblastic leukemia. Leukemia 2000;14(5):783–5.

57. Chessells JM, Bailey C, Richards SM. Intensification of treatment and survival in all children with lymphoblastic leukaemia: results of UK Medical Research Council trial UKALL X. Medical Research Council Working Party on Childhood Leukaemia. Lancet 1995;345(8943):143–8.

58. Evans WE, Relling MV, Rodman JH, et al. Conventional compared with individualized chemotherapy for childhood acute lymphoblastic leukemia. N Engl J Med 1998;338(8):499–505.

59. Nachman JB, Sather HN, Sensel MG, et al. Augmented post-induction therapy for children with high-risk acute lymphoblastic leukemia and a slow response to initial therapy. N Engl J Med 1998;338(23):1663–71.

60. Gaynon PS, Trigg ME, Heerema NA, et al. Children's Cancer Group trials in childhood acute lymphoblastic leukemia: 1983-1995. Leukemia 2000;14(12): 2223–33.

61. Pui CH, Sandlund JT, Pei D, et al. Improved outcome for children with acute lymphoblastic leukemia: results of Total Therapy Study XIIIB at St Jude Children's Research Hospital. Blood 2004;104(9):2690–6.

62. Loh ML, Goldwasser MA, Silverman LB, et al. Prospective analysis of TEL/AML1-positive patients treated on Dana-Farber Cancer Institute Consortium Protocol 95-01. Blood 2006;107(11):4508–13.

63. Camitta B, Leventhal B, Lauer S, et al. Intermediate-dose intravenous methotrexate and mercaptopurine therapy for non-T, non-B acute lymphocytic leukemia of childhood: a Pediatric Oncology Group study. J Clin Oncol 1989; 7(10):1539–44.

64. Camitta B, Mahoney D, Leventhal B, et al. Intensive intravenous methotrexate and mercaptopurine treatment of higher-risk non-T, non-B acute lymphocytic leukemia: a Pediatric Oncology Group study. J Clin Oncol 1994;12(7):1383–9.

65. Land VJ, Shuster JJ, Crist WM, et al. Comparison of two schedules of intermediate-dose methotrexate and cytarabine consolidation therapy for childhood B-precursor cell acute lymphoblastic leukemia: a Pediatric Oncology Group study. J Clin Oncol 1994;12(9):1939–45.

66. Pui CH, Boyett JM, Rivera GK, et al. Long-term results of Total Therapy studies 11, 12 and 13A for childhood acute lymphoblastic leukemia at St Jude Children's Research Hospital. Leukemia 2000;14(12):2286–94.

67. Pui CH, Sallan S, Relling MV, et al. International childhood acute lymphoblastic leukemia workshop: Sausalito, CA, 30 November–1 December 2000. Leukemia 2001;15(5):707–15.

68. Galpin AJ, Schuetz JD, Masson E, et al. Differences in folylpolyglutamate synthetase and dihydrofolate reductase expression in human B-lineage versus T-lineage leukemic lymphoblasts: mechanisms for lineage differences in methotrexate polyglutamylation and cytotoxicity. Mol Pharmacol 1997;52(1):155–63.

69. Panetta JC, Yanishevski Y, Pui CH, et al. A mathematical model of in vivo methotrexate accumulation in acute lymphoblastic leukemia. Cancer Chemother Pharmacol 2002;50(5):419–28.

70. Masson E, Relling MV, Synold TW, et al. Accumulation of methotrexate polyglutamates in lymphoblasts is a determinant of antileukemic effects in vivo. A rationale for high-dose methotrexate. J Clin Invest 1996;97(1):73–80.

71. Kager L, Cheok M, Yang W, et al. Folate pathway gene expression differs in subtypes of acute lymphoblastic leukemia and influences methotrexate pharmacodynamics. J Clin Invest 2005;115(1):110–7.

72. Hutchinson RJ, Gaynon PS, Sather H, et al. Intensification of therapy for children with lower-risk acute lymphoblastic leukemia: long-term follow-up of patients treated on Children's Cancer Group Trial 1881. J Clin Oncol 2003;21(9):1790–7.

73. Lange BJ, Bostrom BC, Cherlow JM, et al. Double-delayed intensification improves event-free survival for children with intermediate-risk acute lymphoblastic leukemia: a report from the Children's Cancer Group. Blood 2002; 99(3):825–33.

74. Cassileth PA, Andersen JW, Bennett JM, et al. Adult acute lymphocytic leukemia: the Eastern Cooperative Oncology Group experience. Leukemia 1992;6(Suppl):2178–81.

75. Riehm H, Gadner H, Henze G, et al. Results and significance of six randomized trials in four consecutive ALL-BFM studies. Haematol Blood Transfus 1990;33: 439–50.

76. Cuttner J, Mick R, Budman DR, et al. Phase III trial of brief intensive treatment of adult acute lymphocytic leukemia comparing daunorubicin and mitoxantrone: a CALGB Study. Leukemia 1991;5(5):425–31.

77. Toyoda Y, Manabe A, Tsuchida M, et al. Six months of maintenance chemotherapy after intensified treatment for acute lymphoblastic leukemia of childhood. J Clin Oncol 2000;18(7):1508–16.

78. Duration and intensity of maintenance chemotherapy in acute lymphoblastic leukaemia: overview of 42 trials involving 12 000 randomised children. Childhood ALL Collaborative Group. Lancet 1996;347(9018):1783–8.

79. Sather H, Miller D, Nesbit M, et al. Differences in prognosis for boys and girls with acute lymphoblastic leukaemia. Lancet 1981;1(8223):739–43.

80. Duration of chemotherapy in childhood acute lymphoblastic leukaemia. The medical research council's working party on leukaemia in childhood. Med Pediatr Oncol 1982;10(5):511–20.

81. Lennard L, Lilleyman JS, Van LJ, et al. Genetic variation in response to 6-mercaptopurine for childhood acute lymphoblastic leukaemia. Lancet 1990; 336(8709):225–9.

82. Whitehead VM, Vuchich MJ, Lauer SJ, et al. Accumulation of high levels of methotrexate polyglutamates in lymphoblasts from children with hyperdiploid (greater than 50 chromosomes) B-lineage acute lymphoblastic leukemia: a Pediatric Oncology Group study. Blood 1992;80(5):1316–23.

83. Schmiegelow K, Schroder H, Gustafsson G, et al. Risk of relapse in childhood acute lymphoblastic leukemia is related to RBC methotrexate and mercaptopurine metabolites during maintenance chemotherapy. Nordic Society for Pediatric Hematology and Oncology. J Clin Oncol 1995;13(2):345–51.

84. Chessells JM, Harrison G, Lilleyman JS, et al. Continuing (maintenance) therapy in lymphoblastic leukaemia: lessons from MRC UKALL X. Medical Research Council Working Party in Childhood Leukaemia. Br J Haematol 1997;98(4): 945–51.

85. Relling MV, Hancock ML, Boyett JM, et al. Prognostic importance of 6-mercaptopurine dose intensity in acute lymphoblastic leukemia. Blood 1999;93(9):2817–23.

86. Schmiegelow K, Glomstein A, Kristinsson J, et al. Impact of morning versus evening schedule for oral methotrexate and 6-mercaptopurine on relapse risk for children with acute lymphoblastic leukemia. Nordic Society for Pediatric Hematology and Oncology (NOPHO). J Pediatr Hematol Oncol 1997;19(2): 102–9.

87. Rivard GE, Lin KT, Leclerc JM, et al. Milk could decrease the bioavailability of 6-mercaptopurine. Am J Pediatr Hematol Oncol 1989;11(4):402–6.

88. Farrow AC, Buchanan GR, Zwiener RJ, et al. Serum aminotransferase elevation during and following treatment of childhood acute lymphoblastic leukemia. J Clin Oncol 1997;15(4):1560–6.

89. Evans WE, Horner M, Chu YQ, et al. Altered mercaptopurine metabolism, toxic effects, and dosage requirement in a thiopurine methyltransferase-deficient child with acute lymphocytic leukemia. J Pediatr 1991;119(6):985–9.

90. Relling MV, Hancock ML, Rivera GK, et al. Mercaptopurine therapy intolerance and heterozygosity at the thiopurine S-methyltransferase gene locus. J Natl Cancer Inst 1999;91(23):2001–8.

91. Pui CH, Relling MV. Topoisomerase II inhibitor-related acute myeloid leukaemia. Br J Haematol 2000;109:13–23.

92. Relling MV, Rubnitz JE, Rivera GK, et al. High incidence of secondary brain tumours after radiotherapy and antimetabolites. Lancet 1999;354(9172):34–9.

93. Evans WE, Relling MV. Moving towards individualized medicine with pharmacogenomics. Nature 2004;429(6990):464–8.

94. Relling MV, Dervieux T. Pharmacogenetics and cancer therapy. Nat Rev Cancer 2001;1(2):99–108.

95. Jacobs SS, Stork LC, Bostrom BC, et al. Substitution of oral and intravenous thioguanine for mercaptopurine in a treatment regimen for children with standard risk acute lymphoblastic leukemia: a collaborative Children's Oncology Group/ National Cancer Institute pilot trial (CCG-1942). Pediatr Blood Cancer 2007; 49(3):250–5.

96. Harms DO, Gobel U, Spaar HJ, et al. Thioguanine offers no advantage over mercaptopurine in maintenance treatment of childhood ALL: results of the randomized trial COALL-92. Blood 2003;102(8):2736–40.

97. Vora A, Mitchell CD, Lennard L, et al. Toxicity and efficacy of 6-thioguanine versus 6-mercaptopurine in childhood lymphoblastic leukaemia: a randomised trial. Lancet 2006;368(9544):1339–48.

98. Lennard L, Richards S, Cartwright CS, et al. The thiopurine methyltransferase genetic polymorphism is associated with thioguanine-related veno-occlusive disease of the liver in children with acute lymphoblastic leukemia. Clin Pharmacol Ther 2006;80(4):375–83.

99. Conter V, Valsecchi MG, Silvestri D, et al. Pulses of vincristine and dexamethasone in addition to intensive chemotherapy for children with intermediate-risk acute lymphoblastic leukaemia: a multicentre randomised trial. Lancet 2007; 369(9556):123–31.

100. Pui CH, Howard SC. Current management and challenges of malignant disease in the CNS in paediatric leukaemia. Lancet Oncol 2008;9(3):257–68.

101. Conter V, Schrappe M, Arico M, et al. Role of cranial radiotherapy for childhood T-cell acute lymphoblastic leukemia with high WBC count and good response to prednisone. Associazione Italiana Ematologia Oncologia Pediatrica and the Berlin-Frankfurt-Munster groups. J Clin Oncol 1997;15(8):2786–91.

102. Mahmoud HH, Rivera GK, Hancock ML, et al. Low leukocyte counts with blast cells in cerebrospinal fluid of children with newly diagnosed acute lymphoblastic leukemia. N Engl J Med 1993;329(5):314–9.

103. Gajjar A, Harrison PL, Sandlund JT, et al. Traumatic lumbar puncture at diagnosis adversely affects outcome in childhood acute lymphoblastic leukemia. Blood 2000;96(10):3381–4.

104. Burger B, Zimmermann M, Mann G, et al. Diagnostic cerebrospinal fluid examination in children with acute lymphoblastic leukemia: significance of low leukocyte counts with blasts or traumatic lumbar puncture. J Clin Oncol 2003;21(2):184–8.

105. te Loo DM, Kamps WA, van der Does-van den Berg A, et al. Prognostic significance of blasts in the cerebrospinal fluid without pleiocytosis or a traumatic lumbar puncture in children with acute lymphoblastic leukemia: experience of the Dutch Childhood Oncology Group. J Clin Oncol 2006;24(15):2332–6.

106. Howard SC, Gajjar A, Ribeiro RC, et al. Safety of lumbar puncture for children with acute lymphoblastic leukemia and thrombocytopenia. JAMA 2000;284(17):2222–4.

107. Blaney SM, Poplack DG, Godwin K, et al. Effect of body position on ventricular CSF methotrexate concentration following intralumbar administration. J Clin Oncol 1995;13(1):177–9.

108. Matloub Y, Lindemulder S, Gaynon PS, et al. Intrathecal triple therapy decreases central nervous system relapse but fails to improve event-free survival when compared with intrathecal methotrexate: results of the Children's Cancer Group (CCG) 1952 study for standard-risk acute lymphoblastic leukemia, reported by the Children's Oncology Group. Blood 2006;108(4):1165–73.

109. Pui CH, Cheng C, Leung W, et al. Extended follow-up of long-term survivors of childhood acute lymphoblastic leukemia. N Engl J Med 2003;349(7):640–9.

110. Hijiya N, Hudson MM, Lensing S, et al. Cumulative incidence of secondary neoplasms as a first event after childhood acute lymphoblastic leukemia. JAMA 2007;297(11):1207–15.

111. Waber DP, Turek J, Catania L, et al. Neuropsychological outcomes from a randomized trial of triple intrathecal chemotherapy compared with 18 Gy cranial radiation as CNS treatment in acute lymphoblastic leukemia: findings from Dana-Farber Cancer Institute ALL Consortium Protocol 95-01. J Clin Oncol 2007;25(31):4914–21.

112. Hilden JM, Dinndorf PA, Meerbaum SO, et al. Analysis of prognostic factors of acute lymphoblastic leukemia in infants: report on CCG 1953 from the Children's Oncology Group. Blood 2006;108(2):441–51.

113. Pui C, Campana D, Pei D, Bowman W, Sandlund J, Kaste S, et al. Treatment of childhood acute lymphoblastic leukemia without prophylactic cranial irradiation. N Engl J Med 2009;360(26):2730–41.

114. Stam J. Thrombosis of the cerebral veins and sinuses. N Engl J Med 2005;352(17):1791–8.

115. Laningham FH, Kun LE, Reddick WE, et al. Childhood central nervous system leukemia: historical perspectives, current therapy, and acute neurological sequelae. Neuroradiology 2007;49(11):873–88.

116. Schultz K, Bowman W, Aledo A, Slayton W, Sather H, Devidas M, et al. Improved early event free survival with imatinib in Philadelphia chromosome-positive acute lymphoblastic leukemia: a Children's Oncology Study. J Clin Oncol, in press.

117. Schrauder A, Reiter A, Gadner H, et al. Superiority of allogeneic hematopoietic stem-cell transplantation compared with chemotherapy alone in high-risk childhood T-cell acute lymphoblastic leukemia: results from ALL-BFM 90 and 95. J Clin Oncol 2006;24(36):5742–9.

118. Moricke A, Reiter A, Zimmermann M, et al. Risk-adjusted therapy of acute lymphoblastic leukemia can decrease treatment burden and improve survival: treatment results of 2169 unselected pediatric and adolescent patients enrolled in the trial ALL-BFM 95. Blood 2008;111(9):4477–89.

119. Gruber F, Mustjoki S, Porkka K. Impact of tyrosine kinase inhibitors on patient outcomes in Philadelphia chromosome-positive acute lymphoblastic leukaemia. Br J Haematol 2009;145(5):581–97.

120. Gandemer V, Auclerc MF, Perel Y, et al. Impact of age, leukocyte count and day 21-bone marrow response to chemotherapy on the long-term outcome of children with philadelphia chromosome-positive acute lymphoblastic leukemia in the pre-imatinib era: results of the FRALLE 93 study. BMC Cancer 2009;9:14.

121. Thomas DA, Faderl S, Cortes J, et al. Treatment of Philadelphia chromosome-positive acute lymphocytic leukemia with hyper-CVAD and imatinib mesylate. Blood 2004;103(12):4396–407.

122. Yanada M, Takeuchi J, Sugiura I, et al. High complete remission rate and promising outcome by combination of imatinib and chemotherapy for newly diagnosed BCR-ABL-positive acute lymphoblastic leukemia: a phase II study by the Japan Adult Leukemia Study Group. J Clin Oncol 2006;24(3):460–6.

123. Pui CH, Jeha S. New therapeutic strategies for the treatment of acute lymphoblastic leukaemia. Nat Rev Drug Discov 2007;6(2):149–65.

124. Thomas DA, O'Brien S, Jorgensen JL, et al. Prognostic significance of CD20 expression in adults with de novo precursor B-lineage acute lymphoblastic leukemia. Blood 2009;113(25):6330–7.

125. Jeha S, Behm F, Pei D, et al. Prognostic significance of CD20 expression in childhood B-cell precursor acute lymphoblastic leukemia. Blood 2006; 108(10):3302–4.

126. Gokbuget N, Hoelzer D. Novel antibody-based therapy for acute lymphoblastic leukaemia. Best Pract Res Clin Haematol 2006;19(4):701–13.

127. Raetz EA, Cairo MS, Borowitz MJ, et al. Chemoimmunotherapy reinduction with epratuzumab in children with acute lymphoblastic leukemia in marrow relapse: a Children's Oncology Group Pilot Study. J Clin Oncol 2008;26(22):3756–62.

128. Pastan I, Hassan R, FitzGerald DJ, et al. Immunotoxin therapy of cancer. Nat Rev Cancer 2006;6(7):559–65.

Cytogenetics and Molecular Genetics of Acute Lymphoblastic Leukemia

Krzysztof Mrózek, MD, PhD[a],*, David P. Harper, MD[b,c],
Peter D. Aplan, MD[d]

KEYWORDS

- Acute lymphoblastic leukemia • Gene mutations
- Chromosome aberrations • Human • Prognosis

Acute lymphoblastic leukemia (ALL) is a neoplastic disease characterized by clonal expansion of leukemic cells in the bone marrow (BM), lymph nodes, thymus, or spleen. ALL is a genetic disease because most patients harbor acquired genetic alterations (somatic mutations) that contribute to the increased proliferation, prolonged survival, or impaired differentiation of the lymphoid hematopoietic progenitors. In most, but not all, patients diagnosed with ALL, one or more of these genetic alterations are in the form of nonrandom numerical or structural chromosome aberrations that can be detected microscopically.[1,2] The application of contemporary genome-wide molecular analyses continues to reveal many additional genetic rearrangements that are not detectable cytogenetically.[3]

Several of the ALL-specific chromosome aberrations and their molecular counterparts have been included in the 2008 World Health Organization (WHO) Classification of Tumours of Haematopoietic and Lymphoid Tissues (**Table 1**), and together with

K Mrózek and DP Harper contributed equally to this work. The authors have no conflicting financial interests to disclose. This research was supported in part by the Intramural Research Program of the NIH, NCI, and NCI grants CA101140 and CA16058, and The Coleman Leukemia Research Foundation.

[a] Division of Hematology and Oncology, Department of Internal Medicine, Comprehensive Cancer Center, James Cancer Hospital, The Ohio State University, Room 1248B, 300 West Tenth Avenue, Columbus, OH 43210-1228, USA
[b] Genetics Branch, Center for Cancer Research, National Cancer Institute, 8901 Wisconsin Avenue, Bethesda, MD 20889-5105, USA
[c] Department of Pediatrics, Uniformed Services University of the Health Sciences, 4301 Jones Bridge Road, Bethesda, MD 20814, USA
[d] Genetics Branch, Center for Cancer Research, National Cancer Institute, Navy 8, Rm 5101, 8901 Wisconsin Avenue, Bethesda, MD 20889-5105, USA
* Corresponding author.
E-mail address: krzysztof.mrozek@osumc.edu (K. Mrózek).

Hematol Oncol Clin N Am 23 (2009) 991–1010
doi:10.1016/j.hoc.2009.07.001
0889-8588/09/$ – see front matter © 2009 Elsevier Inc. All rights reserved.

Table 1
World Health Organization classification of acute lymphoblastic leukemia
Category in WHO Classification
PRECURSOR LYMPHOID NEOPLASMS
B lymphoblastic leukemia/lymphoma
B lymphoblastic leukemia/lymphoma, NOS
B lymphoblastic leukemia/lymphoma with recurrent genetic abnormalities
B lymphoblastic leukemia/lymphoma with t(9;22)(q34;q11.2); *BCR-ABL1*
B lymphoblastic leukemia/lymphoma with t(v;11q23); *MLL* rearranged
B lymphoblastic leukemia/lymphoma with t(12;21)(p13;q22); *TEL-AML1 (ETV6-RUNX1)*
B lymphoblastic leukemia/lymphoma with hyperdiploidy
B lymphoblastic leukemia/lymphoma with hypodiploidy (hypodiploid ALL)
B lymphoblastic leukemia/lymphoma with t(5;14)(q31;q32); *IL3-IGH*
B lymphoblastic leukemia/lymphoma with t(1;19)(q23;p13.3); *E2A-PBX1 (TCF3-PBX1)*
T lymphoblastic leukemia/lymphoma

Data from Swerdlow SH, Campo E, Harris NL, et al, editors. WHO classification of tumours of haematopoietic and lymphoid tissues. Lyon, France: IARC; 2008.

morphology, cytochemistry, immunophenotype, and clinical characteristics are being used to define individual disease entities within B-lineage ALL (B-ALL).[4] Although several specific recurrent chromosome aberrations and gene mutations also occur in T-lineage ALL (T-ALL), at present they are not used to delineate separate entities within T-ALL.[5]

Notably, cytogenetic and, increasingly, molecular genetic findings at diagnosis constitute important, independent prognostic factors in childhood and adult ALL.[6–17] Accordingly, cytogenetic and molecular analyses are considered obligatory for analyzing outcomes of many clinical trials, and detection of specific chromosome aberrations or their molecular equivalents, such as t(9;22)(q34;q11.2) and *BCR-ABL1*, is used to assign ALL patients to specific targeted therapy.[18] In the first part of this article, the cytogenetic methodology is briefly described, followed by a summary of major cytogenetic findings and their clinical relevance in ALL. In the second part, modern molecular techniques and their application in the research on genetics and epigenetics of ALL are reveiwed.

CYTOGENETICS
Standard Cytogenetic Analysis

This technique reveals all microscopically detectable chromosome aberrations occurring simultaneously in leukemic cells, regardless of whether these aberrations are numerical or structural, or, in the case of the latter, balanced or unbalanced. To obtain analyzable metaphase cells, pretreatment samples are subjected to unstimulated short-term (24- or 48-hour) cultures in vitro, at the end of which the cells are treated with a compound that arrests dividing cells in metaphase (eg, colcemide), hypotonic solution, and repeated changes of fixative solution. Thereafter, microscope slides containing metaphase spreads are made, appropriately aged, stained using banding techniques (most often G-banding), and analyzed under a microscope. Twenty or more metaphase cells are usually analyzed. In cases with an abnormal karyotype, analysis of less than 20 cells can be acceptable, but for a case to be reliably determined as cytogenetically normal, an analysis of at least 20 karyotypes from a BM sample is required.[19] To be considered relevant, the identified chromosome aberrations must be clonal, that is, present in a minimum of two metaphase cells in the case of an identical structural aberration and gain of the same structurally intact chromosome (trisomy), or in at least three cells in the case of a missing chromosome (monosomy).[20]

Fluorescence in Situ Hybridization

Many chromosome aberrations recurrent in ALL can also be detected using molecular-cytogenetic techniques, such as fluorescence in situ hybridization (FISH). This method employs cDNA or genomic DNA fragments (probes) complementary to specific sequences in the human genome that are labeled with fluorochromes and hybridized to fixed metaphase chromosomes or interphase nuclei. The locations of the fluorescent signals are then visualized using a fluorescence microscope. Several types of probes are available including (1) centromeric probes consisting of chromosome-specific DNA repeats (satellite DNA), which are useful for detection of numerical aberrations such as trisomies and monosomies; (2) whole chromosome painting (WCP) probes containing numerous unique DNA sequences capable of binding to the entire length of specific chromosomes, which allow the identification of individual chromosomes or their parts participating in structural aberrations in metaphase cells; and (3) locus-specific probes hybridizing to particular sequences within individual genes, which are used to detect recurrent structural abnormalities such as translocations, inversions, or deletions.[21]

FISH and molecular genetic techniques such as reverse transcriptase polymerase chain reaction (RT-PCR), are especially valuable in patients for whom standard cytogenetic analysis yields no analyzable metaphase cells or only a few cells of poor quality. They are also essential for identification of cytogenetically cryptic abnormalities, a prime example of which is t(12;21)(p13;q22), a translocation that involves the juxtaposition of similarly banded regions and thus cannot be discerned reliably in G-banded preparations.[22] In addition, FISH and RT-PCR are invaluable for detection or confirmation of suspected variants of recurrent aberrations, such as cryptic insertions between seemingly intact chromosomes 9 and 22 leading to the BCR-ABL1 gene fusion,[23] which in most ALL patients is generated by the typical t(9;22)(q34;q11.2).

Multicolor Fluorescence in Situ Hybridization

In a portion of ALL patients, cytogenetic preparations are of suboptimal quality, with poor chromosome morphology and indistinct banding, making the interpretation of karyotypes difficult. In these and some good quality cases, the karyotype may contain aberrations unrecognizable using G-banding, for example, marker or certain ring chromosomes, or only partially recognizable, such as an unidentified chromosome segment attached to a known chromosome, usually designated "add". Analysis of such cases can be greatly aided by application of multicolor FISH techniques. Spectral karyotyping (SKY) and multiplex FISH (M-FISH) use WCP probes specific for each of the 22 pairs of autosomal chromosomes and the sex chromosomes X and Y, and allow simultaneous display of all chromosome pairs in different colors. Studies of pediatric ALL that applied SKY or M-FISH, complemented in some instances by FISH with locus-specific probes, identified cryptic translocations, and revealed the origin and chromosomal composition of marker and derivative chromosomes.[24–27] In ALL patients with high hyperdiploidy with poor chromosome morphology, SKY allowed accurate characterization of all numerical aberrations and of the chromosomal origin of segments involved in interchromosomal structural rearrangements.[28] In patients with t(12;21), SKY revealed nonrandom unbalanced translocations of chromosome 6.[29] Nordgren and colleagues[25] concluded that although in most instances the combination of standard cytogenetic analysis and interphase FISH was sufficient for the detection of prognostically relevant chromosome aberrations, SKY (and M-FISH) can greatly improve the accuracy of karyotype interpretation, especially in patients with complex chromosome rearrangements.

Success Rates of Cytogenetic Analyses and Rates of Aberration Detection in Acute Lymphoblastic Leukemia

Meaningful results of standard cytogenetic analysis can be obtained in most patients with ALL. In large studies of adult ALL, between 70% and 75% of samples analyzed cytogenetically were deemed successful.[13–15,19] In one-third of cases with results described as unsuccessful, the sample processed cytogenetically yielded no, or only a few, analyzable mitotic cells, whereas in the remaining cases, the karyotypes were obtained but were considered to be of too poor quality to allow unambiguous interpretation.[15,19] Higher success rates, 83% and 91%, were reported by 2 large studies of childhood ALL.[9,30] Importantly, BM samples are preferable to blood samples because the latter had a significantly higher rate of unacceptable cytogenetic results compared with BM.[11,14] As shown in a large cooperative UK Cancer Cytogenetics Group (UKCCG) study of more than 2300 pediatric ALL patients, the success rate can be increased by the use of interphase FISH with probes capable of detecting prognostically relevant chromosome abnormalities from 83% when only G-banding was applied to 91% when interphase FISH was carried out on the fixed cell suspensions used for cytogenetic analysis.[30]

Among successfully analyzed patients, at least one clonal aberration has been detected in 60% to 79% of adults,[13–15,19] and 57% to 82% of children[9,30,31] with ALL. In general, the rates of aberration detection were higher in more recent series compared with the earliest ones,[14,19] and, as mentioned before, they can be further increased by the use of FISH and SKY.

Prognostic Relevance of Cytogenetics in Acute Lymphoblastic Leukemia

The first major study demonstrating the independent prognostic significance of cytogenetic findings at diagnosis in ALL was the Third International Workshop on Chromosomes in Leukemia.[6,7,10] Subsequent studies confirmed the Workshop's results and refined them by providing data on clinical relevance of further recurrent aberrations and elucidating the molecular basis and biologic consequences of many of these aberrations. **Table 2** summarizes the incidence and prognostic impact of the major cytogenetic findings in childhood and adult ALL.

High hyperdiploidy (ie, karyotypes containing modal chromosome number of 51–67 chromosomes) defines one of the largest cytogenetic subsets of childhood ALL, comprising 25% to 30% of patients with B-ALL.[32] High hyperdiploidy is less frequent in adult ALL, being seen in 2% to 10% of patients,[8,14] and it is rare in T-ALL. The distribution of specific chromosome gains is nonrandom, with the most often gained chromosomes 21, X, 14, 6, 18, 4, 17 and 10, each of which is gained in more than 50% of hyperdiploid ALL patients, followed by chromosomes 8, 5, 11, and 12, gains of which occur more often in patients with 57 or more chromosomes.[52] The prognosis of children with high hyperdiploidy is excellent, with CR rates approaching 100% in some studies, the 5-year event-free survival (EFS) rates between 71% and 83%[9,33,34,36] and 5-year overall survival (OS) rates of approximately 90%.[34,36] Outcome of adults with high hyperdiploidy has been improved in some,[8,14] but not all,[12,13] studies in relation to other cytogenetic groups, but it is not comparable to the excellent outcome of children with high hyperdiploidy. In the latter age group, prognosis may also be influenced by specific cytogenetic features of the hyperdiploid karyotype. Patients with the concurrent presence of +4, +10 and +17 have been reported to have especially favorable prognosis,[53] as were those with +4 and +18 in another study.[36] On the other hand, the rare patients with recurrent translocations, such as t(9;22)(q34;q11), t(1;19)(q23;p13) or translocations involving 11q23, have outcomes similar to nonhyperdiploid patients with these aberrations,[36,37] and thus are often excluded from the high hyperdiploidy category. Approximately one-half of the high hyperdiploid patients harbor other structural aberrations, such as duplications and gains of 1q, del(6q) or i(17)(q10), but their presence does not seem to influence prognosis,[36,54] with a possible exception of prognostically adverse i(17)(q10).[54] Because hyperdiploid leukemic cells sometimes fail to proliferate in culture, ALL patients with unsuccessful cytogenetic analysis or those with normal karyotypes should be analyzed using FISH with centromeric probes, flow cytometry to measure DNA index, or single nucleotide polymorphism (SNP) genomic microarray.[30,32,55]

Another large cytogenetic subset of pediatric ALL is characterized by the presence of a cryptic t(12;21)(p13;q22)/ETV6-RUNX1(TEL-AML1). Although this translocation, detectable using FISH or RT-PCR, occurs in approximately 25% of children with pre-B-ALL,[34,39] it is almost nonexistent in adult ALL. The prognosis of children with t(12;21) is excellent, both among patients with standard-risk and those with high-risk ALL according to the National Cancer Institute (NCI) criteria, with 94% of the patients experiencing rapid early responses to therapy.[34,39] Three-fourths of t(12;21) patients harbor additional genetic changes, most often deletions of 12p with loss of the second copy of ETV6 gene (in 55%–70% of patients), +21 (in 15%–20%) and an extra der(21)t(12;21) (in 10%–15%).[35,56] Stams and colleagues[56] reported that disease-free survival (DFS) of patients with +der(21)t(12;21) and those without secondary aberrations was worse than DFS of patients with del(12p) and +21, whereas in a study of Attarbaschi and colleagues[35] worse EFS was associated with a secondary deletion of nontranslocated ETV6 allele. Further studies are needed to clarify the prognostic role of secondary aberrations in B-ALL patients with t(12;21).

The most frequent abnormality among adults with ALL is the Philadelphia chromosome (Ph), that is t(9;22)(q34;q11.2)/BCR-ABL1, which is detected in 11% to 29% of patients.[8,11–15] In contrast, t(9;22) is rare in children (1%–3%).[9,31,43] With rare exceptions,[13,14] Ph+ patients are diagnosed with B-ALL. Prognosis of adults and children treated with standard chemotherapy is poor, with less than 5% of adults being cured.[18] The only potentially curative therapy is allogeneic hematopoietic stem cell transplantation (HSCT), although this procedure is associated with increased treatment-related mortality.[57] Administration of imatinib as part of induction therapy resulted in higher rates of complete remission (CR) and improved survival of patients who underwent transplantation,[58,59] although patients receiving imatinib may develop resistance to the drug and relapse. Other tyrosine kinase inhibitors (eg, dasatinib) that may overcome the mechanisms of resistance are currently being tested.[18] Approximately two-thirds of newly diagnosed patients harbor one or more secondary chromosome aberrations in addition to t(9;22), most frequently an extra copy of der(22)t(9;22), −7 or loss of 7p arm, an abnormality of 9p, +21, +8, and +X. High hyperdiploidy is detected in approximately 15% of Ph+ patients.[14,44,60] The presence of secondary aberrations as such, regardless of type, compared with a sole t(9;22), did not affect prognosis in pediatric[44] or adult[60] studies in the pre-imatinib era, but it was found to be an independent, adverse prognostic factor in adult Japanese patients receiving imatinib as part of their treatment.[61] In that latter study,[61] both +der(22)t(9;22) and abnormalities of 9p had a negative impact on disease-free survival. Abnormal 9p also portended worse outcome in

Table 2
Major chromosome aberrations in pediatric and adult acute lymphoblastic leukemia: frequency and prognostic significance

Chromosome Aberration/Genes Involved	Children		Adults	
	Frequency	Clinical Outcome	Frequency	Clinical Outcome
High hyperdiploidy	23%–30%[9,32–35]	Favorable[9,33,34,36,37]	7%–8%[8,11,13,14]	Favorable[8,11,14] Intermediate[13]
Hypodiploidy	6%[9]	Intermediate for patients with 45 chromosomes[38] Adverse for patients with <45 chromosomes[38] Intermediate for patients with <46 chromosomes[9]	7%–8%[8,11,15]	Adverse[8,11]
Near-haploidy	0.4%–0.7%[9]	Adverse[9,38]	Rare	Not determined
t(12;21)(p13;q22)/ETV6-RUNX1 (TEL-AML1)	22%–26%[34,39,40]	Favorable[34,39,40]	0%–4%[41,42]	Not determined
t(9;22)(q34;q11.2)/BCR-ABL1	1%–3%[9,43]	Adverse[9,34,37,44]	11%–29%[8,11–15]	Adverse[8,11–15]
t(4;11)(q21;q23)/MLL-AFF1(AF4)	1%–2%[9,37] 55% of infants[45]	Adverse[9,37,45]	4%–9%[8,11–14]	Adverse[8,11–14]
t(1;19)(q23;p13.3)/der(19)t(1;19)(q23;p13.3)/TCF3(E2A)-PBX1	1%–6%[9,37,46,47]	Favorable[9] Intermediate[37,46]	1%–3%[8,11,13,14,48]	Favorable[48] Intermediate[14] Adverse[8,13]
t(10;14)(q24;q11)/TCRA/TCRD-TLX1 (HOX11)	Rare	Not determined	0.6%–3%[8,12,13]	Favorable[8,11] Intermediate[14]
del(6q)	6%–9%[9,49]	Not prognostic[9,49]	3%–7%[8,11–14]	Intermediate[8,13,14]
Abnormal 9p	7%–11%[9,50]	Not prognostic[9] Adverse[50]	5%–15%[8,11,12,14]	Favorable[14] Relatively favorable[12,13] Intermediate[8,11]
Abnormal 12p	3%–9%[9,37,51]	Not prognostic[9,37,51]	4%–5%[8,11,12,14]	Favorable[11,12]
Normal karyotype (no aberration detected)	31%–42%[9,37,38]	Relatively favorable[37,38]	15%–34%[8,11–14]	Relatively favorable[8,12–14] Intermediate[8,14]

other studies,[44,57,62] whereas +der(22)t(9;22) conferred a poor prognosis in some[60] but a better outcome in other[57] studies. Notably, half of the patients with +der(22)t(9;22) analyzed by Fielding and colleagues[57] also had high hyperdiploidy, which was suggested to confer improved outcome in adult[62] and pediatric[44] series. The presence of secondary −7 was associated with lower CR rates in the pre-imatinib era;[60,62] it is unclear if this is also the case in Ph+ patients treated with imatinib.

Translocations involving band 11q23/MLL are detected in two-thirds of infants with ALL.[45] Their incidence in older children and adults is much lower, 1% to 2% and 4% to 9%, respectively.[8,9,11–14,37] By far the most common among 11q23 rearrangements is t(4;11)(q21;q23)/MLL-AFF1(AF4), detected in more than 50% of patients, followed by t(11;19)(q23;p13.3)/MLL-MLLT1(ENL) and, less commonly, t(9;11)(p22;q23)/MLL-MLLT3(AF9), t(10;11)(p13-15;q14-21)/MLL-MLLT10(AF10), and others.[45,63] The t(4;11) predicts a poor prognosis in children and adults, with particularly dismal outcome in patients with a poor early response to prednisone, infants aged less than 3 months and older adults.[8,11–14,64,65] The outcome of patients with t(11;19) is also generally poor, especially in infants less than 1 year of age. In older children with t(11;19), those with T-ALL had a better outcome than patients with B-ALL.[64] Secondary aberrations are detected in one-third of patients with t(4;11), the most frequent of which are +X, abnormalities of 7p [including i(7)(q10)] and 9p and +8.[63,65] Similarly, secondary chromosomal abnormalities are detected in one-half of patients with t(11;19) who most often carry secondary +X, +8 and del(6q).[63] A large multi-institutional study has conclusively shown that secondary aberrations do not affect prognosis of infants or older children with ALL and t(4;11), t(11;19)(q23;p13.3), or other 11q23 translocations, which were analyzed as 1 group.[63]

Translocation (1;19)(q23;p13.3)/TCF3(E2A)-PBX1 occurs in 1% to 3% of adult [8,11,13,14,48] and 1% to 6% pediatric ALL,[9,37,46,47] and can be in either balanced or unbalanced form, as der(19)t(1;19) with two normal chromosomes 1. Most patients have pseudodiploid karyotypes, and almost all are diagnosed with pre–B-ALL. Outcome of patients with t(1;19) is controversial. In adult studies it was reported as poor,[8,13] relatively favorable[11] or not different from the outcome of Ph-negative patients without t(1;19).[14] In pediatric series, the initially unfavorable prognosis, especially for the patients with balanced t(1;19),[46] has been improved by the use of more effective therapies.[43,47] However, t(1;19)/TCF3-PBX1 was found to be an independent risk factor for isolated central nervous system (CNS) relapse in children.[47] A recent study of adult ALL has suggested that prognosis of patients with t(1;19) can be markedly improved by the hyper-CVAD regimen.[48]

Recent studies identified an intrachromosomal amplification of chromosome 21 (iAMP21) as a novel recurrent abnormality in B-ALL.[66–68] Approximately 2% of children and less than 0.5% of adults display iAMP21. In contrast to acute myeloid leukemia (AML), in which similar iAMP21 does not involve the amplification of the RUNX1 gene,[69,70] virtually all ALL patients with iAMP21 show multiple extra copies of RUNX1 in structurally rearranged abnormal chromosomes, which are composed of chromosome 21 material only.[66–68] The outcome is poor, with ALL patients with iAMP21 having a three-fold increased risk of relapse and twice the risk of death compared with those without this abnormality.[68]

Complex karyotype, defined as greater than or equal to three or greater than or equal to 5 chromosome aberrations, is a well-established adverse prognostic factor in AML.[71] Only a few studies have investigated the prognostic significance of a complex karyotype in ALL. Although Wetzler and colleagues[60] did not detect any impact of karyotype complexity (with ≥3 or ≥5 aberrations) on cumulative incidence of relapse or OS of Ph-positive patients, Moorman and colleagues[14] reported that ALL patients with a complex karyotype with greater than or equal to five aberrations who did not harbor an established translocation (4% of adults with ALL) had a significantly inferior EFS and OS, and that complex karyotype was an independent adverse prognostic factor within the Ph-negative patient cohort. This observation requires confirmation.

T-ALL occurs in 16% to 25% of adult[4,8,11–14] and 8% to 15% of childhood ALL.[4,9,37] At diagnosis, the proportion of cytogenetically normal cases is higher in T-ALL than B-ALL, with approximately 50% of T-ALL patients having a normal karyotype. Roughly one-third of T-ALL patients have a translocation involving one of the T cell receptor genes (TCR), with a breakpoint at 14q11 (TCRA/TCRD) or 7q34 (TCRB). The most common of these translocations in adults is t(10;14)(q24;q11.2), which results in overexpression of the TLX1 (HOX11) gene, and is associated with a favorable outcome.[8,12] Detected in 3% to 6% of childhood T-ALL, t(1;14)(p32;q11.2) juxtaposes TCRD and TAL1 (SCL) resulting in overexpression of TAL1. TAL1 overexpression is also brought about by a cryptic interstitial deletion of chromosome 1, which leads to a fusion between the 5′ untranslated region of STIL (formerly known as SIL), and the 5′ untranslated region of TAL1. In pediatric T-ALL, STIL-TAL1 fusion occurs in 16% to 26% of cases, making the combination of the 2 rearrangements involving TAL1 the most frequent abnormality in childhood T-ALL.[72,73] In contrast, the frequency of these rearrangements in adult T-ALL is low.[73] Similarly, a cryptic t(5;14)(q35;q32), juxtaposing TLX3 to BCL11B, occurs in 20% to 30% of pediatric T-ALL, but is less common in adults.[2,74]

A novel genetic phenomenon in T cell ALL, namely cryptic extrachromosomal amplification of a segment from chromosome 9 containing a fusion between ABL1 and NUP214 (nucleoporin) was recently described.[75–77] The amplified NUP214-ABL1 sequences are located on submicroscopic circular extrachromosomal DNA molecules called episomes. NUP214-ABL1 is a constitutively activated tyrosine kinase activating similar pathways as BCR-ABL1, and is sensitive to inhibition with tyrosine kinase inhibitors, especially nilotinib and dasatinib.[78] Notably, essentially all patients harbor rearrangements of TLX1 or TLX3 or their ectopic expression, and most also carry hemi- or homozygous deletions of CDKN2A and CDKN2B, and chromosome aberrations, including +8, t(7;10)(q35;q24) or t(10;14)(q24;q11). In a study of Graux and colleagues,[77] the estimated 5-year OS rate of NUP214-ABL1-positive T-ALL patients was 49% (SD 11%).

MOLECULAR GENETICS
Expression Microarray Analysis

Array-based gene expression profiling (GEP) combines synthesis of cDNA from the entire mRNA transcriptome with DNA array technology to evaluate the entire "transcriptome" of samples. Rather than evaluating changes in copy number or sequence of the nuclear DNA, GEP is used to determine the level at which genes are expressed in samples compared with controls. Sample cDNA is generated from mRNA, labeled with fluorochromes, and subsequently hybridized to chips spotted with probes corresponding to known transcripts. Fluorescent signals are captured and analyzed. The intensity of the signal at each spot corresponds to the amount of cDNA and thus mRNA or expression of the gene targeted by the spot on the probe.

Retrospective studies have demonstrated that expression profiling can be effective in classifying lymphoblastic leukemias into recognized, prognostically important subtypes including BCR-ABL1, TCF3-PBX1, hyperdiploid, 11q23/MLL rearranged, ETV6-RUNX1, and T-ALL.[16,79,80] GEP has also identified a new subtype of ALL without BCR-ABL1 fusion but with a similar expression profile to BCR-ABL1 leukemia.[80] In addition, GEP has shown that lymphoblastic leukemias with MLL rearrangements have a unique gene expression profile separate from other ALL and AML.[81] GEP has been retrospectively used to identify gene expression signatures at diagnosis that were predictive of early response and long-term outcome in NCI-defined high-risk childhood ALL. These profiles were generated from patient samples treated on COG 1961 and then validated in 3 independent cohorts from Pediatric Oncology Group (POG) trials, the German Cooperative Study Group for Childhood ALL (COALL) and the Dutch Childhood Oncology Group (DCOG) protocols. Although the expression profiling correlated with outcome in univariable analysis, they lost significance when known predictors of outcome like age, white blood cell count (WBC), and genotype were accounted for, suggesting that the profiling does not predict outcome beyond previously established prognostic factors in high-risk pediatric precursor B-ALL.[82] However, retrospective GEP in conjunction with flow cytometry, and SNP array analysis have recently been used to identify a subtype of T-ALL (early T cell precursor, ETP-ALL), which has a poor prognosis with standard intensive chemotherapy.[83] It remains to be seen whether augmented therapy, like HSCT in first remission, will benefit patients prospectively identified with ETP-ALL by GEP.

Although expression arrays analyze gene expression, and thus could potentially identify highly differentially expressed genes as target entry points for biologic studies, for the most part expression profiling has been used for classification of leukemias, rather than the identification of genes whose aberrant expression may be important in leukemic transformation. Exceptions include *HOXA9*,[84] *MEIS1*,[85] and *FLT3*[86] in *MLL* leukemias, and the erythropoietin receptor in *ETV6-RUNX1* leukemias.[80]

Array-based Comparative Genomic Hybridization

Array-based comparative genomic hybridization (a-CGH) is a recently developed technology that combines the ability to screen the entire genome like conventional comparative genomic hybridization (CGH) with the ability to detect small variations in DNA copy number. This broad-spectrum, high-resolution technique uses cloned DNA fragments of large size (100–200 kb), or, more recently, long (60–75 nucleotides) oligonucleotides spotted onto a solid matrix. The resolution of this technique is determined by the size of, and distance between, the clones used to construct the array. Test sample and control DNA are labeled with different fluorochromes and then hybridized to the DNA on the array. The fluorescent signals are captured from each spot on the array and analyzed. The fluorescent signal ratio is used to determine gain or loss of test DNA compared with the control DNA at each spot on the array. For example, if test DNA was labeled with a green fluorochrome, and control DNA with a red fluorochrome, a predominantly green signal at a spot would indicate gain of test DNA at that region. A yellow signal would indicate relatively equal amounts of test and control DNA, and a red signal, loss of test DNA at the corresponding region.[87] A-CGH augments traditional karyotyping in the detection of deletions or amplifications smaller than those that can be found by banding techniques, and allows analysis of samples for which metaphase chromosomes are not available. For example, using a tiling path 33 K bacterial artificial chromosome (BAC) array, Kuchinskaya and colleagues[88] detected copy number alterations, several of which were below the resolution of standard G-banding analysis, in approximately 80% of pediatric ALL patients with either a normal karyotype or an unsuccessful cytogenetic analysis. Two other studies reported patterns of genomic imbalances in Down syndrome children with ALL.[89,90]

Single Nucleotide Polymorphism Array Analysis

SNP arrays are oligonucleotide arrays with probes specific for regions flanking SNPs. When labeled genomic DNA from an individual is hybridized to the array, the DNA will bind with greater frequency to the probes that correspond to that individual's SNPs, and those regions of the chip will fluoresce with greater intensity. These chips were designed for genome-wide screens to identify SNP linked to inherited or acquired disease.[3] However, recently, using these types of chips, researchers have been able to identify new leukemia-associated genes by identifying small regions of acquired deletions, amplifications, and uniparental disomy in acute leukemias,[55,91,92] and associated some of these genetic aberrations with high-risk leukemias.[17,93]

Some important general themes are revealed by these studies in addition to the specific genes identified. First, high-resolution analysis of SNP arrays confirms pre-established cytogenetic anomalies and identifies submicroscopic anomalies, including unbalanced chromosome translocations. Thus, some leukemias with unidentified lesions on routine cytogenetic analysis can be shown to have common lesions such as a t(12;21) when evaluated at a higher resolution.[92] In addition, SNP-chip analysis permits more accurate detection of hyperdiploid ALL than the DNA-index method.[55] Second, multiple independent copy number aberrations are present in the leukemic samples, suggesting that multiple complementary genetic lesions are required for leukemic transformation. Third, although there seem to be multiple aberrations in each leukemia, the overall numbers of aberrations are not high. For example, 1 study identified a mean of 6.46 aberrations per leukemia,[91] whereas another study identified a mean of 4.2 for B-ALL and 2.6 for T-ALL.[92] These findings suggest that although multiple mutations are associated with leukemic transformation, marked global genomic instability is not an underlying mechanism leading to leukemic transformation. Multiple studies also showed significant differences in the frequency of aberrations among specific ALL subtypes,[17,91] with average frequencies ranging from 1 in 11q23/*MLL* rearranged leukemias to 11 in hyperdiploid ALL with more than 50 chromosomes.

Finally, the study of submicroscopic aberrations has identified aberrations in several genes involved with B cell differentiation and cell-cycle regulation. Two SNP array studies of pediatric ALL reported frequent deletions or other inactivating mutations in regulators of B cell development, with the paired box gene *PAX5*, mapped to 9p13.2, being the most frequent target in B-precursor leukemias.[91,92] The larger study, which also included resequencing of *PAX5* in the entire cohort, found this gene to be altered in 32% of precursor B-ALLs. Mutations in order of frequency included focal deletions of all or part of *PAX5*, loss of the entire chromosome 9 or deletion of 9p, broad deletions involving *PAX5* and flanking genes, and large 9p deletions involving the 3′ region of *PAX5*. Although various mechanisms were involved, including lack of expression of the altered allele, altered proteins (including 3 different fusion proteins) that lack either the DNA-binding domain or transcriptional-regulatory domain, or promoter mutations, all of the mutations resulted in loss of function of *PAX5*.[91] Additional regulators of B cell development found mutated in both studies include *EBF1* and *IKZF1* (Ikaros). The larger study found frequent mutations in additional transcription factors associated with B cell development including *AIOLOS*, *LEF1*, *RAG1*, and *RAG2*. A third, and larger still, study of pediatric ALL also found *PAX5* frequently mutated but the other genes were not found to be mutated at high frequencies.[55]

In addition to B cell differentiation mutations, SNP arrays confirmed previously known involvement of cell-cycle regulation gene mutations in leukemogenesis. *CDKN2A* located at 9p21.3, encodes $p16^{INK4a}$ and $p14^{ARF}$. This region was frequently mutated in SNP-array studies in leukemia.[55,91,92] *P16* deletion or inactivation was associated with B-ALL and T-ALL, although it was more common in T-ALL.[55,92] *P16* deletion was due to monosomy 9, 9p deletions, submicroscopic deletions, or uniparental disomy of 9p in 1 study.[55] This study also found a high frequency of 12p/ *ETV6* deletions, two-thirds of which were in leukemias with *ETV6/RUNX1*.

More recently, *IKZF1* inactivating mutations (complete deletions, or partial deletions, some of which result in a dominant negative $\triangle$3-6 isoform) have been found by SNP arrays in 84% of ALLs with *BCR-ABL1*, but not in chronic myelogenous leukemia (CML). Additionally, *IKZF1* mutations were found to be acquired at conversion from a chronic phase CML to blast crisis in a small sample in which DNA was available pre- and postconversion.[93] Subsequently, these investigators also found that *IKZF1*-inactivating mutations are associated with poor outcomes in pediatric ALL without *BCR-ABL1*. In two large independent cohorts, one of high-risk ALL (including patients with CNS or testicular disease, 11q23/*MLL* rearrangements, age more than 10 years, or high WBC), and the second consisting of standard and high-risk patients, *IKZF1*-inactivating deletions were associated with minimal residual disease, hematologic relapse, and any relapse. Interestingly, leukemias with *IKZF1* mutations without a *BCR-ABL1* fusion have gene expression signatures similar to *BCR-ABL1*-positive ALL.[17]

Resequencing of Candidate Genes

Resequencing of candidate genes has identified a large number of genes that are frequently mutated in specific subgroups of ALL (**Table 3**). Resequencing requires a priori knowledge of a candidate gene that may be mutated. Once a target gene is identified, primers specific to the gene or suspected region of the gene are used to amplify the gene of interest, which is then sequenced and compared with the known sequence of the gene. Several genes, first identified as targets by SNP arrays, have been shown to also harbor small mutations in ALL samples. Some of these, including *PAX5*,[91] *IKZF1*,[91] and *CDKN2A*,[98] have been further studied by resequencing, with identification of additional mutations in each case. These mutations are typically missense or nonsense mutations, or microdeletions that most commonly result in loss of function of the gene product.

Mutations that result in gain of function or constitutive activation of proteins can also be found by resequencing. Mutations in *FLT3* and multiple genes involved in the RAS/MAPK cascade have been shown to have acquired activating mutations in ALL. *FLT3*-activating mutations are present in up to 15% of ALLs with *MLL* rearrangements.[86] These mutations result in constitutively active FLT3, a membrane receptor tyrosine kinase important for early hematopoietic development. Additionally, *FLT3* mutations have been found in 3% to 10% of unselected cases of ALL, and seem to be associated with the high hyperdiploid subgroup.[96,99,100] *PTPN11*, *KRAS*, and *NRAS* also have activating point mutations in a subset of ALL patients, and are frequently associated with high hyperdiploid leukemia, being present in approximately 7%, 16%, and 17% of patients, respectively.[96,97,99,100] These mutations are usually mutually exclusive, suggesting that a single mutation resulting in constitutive activation of the receptor tyrosine kinase-RAS pathway is sufficient to dysregulate this pathway in leukemogenesis. Together, these mutations are present in approximately 30% of high hyperdiploid pediatric ALLs.[99]

NOTCH1, a gene demonstrated to be important in lymphocyte lineage specification, was first identified as a potential oncogene in T-ALL as a translocation partner in the rare t(7;9)(q34;q34.3), found in less than 1% of T-ALL.[101] Resequencing of functional domains of *NOTCH1* revealed that activating *NOTCH1* mutations are present in most primary pediatric and adolescent T-ALL, with mutations occurring in all of the molecular subtypes of T-ALL.[94] These mutations were found to involve either the heterodimer domain (HD) or the PEST domain of the NOTCH1 protein. Mutations involving

Table 3
Genes commonly mutated in acute lymphoblastic leukemia

Disease[a]	Gene	Function	Approximate Frequency %[b]	References	Comments
B-ALL and T-ALL	CDKN2A/2B	Cell cycle modulator	30 and 70	Mullighan and Downing[3]	Deletions
B-ALL and T-ALL	PAX5	B cell differentiation	30 and 10	Mullighan and Downing[3]	Deletions, deletions in T-ALL are large and typically include CDKN2A
B-ALL and T-ALL	EBF	B cell differentiation	4 and 6	Mullighan and Downing[3]	Deletions
B-ALL and T-ALL	RB1	Cell cycle modulator	4 and 12	Mullighan and Downing[3]	Deletions
T-ALL	NOTCH1	T cell differentiation	56	Weng et al[94], Sulis et al[95]	Activating HD and PEST domain mutations
B-ALL	ETV6	Transcription factor	26	Mullighan and Downing[3]	Deletions, also frequently involved on translocations
B-ALL	NRAS	Ras pathway	17	Case et al[96]	Activating point mutation codons 12, 13, 61
B-ALL	KRAS	Ras pathway	16	Case et al[96]	Activating point mutation codons 12, 13, 61
B-ALL	IKZF1	B cell differentiation	8	Mullighan and Downing[3]	84% of BCR-ABL1 ALL; complete or partial deletions
B-ALL	PTPN11	Ras pathway	7	Tartaglia et al[97]	Activating point mutations exons 3 and 13
B-ALL	E2-2	B cell differentiation	6	Kuiper et al[92]	Deletions
B-ALL	FLT3	Receptor tyrosine kinase	3	Case et al[96], Armstrong et al[86]	Activating ITD or point mutations, 15% of MLL-rearranged ALL

[a] B-ALL includes precursor B-ALL.
[b] Frequencies are only approximate due to variation in sample size and sample selection in different studies.

the HD, which is responsible for stable noncovalent association between the extracellular and transmembrane components of inactivated NOTCH1, produce ligand-independent activation of NOTCH1. Frameshift mutations result in complete or partial loss of the C terminal negative regulatory PEST domain,[94] and increased levels of intracellular NOTCH1 due to impaired degradation of the activated receptor. More recently, a third type of activating NOTCH1 mutation, internal tandem duplication of the juxtamembrane portion, has been identified in 7 of 210 primary T-ALL samples from pediatric and young adult T-ALL patients. Like HD mutations, these result in constitutive ligand-independent activation of NOTCH1.[95]

Epigenetic Changes Associated with Acute Lymphoblastic Leukemia

DNA methylation, a type of reversible epigenetic regulation that typically results in downregulation of genes, is prevalent in cancer. Single gene and genome-wide analyses have revealed that aberrant DNA methylation is common in adult and pediatric ALL. Methylation of multiple gene promoters leads to downregulation of tumor suppressor genes or pathways; one of the best described is the methylation and loss of expression of CDKN2A and CDKN2B.[102]

Timing of Mutations Associated with Acute Lymphoblastic Leukemia

Although little is known about proximate causes of small point mutations associated with ALL, the timing of some gross chromosomal rearrangements can be identified in certain cases of childhood ALL. Studies of monozygotic twins with leukemia have used clone-specific gene rearrangements, such as unique breakpoint regions in MLL or ETV6-RUNX1 fusions, or unique immunoglobin heavy chain or TCR gene rearrangements, to demonstrate that leukemias in each twin developed from a single identical clone. In all likelihood, the leukemia initially developed in one twin in utero, and subsequently metastasized via the shared placental circulation to the second twin.[103] Guthrie cards (absorbent cards onto which neonatal blood spots are collected for metabolic or genetic screening) have been retrospectively evaluated in pediatric leukemia patients. These studies revealed that all studied ALLs with MLL-AFF1 fusions, most with ETV6-RUNX1 fusions, some hyperdiploid, and some with TCF3-PBX1 fusions develop prenatally.[104]

Perspectives for the Future

Recently, the entire genome of leukemic cells from a cytogenetically normal AML sample was sequenced and compared with the patient's constitutional genome established from a skin biopsy. Although the entire genome was sequenced, the initial report focused on analysis of known gene coding sequences. Ten single-nucleotide variants were found in the leukemic cells compared with the skin cells, and 8 of these were in genes not previously associated with AML.[105] Although in its infancy, rapid advances in high throughput "next generation sequencing" suggest that whole genome sequencing of ALL samples may become rapidly available and contribute to risk stratification in the not too distant future.

ACKNOWLEDGEMENTS

The authors thank Warren Pear, Martin Carroll, Michael Kuehl, Chris Slape, Dave Caudell, Rachel Novak, Sarah Beachy, and Sheryl Gough for thoughtful discussions, and Clara D. Bloomfield for her constant help and encouragement.

REFERENCES

1. Johansson B, Mertens F, Mitelman F. Clinical and biological importance of cytogenetic abnormalities in childhood and adult acute lymphoblastic leukemia. Ann Med 2004;36(7):492–503.
2. Mrózek K, Heerema NA, Bloomfield CD. Cytogenetics in acute leukemia. Blood Rev 2004;18(2):115–36.
3. Mulligan CG, Downing JR. Global genomic characterization of acute lymphoblastic leukemia. Semin Hematol 2009;46(1):3–15.
4. Swerdlow SH, Campo E, Harris NL, et al, editors. WHO classification of tumours of haematopoietic and lymphoid tissues. Lyon, France: IARC; 2008. p. 157–75.
5. Vardiman JW, Thiele J, Arber DA, et al. The 2008 revision of the World Health Organization (WHO) classification of myeloid neoplasms and acute leukemia: rationale and important changes. Blood 2009;114(5):937–51.
6. Third International Workshop on Chromosomes in Leukemia. Clinical significance of chromosomal abnormalities in acute lymphoblastic leukemia. Cancer Genet Cytogenet 1981;4(2):111–37.
7. Bloomfield CD, Goldman AI, Alimena G, et al. Chromosomal abnormalities identify high-risk and low-risk patients with acute lymphoblastic leukemia. Blood 1986;67(2):415–20.
8. The Groupe Français de Cytogénétique Hématologique. Cytogenetic abnormalities in adult acute lymphoblastic leukemia: correlations with hematologic findings outcome. A collaborative study of the Group Français de Cytogénétique Hématologique. Blood 1996;87(8):3135–42.
9. Chessels JM, Swansbury GJ, Reeves B, et al. Cytogenetics and prognosis in childhood lymphoblastic leukaemia: results of MRC UKALL X. Br J Haematol 1997;99(1):93–100.
10. Bloomfield CD, Secker-Walker LM, Goldman AI, et al. Six-year follow-up of the clinical significance of karyotype in acute lymphoblastic leukemia. Cancer Genet Cytogenet 1989;40(2):171–85.
11. Secker-Walker LM, Prentice HG, Durrant J, et al. Cytogenetics adds independent prognostic information in adults with acute lymphoblastic leukaemia on MRC trial UKALL XA. Br J Haematol 1997;96(3):601–10.
12. Wetzler M, Dodge RK, Mrózek K, et al. Prospective karyotype analysis in adult acute lymphoblastic leukemia: the Cancer and Leukemia Group B experience. Blood 1999;93(11):3983–93.
13. Mancini M, Scappaticci D, Cimino G, et al. A comprehensive genetic classification of adult acute lymphoblastic leukemia (ALL): analysis of the GIMEMA 0496 protocol. Blood 2005;105(9):3434–41.
14. Moorman AV, Harrison CJ, Buck GA, et al. Karyotype is an independent prognostic factor in adult acute lymphoblastic leukemia (ALL): analysis of cytogenetic data from patients treated on the Medical Research Council (MRC) UKALLXII/Eastern Cooperative Oncology Group (ECOG) 2993 trial. Blood 2007;109(8):3189–97.
15. Pullarkat V, Slovak ML, Kopecky KJ, et al. Impact of cytogenetics on the outcome of adult acute lymphoblastic leukemia: results of Southwest Oncology Group 9400 study. Blood 2008;111(5):2563–72.
16. Yeoh E-J, Ross ME, Shurtleff SA, et al. Classification, subtype discovery, and prediction of outcome in pediatric acute lymphoblastic leukemia by gene expression profiling. Cancer Cell 2002;1(2):133–43.

17. Mullighan CG, Su X, Zhang J, et al. Deletion of *IKZF1* and prognosis in acute lymphoblastic leukemia. N Engl J Med 2009;360(5):470–80.
18. Stock W. Advances in the treatment of Philadelphia chromosome-positive acute lymphoblastic leukemia. Clin Adv Hematol Oncol 2008;6(7):487–8.
19. Mrózek K, Carroll AJ, Maharry K, et al. Central review of cytogenetics is necessary for cooperative group correlative and clinical studies of adult acute leukemia: the Cancer and Leukemia Group B experience. Int J Oncol 2008; 33(2):239–44.
20. Mitelman F, editor. ISCN 1995: An international system for human cytogenetic nomenclature 1995. Basel, Switzerland: S Karger; 1995. p. 78.
21. Raimondi SC. Fluorescence in situ hybridization: molecular probes for diagnosis of pediatric neoplastic diseases. Cancer Invest 2000;18(2):135–47.
22. Romana SP, Le Coniat M, Berger R. t(12;21): a new recurrent translocation in acute lymphoblastic leukemia. Genes Chromosomes Cancer 1994;9(3):186–91.
23. Robinson HM, Martineau M, Harris RL, et al. Derivative chromosome 9 deletions are a significant feature of childhood Philadelphia chromosome positive acute lymphoblastic leukaemia. Leukemia 2005;19(4):564–71.
24. Mathew S, Rao PH, Dalton J, et al. Multicolor spectral karyotyping identifies novel translocations in childhood acute lymphoblastic leukemia. Leukemia 2001;15(3):468–72.
25. Nordgren A, Heyman M, Sahlén S, et al. Spectral karyotyping and interphase FISH reveal abnormalities not detected by conventional G-banding. Implications for treatment stratification of childhood acute lymphoblastic leukaemia: detailed analysis of 70 cases. Eur J Haematol 2002;68(1):31–41.
26. Poppe B, Cauwelier B, Van Limbergen H, et al. Novel cryptic chromosomal rearrangements in childhood acute lymphoblastic leukemia detected by multiple color fluorescent in situ hybridization. Haematologica 2005;90(9):1179–85.
27. Karst C, Gross M, Haase D, et al. Novel cryptic chromosomal rearrangements detected in acute lymphoblastic leukemia detected by application of new multicolor fluorescent in situ hybridization approaches. Int J Oncol 2006;28(4):891–7.
28. Nordgren A, Farnebo F, Johansson B, et al. Identification of numerical and structural chromosome aberrations in 15 high hyperdiploid childhood acute lymphoblastic leukemias using spectral karyotyping. Eur J Haematol 2001;66(5):297–304.
29. Betts DR, Stanchescu R, Niggli FK, et al. SKY reveals a high frequency of unbalanced translocations involving chromosome 6 in t(12;21)-positive acute lymphoblastic leukemia. Leuk Res 2008;32(1):39–43.
30. Harrison CJ, Moorman AV, Barber KE, et al. Interphase molecular cytogenetic screening for chromosomal abnormalities of prognostic significance in childhood acute lymphoblastic leukaemia: a UK Cancer Cytogenetics Group Study. Br J Haematol 2005;129(4):520–30.
31. Forestier E, Johansson B, Borgström G, et al. Cytogenetic findings in a population-based series of 787 childhood acute lymphoblastic leukemias from the Nordic countries. Eur J Haematol 2000;64(3):194–200.
32. Paulsson K, Johansson B. High hyperdiploid childhood acute lymphoblastic leukemia. Genes Chromosomes Cancer 2009;48(8):637–60.
33. Heerema NA, Sather HN, Sensel MG, et al. Prognostic impact of trisomies of chromosomes 10, 17, and 5 among children with acute lymphoblastic leukemia and high hyperdiploidy (>50 chromosomes). J Clin Oncol 2000; 18(9):1876–87.
34. Forestier E, Heyman M, Andersen MK, et al. Outcome of *ETV6/RUNX1*-positive childhood acute lymphoblastic leukaemia in the NOPHO-ALL-1992

protocol: frequent late relapses but good overall survival. Br J Haematol 2008; 140(6):665–72.

35. Attarbaschi A, Mann G, König M, et al. Incidence and relevance of secondary chromosome abnormalities in childhood *TEL/AML1+* acute lymphoblastic leukemia: an interphase FISH analysis. Leukemia 2004;18(10):1611–6.

36. Moorman AV, Richards SM, Martineau M, et al. Outcome heterogeneity in childhood high-hyperdiploid acute lymphoblastic leukemia. Blood 2003;102(8):2756–62.

37. Forestier E, Johansson B, Gustafsson G, et al. Prognostic impact of karyotypic findings in childhood acute lymphoblastic leukaemia: a Nordic series comparing two treatment periods. Br J Haematol 2000;110(1):147–53.

38. Heerema NA, Nachman JB, Sather HN, et al. Hypodiploidy with less than 45 chromosomes confers adverse risk in childhood acute lymphoblastic leukemia: a report from the Children's Cancer Group. Blood 1999;94(12):4036–45.

39. Rubnitz JE, Wichlan D, Devidas M, et al. Prospective analysis of *TEL* gene rearrangements in childhood acute lymphoblastic leukemia: a Children's Oncology Group Study. J Clin Oncol 2008;26(13):2186–91.

40. Loh ML, Goldwasser MA, Silverman LB, et al. Prospective analysis of *TEL/AML1-* positive patients treated on Dana-Farber Cancer Institute Consortium Protocol 95-01. Blood 2006;107(11):4508–13.

41. Shih LY, Chou TB, Liang DC, et al. Lack of *TEL-AML1* fusion transcript resulting from a cryptic t(12;21) in adult B lineage acute lymphoblastic leukemia in Taiwan. Leukemia 1996;10(9):1456–8.

42. Jabbar Al-Obaidi MS, Martineau M, Bennett CF, et al. *ETV6/AML1* fusion by FISH in adult acute lymphoblastic leukemia. Leukemia 2002;16(4):669–74.

43. Schultz KR, Pullen DJ, Sather HN, et al. Risk- and response-based classification of childhood B-precursor acute lymphoblastic leukemia: a combined analysis of prognostic markers from the Pediatric Oncology Group (POG) and Children's Cancer Group (CCG). Blood 2007;109(3):926–35.

44. Heerema NA, Harbott J, Galimberti S, et al. Secondary cytogenetic aberrations in childhood Philadelphia chromosome positive acute lymphoblastic leukemia are nonrandom and may be associated with outcome. Leukemia 2004;18(4):693–702.

45. Chessells JM, Harrison CJ, Kempski H, et al. Clinical features, cytogenetics and outcome in acute lymphoblastic and myeloid leukaemia of infancy: report from the MRC Childhood Leukaemia working party. Leukemia 2002;16(5):776–84.

46. Uckun FM, Sensel MG, Sather HN, et al. Clinical significance of translocation t(1;19) in childhood acute lymphoblastic leukemia in the context of contemporary therapies: a report from the Children's Cancer Group. J Clin Oncol 1998; 16(2):527–35.

47. Jeha S, Pei D, Raimondi SC, et al. Increased risk for CNS relapse in pre-B cell leukemia with the t(1;19)/*TCF3-PBX1*. Leukemia, 2009;23(8):1406–9.

48. Garg R, Kantarjian H, Thomas D, et al. Adults with acute lymphoblastic leukemia and translocation (1;19) abnormality have a favorable outcome with hyperfractionated cyclophosphamide, vincristine, doxorubicin, and dexamethasone alternating with methotrexate and high-dose cytarabine chemotherapy. Cancer 2009;115(10):2147–54.

49. Heerema NA, Sather HN, Sensel MG, et al. Clinical significance of deletions of chromosome arm 6q in childhood acute lymphoblastic leukemia: a report from the Children's Cancer Group. Leuk Lymphoma 2000;36(5–6):467–78.

50. Heerema NA, Sather HN, Sensel MG, et al. Association of chromosome arm 9p abnormalities with adverse risk in childhood acute lymphoblastic leukemia: a report from the Children's Cancer Group. Blood 1999;94(5):1537–44.

51. Heerema NA, Sather HN, Sensel MG, et al. Prognostic significance of cytogenetic abnormalities of chromosome arm 12p in childhood acute lymphoblastic leukemia: a report from the Children's Cancer Group. Cancer 2000;88:1945–54.

52. Heerema NA, Raimondi SC, Anderson JR, et al. Specific extra chromosomes occur in a modal number dependent pattern in pediatric acute lymphoblastic leukemia. Genes Chromosomes Cancer 2007;46(7):684–93.

53. Sutcliffe MJ, Shuster JJ, Sather HN, et al. High concordance from independent studies by the Children's Cancer Group (CCG) and Pediatric Oncology Group (POG) associating favorable prognosis with combined trisomies 4,10, and 17 in children with NCI Standard-Risk B-precursor Acute Lymphoblastic Leukemia: a Children's Oncology Group (COG) initiative. Leukemia 2005;19:734–40.

54. Raimondi SC, Pui C-H, Hancock ML, et al. Heterogeneity of hyperdiploid (51–67) childhood acute lymphoblastic leukemia. Leukemia 1996;10(2):213–24.

55. Kawamata N, Ogawa S, Zimmermann M, et al. Molecular allelokaryotyping of pediatric acute lymphoblastic leukemias by high-resolution single nucleotide polymorphism oligonucleotide genomic microarray. Blood 2008;111(2):776–84.

56. Stams WAG, Beverloo HB, den Boer ML, et al. Incidence of additional genetic changes in the *TEL* and *AML1* genes in DCOG and COALL-treated t(12;21)-positive pediatric ALL, and their relation with drug sensitivity and clinical outcome. Leukemia 2006;20(3):410–6.

57. Fielding AK, Rowe JM, Richards SM, et al. Prospective outcome data on 267 unselected adult patients with Philadelphia chromosome-positive acute lymphoblastic leukemia confirms superiority of allogeneic transplantation over chemotherapy in the pre-imatinib era: results from the international ALL trial MRC UKALLXII/ECOG2993. Blood 2009;113(19):4489–96.

58. Thomas DA, Faderl S, Cortes J, et al. Treatment of Philadelphia chromosome-positive acute lymphocytic leukemia with hyper-CVAD and imatinib mesylate. Blood 2004;103(12):4396–407.

59. Yanada M, Takeuchi J, Sugiura I, et al. High complete remission rate and promising outcome by combination of imatinib and chemotherapy for newly diagnosed *BCR-ABL*-positive acute lymphoblastic leukemia: a phase II study by the Japan Adult Leukemia Study Group. J Clin Oncol 2006;24(3):460–6.

60. Wetzler M, Dodge RK, Mrózek K, et al. Additional cytogenetic abnormalities in adults with Philadelphia chromosome-positive acute lymphoblastic leukaemia: a study of the Cancer and Leukaemia Group B. Br J Haematol 2004;124(3):275–88.

61. Yanada M, Takeuchi J, Sugiura I, et al. Karyotype at diagnosis is the major prognostic factor predicting relapse-free survival for patients with Philadelphia chromosome-positive acute lymphoblastic leukemia treated with imatinib-combined chemotherapy. Haematologica 2008;93(2):287–90.

62. Rieder H, Ludwig WD, Gassmann W, et al. Prognostic significance of additional chromosome abnormalities in adult patients with Philadelphia chromosome positive acute lymphoblastic leukaemia. Br J Haematol 1996;95(4):678–91.

63. Moorman AV, Raimondi SC, Pui C-H, et al. No prognostic effect of additional chromosomal abnormalities in children with acute lymphoblastic leukemia and 11q23 abnormalities. Leukemia 2005;19(4):557–63.

64. Pui C-H, Chessells JM, Camitta B, et al. Clinical heterogeneity in childhood acute lymphoblastic leukemia with 11q23 rearrangements. Leukemia 2003;17(4):700–6.

65. Johansson B, Moorman AV, Haas OA, et al. Hematologic malignancies with t(4;11)(q21;q23) - a cytogenetic, morphologic, immunophenotypic and clinical study of 183 cases. Leukemia 1998;12(5):779–87.

66. Harewood L, Robinson H, Harris R, et al. Amplification of *AML1* on a duplicated chromosome 21 in acute lymphoblastic leukemia: a study of 20 cases. Leukemia 2003;17(3):547–53.
67. Strefford JC, van Delft FW, Robinson HM, et al. Complex genomic alterations and gene expression in acute lymphoblastic leukemia with intrachromosomal amplification of chromosome 21. Proc Natl Acad Sci U S A 2006;103(21):8167–72.
68. Moorman AV, Richards SM, Robinson HM, et al. Prognosis of children with acute lymphoblastic leukemia (ALL) and intrachromosomal amplification of chromosome 21 (iAMP21). Blood 2007;109(6):2327–30.
69. Mrózek K, Heinonen K, Theil KS, et al. Spectral karyotyping in patients with acute myeloid leukemia and a complex karyotype shows hidden aberrations, including recurrent overrepresentation of 21q, 11q, and 22q. Genes Chromosomes Cancer 2002;34(2):137–53.
70. Baldus CD, Liyanarachchi S, Mrózek K, et al. Acute myeloid leukemia with complex karyotypes and abnormal chromosome 21: amplification discloses overexpression of *APP, ETS2*, and *ERG* genes. Proc Natl Acad Sci U S A 2004;101(11):3915–20.
71. Mrózek K. Cytogenetic, molecular genetic, and clinical characteristics of acute myeloid leukemia with a complex karyotype. Semin Oncol 2008;35(4):365–77.
72. Aplan PD, Lombardi DP, Reaman GH, et al. Involvement of the putative hematopoietic transcription factor SCL in T-cell acute lymphoblastic leukemia. Blood 1992;79(5):1327–33.
73. Stock W, Westbrook CA, Sher DA, et al. Low incidence of *TAL1* gene rearrangements in adult acute lymphoblastic leukemia: a Cancer and Leukemia Group B Study (8762). Clin Cancer Res 1995;1(4):459–63.
74. Bernard OA, Busson-LeConiat M, Ballerini P, et al. A new recurrent and specific cryptic translocation, t(5;14)(q35;q32), is associated with expression of the Hox11L2 gene in T acute lymphoblastic leukemia. Leukemia 2001;15(10): 1495–504.
75. Barber KE, Martineau M, Harewood L, et al. Amplification of the *ABL* gene in T-cell acute lymphoblastic leukemia. Leukemia 2004;18(6):1153–6.
76. Graux C, Cools J, Melotte C, et al. Fusion of *NUP214* to *ABL1* on amplified episomes in T-cell acute lymphoblastic leukemia. Nat Genet 2004;36(10): 1084–9.
77. Graux C, Stevens-Kroef M, Lafage M, et al. Heterogeneous patterns of amplification of the *NUP214-ABL1* fusion gene in T-cell acute lymphoblastic leukemia. Leukemia 2009;23(1):125–33.
78. Quintás-Cardama A, Tong W, Manshouri T, et al. Activity of tyrosine kinase inhibitors against human *NUP214-ABL1*-positive T cell malignancies. Leukemia 2008; 22(6):1117–24.
79. Ross ME, Zhou X, Song G, et al. Classification of pediatric acute lymphoblastic leukemia by gene expression profiling. Blood 2003;102(8):2951–9.
80. Den Boer ML, van Slegtenhorst M, De Menezes RX, et al. A subtype of childhood acute lymphoblastic leukaemia with poor treatment outcome: a genome-wide classification study. Lancet Oncol 2009;10(2):125–34.
81. Armstrong SA, Staunton JE, Silverman LB, et al. *MLL* translocations specify a distinct gene expression profile that distinguishes a unique leukemia. Nat Genet 2002;30(1):41–7.
82. Bhojwani D, Kang H, Menezes RX, et al. Gene expression signatures predictive of early response and outcome in high-risk childhood acute lymphoblastic leukemia: a Children's Oncology Group Study. J Clin Oncol 2008;26(27):4376–84.

83. Coustan-Smith E, Mullighan CG, Onciu M, et al. Early T-cell precursor leukaemia: a subtype of very high-risk acute lymphoblastic leukaemia. Lancet Oncol 2009; 10(2):147–56.
84. Faber J, Krivtsov AV, Stubbs MC, et al. HOXA9 is required for survival in human *MLL*-rearranged acute leukemias. Blood 2009;113(11):2375–85.
85. Kumar AR, Li Q, Hudson WA, et al. A role for MEIS1 in *MLL*-fusion gene leukemia. Blood 2009;113(8):1756–8.
86. Armstrong SA, Kung AL, Mabon ME, et al. Inhibition of FLT3 in MLL: validation of a therapeutic target identified by gene expression based classification. Cancer Cell 2003;3(2):173–83.
87. Oostlander AE, Meijer GA, Ylstra B. Microarray-based comparative genomic hybridization and its applications in human genetics. Clin Genet 2004;66(6): 488–95.
88. Kuchinskaya E, Heyman M, Nordgren A, et al. Array-CGH reveals hidden gene dose changes in children with acute lymphoblastic leukaemia and a normal or failed karyotype by G-banding. Br J Haematol 2008;140(5):572–7.
89. Lo KC, Chalker J, Strehl S, et al. Array comparative genome hybridization analysis of acute lymphoblastic leukaemia and acute megakaryoblastic leukaemia in patients with Down syndrome. Br J Haematol 2008;142(6):934–45.
90. Lundin C, Davidsson J, Hjorth L, et al. Tiling resolution array-based comparative genomic hybridisation analyses of acute lymphoblastic leukaemias in children with Down syndrome reveal recurrent gain of 8q and deletions of 7p and 9p. Br J Haematol 2009;146(1):113–5.
91. Mullighan CG, Goorha S, Radtke I, et al. Genome-wide analysis of genetic alterations in acute lymphoblastic leukemia. Nature 2007;446(7137):758–64.
92. Kuiper RP, Schoenmakers EFPM, van Reijmersdal SV, et al. High-resolution genomic profiling of childhood ALL reveals novel recurrent genetic lesions affecting pathways involved in lymphocyte differentiation and cell cycle progression. Leukemia 2007;21(6):1258–66.
93. Mullighan CG, Miller CB, Radtke I, et al. *BCR-ABL1* lymphoblastic leukaemia is characterized by the deletion of Ikaros. Nature 2008;453(7191):110–4.
94. Weng AP, Ferrando AA, Lee W, et al. Activating mutations of *NOTCH1* in human T cell acute lymphoblastic leukemia. Science 2004;306(5694):269–71.
95. Sulis ML, Williams O, Palomero T, et al. NOTCH1 extracellular juxtamembrane expansion mutations in T-ALL. Blood 2008;112(3):733–40.
96. Case M, Matheson E, Minto L, et al. Mutation of genes affecting the RAS pathway is common in childhood acute lymphoblastic leukemia. Cancer Res 2008;68(16):6803–9.
97. Tartaglia M, Martinelli S, Cazzaniga G, et al. Genetic evidence for lineage-related and differentiation stage-related contribution of somatic *PTPN11* mutations to leukemogenesis in childhood acute leukemia. Blood 2004;104(2):307–13.
98. Sulong S, Moorman AV, Irving JA, et al. A comprehensive analysis of the *CDKN2A* gene in childhood acute lymphoblastic leukemia reveals genomic deletion, copy number neutral loss of heterozygosity, and association with specific cytogenetic subgroups. Blood 2009;113(1):100–7.
99. Paulsson K, Horvat A, Strömbeck B, et al. Mutations of *FLT3, NRAS, KRAS,* and *PTPN11* are frequent and possibly mutually exclusive in high hyperdiploid childhood acute lymphoblastic leukaemia. Genes Chromosomes Cancer 2008;47(1): 26–33.
100. Yamamoto T, Isomura M, Xu Y, et al. PTPN11, RAS and FLT3 mutations in childhood acute lymphoblastic leukemia. Leuk Res 2006;30(9):1085–9.

101. Ellisen LW, Bird J, West DC, et al. *TAN*-1, the human homolog of the Drosophila *Notch* gene, is broken by chromosomal translocations in T lymphoblastic neoplasms. Cell 1991;66(4):649–61.
102. Garcia-Manero G, Yang H, Kuang S-Q, et al. Epigenetics of acute lymphocytic leukemia. Semin Hematol 2009;46(1):24–32.
103. Greaves MF, Maia AT, Wiemels JL, et al. Leukemia in twins: lessons in natural history. Blood 2003;102(7):2321–33.
104. Greaves MF, Wiemels J. Origins of chromosome translocations in childhood leukemia. Nat Rev Cancer 2003;3(9):639–49.
105. Ley TJ, Mardis ER, Ding L, et al. DNA sequencing of a cytogenetically normal acute myeloid leukemia genome. Nature 2008;456(7218):66–72.

Allogeneic Hematopoietic Cell Transplantation for Acute Lymphoblastic Leukemia in Adults

Stephen J. Forman, MD[a,b],*

KEYWORDS

- Acute lymphoblastic leukemia • Graft versus leukemia
- Minimal residual disease
- Philadelphia chromosome positive ALL
- Precursor B cell ALL • Precursor T cell ALL
- Total body irradiation • Reduced intensity transplant

Acute lymphoblastic leukemia (ALL) is a hematologic malignancy of the bone marrow characterized by the rapid proliferation and subsequent accumulation of immature lymphocytes. ALL accounts for 20% of all acute leukemias that are seen in adults over the age of 20 years. In the past 2 decades, there has been substantial improvement in the understanding of the molecular biology of the disease and in the management of adult patients who have this disorder. The success of therapy in children with ALL has continued to fuel the quest for similar success in adults using the same principles that guide therapy in children, namely intensive induction and consolidation, maintenance therapy and prevention of disease in extramedullary sites such as the central nervous system (CNS). However, except for some studies focusing on the treatment of young adults, most adult patients will relapse and succumb to their disease. Transplantation has been used in the treatment of patients with high-risk disease and in those who have suffered a relapse. Laboratory and clinical studies are beginning to refine the decisions concerning both the indication and timing of allogeneic hematopoietic cell transplantation (HCT). This article reviews the biology of adult ALL, the relationship of specific disease characteristics to the natural history

[a] Department of Hematology and Hematopoietic Cell Transplantation, City of Hope National Medical Center, 1500 E. Duarte Road, Duarte, CA 91010, USA
[b] Clinical Research, Department of Cancer Immunotherapeutics & Tumor Immunology, City of Hope Comprehensive Cancer Center, 1500 E. Duarte Road, Duarte, CA 91010, USA
* Corresponding author. Department of Hematology and Hematopoietic Cell Transplantation, City of Hope National Medical Center, 1500 E. Duarte Road, Duarte, CA 91010.
E-mail address: sforman@coh.org

Hematol Oncol Clin N Am 23 (2009) 1011–1031
doi:10.1016/j.hoc.2009.07.006
0889-8588/09/$ – see front matter © 2009 Elsevier Inc. All rights reserved.
hemonc.theclinics.com

of the disease and the role of allogeneic HCT in the management of adult patients with this disease.

PROGNOSTIC FACTORS IN ACUTE LYMPHOBLASTIC LEUKEMIA

The major prognostic factors for achieving an initial complete remission (CR) are advancing age and Philadelphia chromosome positive (Ph+) ALL. These prognostic factors are of even greater importance in predicting the durability of remission and survival, and are used to assess the need for allogeneic HCT. **Table 1** presents some of the generally accepted adverse prognostic factors for remission duration in adult ALL that have been identified in previous clinical trials, and are often used in determining a patient's risk of relapse and the decision to pursue allogeneic transplant.

ROLE OF MINIMAL RESIDUAL DISEASE

In addition to age, cytogenetic analysis at the time of diagnosis, the most important prognostic factor, and a direct reflection of sensitivity to chemotherapy, is the rapid achievement of a CR. Thus, a slower time to achieving a remission is an indicator of relative chemoresistance, similar to what has been observed in pediatric patients. Those patients who take more than one cycle of induction chemotherapy or take longer than 4 weeks to achieve remission have a poor long-term prognosis and a shorter remission duration.[1–3]

A more quantitative approach to assess the response of an individual patient to chemotherapy is the measurement of minimal residual disease at various time points after therapy (see the article by Campana elsewhere in this issue for a detailed review of minimal residual disease (MRD) monitoring in ALL). Quantitative assessment of tumor cell kill is emerging as an independent prognostic factor that reflects the resistance of the cells to chemotherapy and allows potential individualization of treatment.[4,5] The assessment allows the identification of potential patients at high risk for relapse despite achieving a morphologic remission and who may benefit from early HCT. Studies are being performed to determine the most predictive time point for measurement. It seems that after consolidation, a high level of MRD at 10^{-4} is associated with a high risk of disease relapse, with a rising level of MRD on treatment also portending relapse.[6,7] In some studies, a high level of MRD after induction and consolidation has been identified

Table 1			
High-risk features in adult acute lymphoblastic leukemia			
	All	**B-Precursor**	**T-ALL**
At diagnosis			
High WBC		>30,000/µl (20–50)	>100,000
Subtype		Pro B	Early T
		CD10-neg pre-B	Mature T
Cytogenetics/	Complex	t(9;22)/BCR-ABL	BAALC+
Molecular genetics	Karyotype	t(4;11)/ALL1-AF4 (pro B)	HOX11L2
		T(1;19)	EGR+
During course	Time to CR (>4 weeks), more than 1 cycle to CR		
	MRD persistence (molecular failure)		
	MRD reappearance (molecular relapse)		
Age	>35		

Abbreviation: WBC, white blood cell count.

as a high-risk feature despite the achievement of a morphologic remission and the absence of high-risk cytogenetics.[6,7] Conversely, patients who are sensitive to chemotherapy and achieve a low level of MRD (nondetectable) may identify a group of patients who do not need transplantation in first remission or can wait until there is clear evidence of relapse.[6,7] It also remains to be determined what the benefit of HCT may be in patients who are in first remission, but have evidence of a new factor that defines high-risk disease, that is, high MRD. At the present time, MRD measurement has certain limitations related to the technical procedure, which is time consuming, expensive and requires a specialized laboratory to conduct the studies. The testing also involves multiple evaluations with either immunophenotypic flow cytometry analysis or molecular analysis with patient-specific probes for gene rearrangements. Thus, the future of treatment of adult patients with ALL in first remission may be refined to determine those patients who are unlikely to benefit from further chemotherapy and should be considered for transplantation during first remission or whose prognosis is excellent and can be spared the risk and late effects of transplant.

ALLOGENEIC HEMATOPOIETIC CELL TRANSPLANTATION IN FIRST COMPLETE REMISSION OF ACUTE LYMPHOBLASTIC LEUKEMIA

Allogeneic HCT in first CR has generally been reserved for those patients who present with poor risk features, such as those described earlier. In several phase 2 studies, patients with high-risk disease treated with allogeneic HCT had disease-free survival (DFS) longer than would have been predicted, especially those with Ph+ ALL. Depending on the risk factors present at diagnosis in an individual patient, standard chemotherapy leads to continued remissions ranging from less than 10% to more than 50%.[8,9] Studies indicate that HCT offers some groups of high-risk patients long-term disease survival rates of between 40% and 60%.[10–16] At the City of Hope and Stanford University, two series of patients with high-risk features who underwent allogeneic HCT in first CR have been recently updated. Selection criteria included white blood cell count (WBC) >25,000/µl, chromosomal translocations t(9;22), t(4;11), t(8;14); age older than 30 years; extramedullary disease at the time of diagnosis; and/or requiring more than 4 weeks to achieve a CR. Two-thirds of the patients had at least one risk factor and the remaining patients had two or more high-risk features at presentation. Most of these patients underwent allogeneic HCT within the first 4 months after achieving a CR. Allogeneic HCT during first remission led to prolonged DFS in this patient population who would otherwise have been expected to fare poorly. At a median follow-up of greater than 5 years, the probability of event-free survival was 64% with a relapse rate of 15% (**Fig. 1**).[17]

The French Group on Therapy for Adult ALL conducted a study comparing chemotherapy to autologous and allogeneic HCT.[8] Although the overall results of treatment did not show a treatment advantage for the group treated with allogeneic HCT, subgroup analysis revealed that those patients with high-risk disease, including patients with a t(9;22) and t(1;19) translocation, had a higher 5-year survival of 44% as opposed to 20% in the other two groups (**Fig. 2**). These trials have supported the strategy of taking patients with high-risk disease to transplant while in first remission. The recently reported EGOG-MRC trial showed that an allogeneic HCT resulted in improved disease control in all adult patients with ALL, but with long-term benefit seen mostly in younger patients with lower risk disease.[18] **Table 2** shows the DFS and response rate for patients on this trial with the risk of relapse reduced following allogeneic HCT when compared with either chemotherapy or autologous HCT, showing the improved outcomes and better leukemia control for those patients undergoing

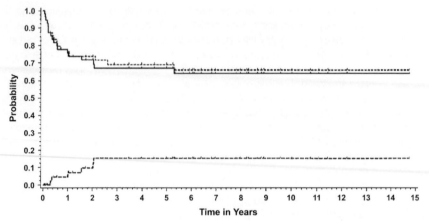

Fig. 1. Probability of event-free survival (EFS), overall survival (OS) and relapse for 55 adult patients with high-risk acute lymphoblastic leukemia transplanted in first remission. (*Modified from* Jamieson CH, Amylon MD, Wong RM, et al. Allogeneic hematopoietic cell transplantation for patients with high-risk acute lymphoblastic leukemia in first or second complete remission using fractionated total-body irradiation and high-dose etoposide: a 15-year experience. Exp Hematol. 2003;31:981–6.)

allogeneic transplant in first remission. **Table 3** shows a comparison of several other trials comparing chemotherapy to HCT. This trial has led to considerable debate about its meaning for patients with ALL, with some advocating early transplant for nearly all patients, whereas others have cautioned a continued individual assessment.

HCT FOR PH$^+$ ALL

Historically, the dismal outcome with chemotherapy has led to trials focusing on the use of allogeneic transplantation for treatment of adult Ph+ ALL. Most have been

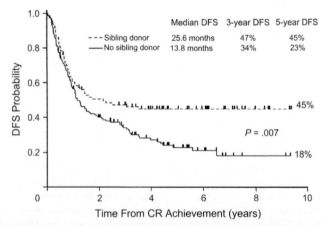

Fig. 2. DFS according to genetic randomization. The group with a sibling donor comprised 100 patients, whereas that with no sibling donor included 159 patients. CR, complete remission. (*Modified from* Thomas X, Boiron JM, Huguet F, et al. Outcome of treatment in adults with acute lymphoblastic leukemia: analysis of the LALA-94 trial. J Clin Oncol. 2004;22:4075–86; with permission.)

Table 2
MRC-ECOG UKALLXII/EC2993: outcome after allogeneic hematopoietic stem cell transplantation in Ph⁻ patients who had donors versus those who did not have donors

	No.	5-Y Overall Survival (%)	5-Y Relapse Rates (%)	2-Y Nonrelapse Mortality (%)
High risk[a]	401			
Donor	171	40	39	39
No donor	230	36	62	12
Standard risk	512			
Donor	218	63	27	20
No donor	294	51	50	7

[a] High risk is defined as age >35 years, WBC >30,000/μL for patients with B cell disease or WBC >100,000/μL for patients with T cell disease, or time to attain CR >4 weeks.

single institution studies using various regimens and the cure rate varies from 30% to 65%, dependent on age and remission status.[19,20] Investigators from City of Hope and Stanford University have analyzed their experience with 79 patients with Ph+ ALL transplanted from human leucocyte antigen (HLA)-identical siblings while in first CR between 1984 and 1997 to determine long-term survival and disease control.[21] All patients but one were conditioned with fractionated total body irradiation (FTBI) (1320 cGy) and high-dose etoposide (60 mg/kg). The 3-year probability of DFS and relapse was 55% and 18%, respectively, with the latest relapse at 27 months. Beyond first remission, HCT is curative in a much smaller minority of patients but remains the treatment of choice (**Fig. 3**).

Table 3
Comparison of several large trials for acute lymphoblastic leukemia CR1 patient outcome

Group Study, Citation	No. of Patients Considered for HCT	Outcome Measure	Chemotherapy (%)	Autologous HCT (%)	Allogeneic HCT (%)	P
MRC-ECOG	913	OS at 5 y	45		53	.02
JALSG-ALL93	142	OS at 6 y	40	–	46	NS
LALA-87	257	OS at 10 y	31		46	.04
LALA-87 high risk	156	OS at 10 y	11		44	.009
LALA-94	259	DFS at 3 y	34		47	.007
LALA-94 high risk	211	OS at 5 y	21	32	51 but median OS not reached	Not stated
GOELAMS 02 high risk	156	OS at 6 y	40 at 6 y		75 at 6 y	.0027
PETHEMA 93 high risk	183	OS at 5 y	49		40	.56

Abbreviations: OS, overall survival; NS, not significant.

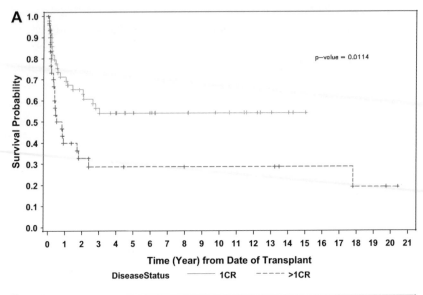

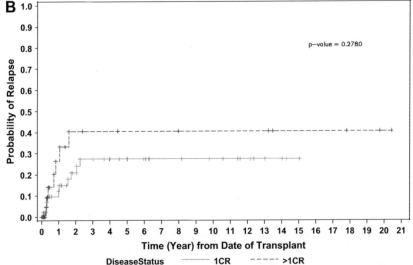

Fig. 3. (*A, B*) Probability of long-term DFS and risk of relapse in 79 patients with Ph+ ALL following allogeneic HCT in first remission and beyond first remission. (*Data from* Laport GG, Alvarnas JC, Palmer JM, et al. Long-term remission of Philadelphia chromosome-positive acute lymphoblastic leukemia after allogeneic hematopoietic cell transplantation from matched sibling donors: a 20-year experience with the fractionated total body irradiation-etoposide regimen. Blood 2008;112:903–9.)

The development of imatinib and other tyrosine kinase inhibitors for the treatment of BCR-ABL positive hematopoietic malignancy has changed the up front treatment strategy and also may affect the outcome after HCT. The feasibility of performing allogeneic HCT after first-line treatment with imatinib plus chemotherapy has been reported.[22] In this series, 29 adult patients who completed induction therapy were treated with allogeneic HCT and the investigators compared their results with 31 patients who had received transplantation in their unit before the availability of imatinib treatment. The data suggest that the risk of relapse was significantly less in the imatinib group (3.5% vs 47.3%) (*P* = .002), potentially reflecting a lower burden of residual disease at the time of HCT and allowing a higher percentage of patients to come to transplantation in a "good" first remission. The results also indicated superiority in DFS (76% vs 38%) (*P*<.001) without much difference in the transplant-related toxicities (**Fig. 4**). Thus, in the same way that imatinib may improve the up front success of induction therapy and potential long-term outcome of patients with Ph+ ALL, entering transplantation with a lower burden of disease may improve the cure rate for such patients. These observations are now the basis for a national trial to determine the outcome of either chemotherapy combined with dasatinib or allogeneic transplant followed by dasatinib. The schema for this trial is shown in **Fig. 5**.

Of additional interest is the follow-up of patients with Ph+ ALL and the impact of the detection of MRD after, rather than before allogeneic HCT. Radich and colleagues reviewed the results of 36 patients with Ph+ ALL who underwent allogeneic HCT and were monitored with sensitive assays of MRD.[23] Seventeen patients were transplanted in relapse and 19 were transplanted in remission. Twenty-three patients had at least one positive BCR-ABL polymerase chain reaction (PCR) assay after transplantation either before a relapse or without subsequent relapse. Ten of these 23 patients relapsed after a positive assay at a median time from first positive PCR assay of 94 days (range 28–416 days). By comparison, only two relapses occurred in the 13 patients with no prior positive PCR assays. The unadjusted relative risk (RR) of relapse associated with a positive PCR assay compared with a negative assay was 5.7. Recent studies have also demonstrated the feasibility of administering imatinib following allogeneic HCT for BCR-ABL positive hematologic malignancy; imatinib can be used either preemptively or to treat any MRD detected after transplant before relapse instead of using donor lymphocyte infusions.[24] This strategy may improve the outcome of high-risk patients with Ph+ ALL and facilitate improved long-term control of disease after HCT. The observation concerning the impact of pretransplant MRD

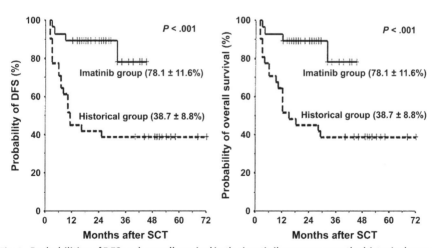

Fig. 4. Probabilities of DFS and overall survival in the imatinib group versus the historical group of patients with Ph+ ALL. Solid line indicates imatinib group: dotted line, historical group. (*From* Lee S, Kim YJ, Min CK, et al. The effect of first-line imatinib therapy on the outcome of allogeneic stem cell transplantation in adults with newly diagnosed Philadelphia chromosome-positive acute lymphoblastic leukemia. Blood 2005;105:3449–57; with permission.)

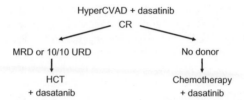

Fig. 5. Design of national trial to determine impact of Dasatinib on outcome after either allogeneic transplant or chemotherapy in adult patients with Ph+ ALL.

suggests that it may be desirable to use second- and third-generation BCR-ABL inhibitors to reduce disease burden before transplant.

RELAPSED OR PRIMARY REFRACTORY ACUTE LYMPHOBLASTIC LEUKEMIA

ALL is refractory to primary chemotherapy in approximately 10% to 15% of patients and allogeneic HCT can sometimes be successfully used to achieve both a remission and long-term control in approximately 20% of such patients. Of patients who do achieve a first CR to primary therapy, approximately 50% to 70% will relapse. Relapsed ALL in an adult is not curable with standard chemotherapy, but remissions are sometimes achieved with reinduction using either a standard vincristine, prednisone, and anthracycline regimen or a cytarabine-based regimen, particularly high-dose cytosine arabinoside (Ara-C) combined with an anthracycline or clofarabine,[25-27] especially in patients with a long first remission. Recent studies confirm that in the absence of HCT, adult patients with relapsed ALL have an extremely poor prognosis regardless of initial remission duration and that transplantation, when feasible, is the only possible curative therapy,[28] an observation confirmed in the MRC-ECOG trial.[29] This study indicated that the DFS after relapse was 7% and included all patients regardless of postrelapse treatment, including transplant.[29] Most patients are unable to achieve a second remission, especially if relapse occurs on treatment. Thus, the optimistic results reported for patients transplanted in second remission are admittedly selective as these are the minority of patients who actually achieve a remission, remain in good condition, and have a suitably matched donor. Available data from the Center for International Blood and Marrow Transplant Research (CIBMTR) show that patients transplanted with an HLA-identical sibling donor for ALL in second CR have approximately a 35% to 40% chance of long-term DFS, whereas those transplanted with disease not in remission have a DFS of only 10% to 20%. **Fig. 6** shows the overall DFS for patients with ALL, depending on their remission status, who underwent allogeneic HCT.[30] As noted earlier in all series, these data do not account for the many patients who suffer a relapse and do not undergo transplantation. Nevertheless, for an adult patient with ALL after a first relapse, allogeneic HCT is the only curative option.

UNRELATED HEMATOPOIETIC CELL TRANSPLANTATION FOR ACUTE LYMPHOBLASTIC LEUKEMIA

Historically, the outcome after transplantation from unrelated donors has been inferior to that observed after matched-sibling transplantation because of increased rates of graft rejection and graft versus host disease (GVHD) resulting from increased alloreactivity in this setting.[31] The National Marrow Donor program (NMDP) reports 5-year DFS of 35% in CR1 in adults and 46% in children, decreasing to 25% and 40%, respectively, in CR2. In the past few years, improved results have been reported from several

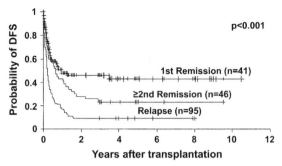

Fig. 6. Long-term survival in patients with ALL demonstrating the impact of remission status on the outcome of transplant. (*Data from* Laport GG, Alvarnas JC, Palmer JM, et al. Long-term remission of Philadelphia chromosome-positive acute lymphoblastic leukemia after allogeneic hematopoietic cell transplantation from matched sibling donors: a 20-year experience with the fractionated total body irradiation-etoposide regimen. Blood 2008;112:903-9.)

single-center studies, reflecting improvements in donor/recipient allele level molecular matching in both class I and II histocompatibility genes, GVHD prophylaxis, and supportive care.[32] An NMDP study showed younger donor and recipient age were associated with significantly improved outcomes. Recent reports suggest equivalent results for high-risk patients from either related or unrelated donors,[33–35] making this a reasonable option for a patient who needs an allogeneic HCT for treatment of their disease.

ROLE OF GRAFT VERSUS LEUKEMIA EFFECT IN PATIENTS WITH ACUTE LYMPHOBLASTIC LEUKEMIA

The low response rate in patients with ALL following donor lymphocyte infusion (DLI) has led to questions about the significance of the graft versus leukemia (GVL) effect in preventing relapse in this disease. The GVL effect is derived from observations of a higher relapse rate after autologous or syngeneic HCT compared with allogeneic HCT, lower incidence of relapse in patients who had GVHD, and increased relapse rates in recipients of T cell–depleted marrow grafts. The most compelling argument for a strong GVL effect in ALL comes from single institution and registry data.[36,37] These studies show consistent decrease in relapse rates in patients who develop GVHD compared with those patients who do not. **Table 4** shows the rate of relapse after HCT for ALL in first CR and the correlation with GVHD. The occurrence of acute, chronic or both forms of GVHD correlated with the best DFS. A study of 192 patients with ALL, most of whom were transplanted in second remission[32] evaluated the probability of relapse among patients without or with GVHD. Relapse was significantly higher in the group that had less than grade II GVHD. In patients without significant GVHD, the actuarial risk of relapse approached 80% versus 40% in those who developed grade II or higher. An evaluation of 1132 patients with T- or B-lineage ALL supports the observation that both acute and chronic GVHD are associated with a decreased risk of relapse in the major immunophenotypes of adult ALL.[38] Recent studies have also demonstrated the beneficial impact of chronic GVHD on reducing relapse in patients undergoing allogeneic HCT for ALL, including Ph+ ALL.[39,40]

Although the data support the importance of a GVL effect in mediating a clinically useful antileukemic response in patients with ALL, the reasons for the limited beneficial effect for patients with relapsed ALL treated with DLI are not clear. The different outcomes may reflect differences in the ability of ALL cells to present antigen targets,

Table 4
Relapse after transplantation for acute lymphoblastic leukemia in CR1

Group	Relapse Probability at 3 Years (%)
Allogeneic, non-T depleted	
No GVHD	44 ± 17
Acute only	17 ± 9
Chronic only	20 ± 19
Both	15 ± 10
Syngeneic	41 ± 32
Allogeneic, T-depleted	34 ± 13

Data from Ref.[37]

an inhibitory microenvironment, the low frequency of T cell precursors reactive with minor antigens presented by ALL cells, the susceptibility of ALL targets to lysis or kinetic differences in the way leukemic cells grow after HCT. Thus, cytoreduction with chemotherapy before infusion of DLI is likely a better strategy for treatment of patients with relapsed ALL. It is for these reasons that HCT after reduced intensity conditioning is of limited effectiveness in patients with ALL who are not in remission. Studies focused on developing antigen-specific T cell immunotherapy for ALL may help augment the GVL activity of donor T cells.[41–46]

REDUCED INTENSITY CONDITIONING FOR TREATMENT OF ACUTE LYMPHOBLASTIC LEUKEMIA

Although many studies have evaluated the role of allogeneic reduced intensity transplantation in patients with myeloid malignancies, multiple myeloma, and low-grade non-Hodgkin lymphoma, there have been fewer studies conducted on patients with ALL. In general, the consensus has been that for patients with ALL, high-dose chemoradiotherapy was required for an improved cure rate, but this approach is of limited use in patients over the age of 45 to 50 years. In addition, an evaluation of outcomes suggests that the graft versus tumor effect is more effective against myeloid malignancies such as acute myelocytic leukemia (AML) and chronic myelocytic leukemia (CML) and B cell malignancies of mature B cells such as low-grade non-Hodgkin lymphoma and multiple myeloma, but less so with a more undifferentiated B cell disease such as pre-B ALL, especially if not in remission.[47–49] Nevertheless, a few small studies have been reported that suggest that there may be a role for reduced intensity allogeneic transplant even in this disease, particularly in older patients, with 34% achieving long-term remission in a report from the European Group for Blood and Marrow Transplantation (EBMT).[47] A recent report of 24 patients with a median age of 47 years, who received an HCT at City of Hope using either related, unrelated, or cord blood donor and a fludarabine/melphalan regimen demonstrated a promising outcome. Of these 24 high-risk patients with poor prognostic features in first remission or undergoing transplant after achieving a second or subsequent remission, an overall and DFS rate of 61% was achieved with a relapse rate of 21%.[50] These results are consistent with reports from the EBMT that showed 52% DFS in patients transplanted in first remission.[51]

The results of the recent UK ALL XII ECOG 2993 study of adult ALL revealed significant transplant-related mortality resulting in no improvement in DFS despite better disease control in patients over the age of 35 years when compared with those receiving chemotherapy consolidation alone. Thus, there is increased interest in the development of clinical trials exploring these reduced intensity approaches in older patients with ALL in remission who would, except for age, be candidates for transplantation based on age, cytogenetics, MRD, and response to initial treatment. The poor outcome of older patients with ALL using either standard chemotherapy or transplant makes this an important consideration for treatment in those patients.

REGIMEN DEVELOPMENT FOR ALLOGENEIC HEMATOPOIETIC CELL TRANSPLANTATION FOR ACUTE LYMPHOBLASTIC LEUKEMIA

Historically, the most commonly used regimen for transplantation of patients with ALL is cyclophosphamide (CY) plus total body irradiation (TBI). Several other different preparative regimens have been developed, each based on substituting a different chemotherapeutic agent for CY in combination with TBI for patients with ALL. High-dose fractionated TBI in combination with high-dose Ara-C has been employed by several centers and, with the exception of a small series of pediatric patients at Case Western Reserve, there has been no significant improvement in DFS with this regimen in recipients of allogeneic HCT from sibling donors.[52,53]

Investigators at Johns Hopkins University approached the problem by conducting trials substituting busulfan (BU) for TBI to decrease the long-term side effects of TBI and to determine the efficacy of high-dose combined alkylating therapy in eliminating leukemic cells.[54,55] These nonradiation-dependent regimens, similar to those used in reduced intensity regimens, have shown activity in the treatment of advanced ALL, suggesting that TBI is not an absolute requirement for successful treatment of ALL by HCT. A retrospective analysis from the CIBMTR found that a conventional CY/TBI regimen was superior to a non–TBI-containing regimen of BU plus CY in children, with a 3-year survival of 55% versus 40% for BU/CY.[56] However, despite these differences in survival, the risk of relapse was similar. A recent study of busulfan, fludarabine and 400 cGy of TBI, which would be considered a high-dose regimen, showed a low transplant-related mortality of 3% and a projected DFS of 65%.[57]

The group at the City of Hope studied the substitution of etoposide (VP16) for CY in combination with fractionated TBI (13.2 Gy) followed by allogeneic HCT.[58] A phase 1 and 2 trial indicated that a VP16 dose of 60 mg/kg is the maximum tolerated dose when combined with a TBI dose of 1320 rad. In that study, 36 patients with ALL were treated, 20 of whom were in relapse. The actual DFS was 57% with a 32% relapse rate, suggesting that the regimen had significant activity in patients with advanced ALL, a result confirmed in a subsequent trial from the Southwest Oncology Group.[59] A subsequent study from City of Hope/Stanford showed a 64% DFS for adult patients undergoing transplantation with this regimen in first CR (see section on Allogeneic transplant for ALL in first remission). The recently completed UK ALL XII/ECOG 2993 Trial, a comparative study of chemotherapy, autologous, and allogeneic HCT, used this regimen for patients in first CR.

A comparative analysis of TBI combined with either cyclophosphamide or etoposide chemotherapy was conducted to determine the relative efficacy of the chemotherapy component in the transplant regimen.[60] The outcomes of 298 patients with ALL in CR1 or CR2 receiving HLA-matched sibling allografts after CY-TBI conditioning were compared with 204 patients receiving etoposide and TBI. In this analysis, 4 groups were compared based on the radiation dose: CY-TBI <13 Gy (n = 217), CY-TBI >13 Gy (n = 81), etoposide-TBI <13 Gy (n = 53), and etoposide-TBI >13 Gy (n = 151). Analyses of relapse, leukemia-free survival (LFS), and overall survival were performed separately for CR1 and CR2 patients. Transplant-related mortality did not differ by conditioning regimen. In CR1, there were also no significant differences in relapse, LFS, or survival by conditioning regimen. In CR2, the outcomes differed among conditioning groups. In comparison with CY-TBI <13 Gy, the risks of relapse, treatment failure (inverse of LFS), and mortality tended to be lower with etoposide (regardless of TBI dose) or with TBI doses >13 Gy. For both CR1 and CR2 patients, causes of death were similar among the groups; disease recurrence accounted for 47% of deaths. These data indicate that for HLA-identical sibling allografts for patients with ALL in CR2, there is an advantage in substituting etoposide for CY or, when CY is used, in increasing the TBI dose to >13 Gy (**Figs. 7** and **8**).

Radioimmunotherapy-Based Transplant Regimens for Acute Lymphoblastic Leukemia

Studies on AML have shown lower relapse rates with higher doses of TBI suggesting that methods that can selectively deliver radiation to sites of leukemia without increasing systemic toxicity might be of benefit to the patient. The use of tumor-reactive monoclonal antibodies (MABs) conjugated with local-acting radionucleotides such as iodine-131 (^{131}I) or yttrium-90 (^{90}Y) are being explored to accomplish the goal of decreased relapse. Initial studies conducted in Seattle on an animal model showed the feasibility of this novel approach, and subsequent phase 1 and 2 studies in patients have been initiated. These studies have demonstrated that initial targeting of marrow and other sites of leukemia could be accomplished using ^{131}I-conjugated MABs. The most recent studies have focused on a MAB reactive with CD45, an antigen that is found on leukemic cells and normal hematopoietic tissue and, unlike CD33, does not internalize after antibody binding. A phase 1 trial of ^{131}I anti-CD45 MAB plus CY and TBI for advanced leukemia was completed.[61] This study focused on the biodistribution and toxicity of escalating doses of targeted radiation combined with 120 mg/kg CY and 12 Gy TBI followed by matched related or autologous HCT. Among 44 patients, 5 had ALL in relapse or refractory disease and 5 were in second or third CR of ALL. Eighty-four percent of the patients had a favorable biodistribution of antibody with a higher estimated radiation absorbed dose to marrow and spleen than in normal tissues. Thirty-four patients received a therapeutic dose of ^{131}I labeled with 76 to 612 mg ^{131}I designed to deliver an estimated radiation absorbed dose to liver of 3.5 to 12.25 Gy. In the group of nine patients treated for ALL, six of whom underwent allogeneic and three autologous HCT, two died of infection, four relapsed and three survived 10, 45 and 57 months after transplantation. This study demonstrated that ^{131}I anti-CD45 antibody can deliver appreciable supplemental doses of radiation to the marrow (approximately 24 Gy) and spleen when combined with conventional fractionated TBI. Estimation of the ultimate benefit to DFS and improved safety of the regimen requires larger phase 2 studies in patients with ALL undergoing transplantation either in remission or in relapse.

Given the efficacy of radiation-based regimens and a dose-response effect of radiation on leukemia, newer approaches to the delivery of radiation to the marrow are also being evaluated to increase the safety and the dose of radiation. Helical tomotherapy, used to focus and intensify local radiation treatment, can be used to treat the major marrow containing bones and offers a potential means to augment the dose of radiation to the marrow without increasing toxicity to other organs. This approach is now being combined with chemotherapy and evaluated in phase 1/2 trials.[62]

MANAGEMENT OF RELAPSE AFTER ALLOGENEIC TRANSPLANT FOR ACUTE LYMPHOBLASTIC LEUKEMIA

Once patients with ALL relapse after HCT, the prognosis is very poor. Similar to the approach in patients with AML and CML, manipulation of the antitumor effect

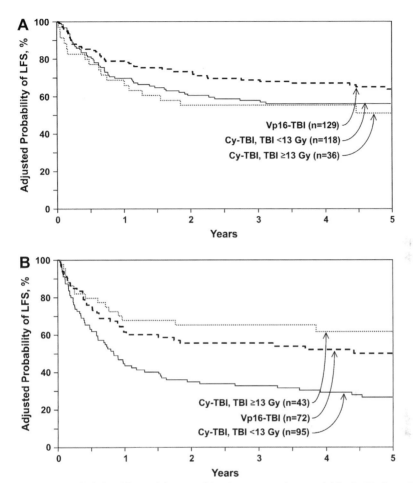

Fig. 7. Adjusted probability (derived from multivariate regression models) of LFS after HLA-identical sibling transplantations for ALL in first (*A*) or second (*B*) complete remission, according to the pretransplantation conditioning regimen (pointwise *P* value at 5 years for CR1 patients: etoposide-TBI versus Cy-TBI <13 Gy, *P* = .21; etoposide-TBI versus Cy-TBI ≥13 Gy, *P* = .17; Cy-TBI <13 Gy versus Cy-TBI ≥13 Gy, *P* = .59; pointwise *P* value at 5 years for CR2 patients: etoposide-TBI versus Cy-TBI <13 Gy, *P* = .002; etoposide-TBI versus Cy-TBI ≥13 Gy, *P* = .23; Cy-TBI <13 Gy versus Cy-TBI ≥13 Gy, *P* < .001). Vp16 indicates etoposide. (*From* Marks DI, Forman SJ, Blume KG, et al. A comparison of cyclophosphamide and total body irradiation with etoposide and total body irradiation as conditioning regimens for patients undergoing sibling allografting for acute lymphoblastic leukemia in first or second complete remission. Biol Blood Marrow Transplant 2006;12:438–53.)

mediated by the donor graft is often employed as a treatment strategy. Unfortunately, in patients with ALL, this therapy has not been as effective as it has been for patients with CML. A report from 25 North American bone marrow transplant programs of 140 patients who received DLI showed that the CR rate was 60% in CML with the responses being higher in patients with cytogenetic and chronic phase relapse compared with those with accelerated phase or blastic phase (75%, 33% and 16%, respectively).[63] The CR rates in relapsed AML and ALL are 15% and 18%, respectively, similar to the blastic phase of CML. In that study, the development of acute

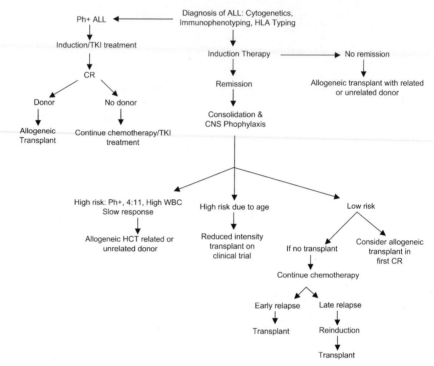

Treatment Algorithm for Adult Patients with ALL

Fig. 8. Suggested treatment and transplant algorithm for adult patients with ALL.

and chronic GVHD following DLI was highly correlated with disease response. In a report from Europe, 40 patients with ALL received DLI as treatment of relapse and of 29 evaluable patients, only 1 achieved CR.[64] Therefore, DLI as a sole therapy seems to have low potential for contributing to a remission and long-term control of disease in patients with relapsed ALL and, if considered, should be a component of a chemotherapy-based treatment program. For those patients with Ph+ ALL, imatinib or dasatinib, either alone or with chemotherapy, is effective in helping some patients achieve another remission, although the duration of the remission is often quite short and DLI should be performed before another relapse occurs.[65]

AUTOLOGOUS HEMATOPOIETIC CELL TRANSPLANTATION FOR ADULT ACUTE LYMPHOBLASTIC LEUKEMIA

There is much less experience with autologous transplantation for ALL and studies have been focused primarily on those patients in either first or second remission who lacked a sibling or unrelated allogeneic donor. Some studies have used the same criteria for autologous transplantation as has been used for allogeneic transplantation based on the idea that the preparative regimen does contribute to the cure of ALL because the allogeneic effect is less potent than in myeloid malignancies. Several groups have reported outcomes for large series of adults with ALL undergoing autologous HCT in first remission.[10,66–68] One study from France reported on 233 such patients with long-term DFS at 41%.[10] The most important prognostic factor was the interval between achieving CR and proceeding to transplant, with those patients being transplanted later having the better DFS. This effect may represent the drop out of high-risk patients who relapse before transplantation or possibly the effect of consolidation therapy in reducing tumor burden administered before HCT. The European Cooperative Group/MRC report on more than 1000 patients indicated a LFS of 36%, whereas the CIBMTR reported a similar plateau at 40%.[66] A long-term outcome analysis from NMDP/CIBMTR suggested equivalent results for autologous or unrelated donor transplants in first or second remission.[69]

One randomized trial evaluated outcomes of adults with ALL in first remission treated with chemotherapy versus autologous transplantation. The French LALA-87 trial allocated patients less than 40 years old with HLA-matched siblings to allogeneic transplantation; the remaining patients received consolidation treatment with modest dose chemotherapy or an autologous transplant.[8] There was a significant drop out rate in the autologous arm caused by early relapse and the long-term follow-up showed no significant difference in overall survival between the two groups, 34% for autologous HCT and 29% for chemotherapy. This difference applied to the standard- and high-risk groups. The ECOG/MRC trial, comparing allogeneic transplant, autologous transplant or chemotherapy in all adult patients with ALL in first remission showed an inferior result for autologous transplantation versus continued chemotherapy,[18] thus further limiting interest in this approach, except possibly as a platform for the study of novel approaches to treat residual disease such as adoptive immunotherapy for central memory T cells genetically modified to recognize antigens on leukemic blasts.[45]

CELL SOURCES FOR HEMATOPOIETIC CELL TRANSPLANTATION

As is true for most patients undergoing allogeneic transplantation, peripheral blood has replaced bone marrow as the hematopoietic cell graft preference. A report from the EBMT presents a retrospective analysis in which the comparison outcome was made for 858 patients, 513 who were in first remission given marrow versus 345 patients who were given blood.[70] Engraftment, as noted in many studies, was faster with peripheral blood but also resulted in an increased risk of chronic GVHD. LFS and overall survival did not differ. In a subsequent retrospective analysis, peripheral blood hematopoietic cells obtained from an unrelated donor were associated with an inferior outcome compared with bone marrow.[71] The incidence of 2-year treatment-related mortality (TRM) in 36 patients receiving blood was 61% compared with 47% in 66 recipients of bone marrow grafts. This resulted in a significantly different 2 year LFS of 32% versus 21% and overall survival of 34% versus 24% ($P = .04$). It appeared that younger patients had significantly lower TRM, but the relapse rates did not differ, indicating a probable similar antileukemic efficacy.

UMBILICAL CORD TRANSPLANTATION

There is considerable interest in exploring the potential of umbilical cord transplant, but there are few data on patients with ALL. In a single institution trial, the comparison was made between hematopoietic cells derived from umbilical cord transplant versus an unrelated donor following high-dose conditioning, which resulted in comparable outcomes.[72] In this study, there were only 16 adult patients with ALL and the diagnosis of ALL predicted a high risk for relapse. A recent report from the University of Minnesota evaluated reduced intensity transplant followed by cord blood transplant in a group of 22 patients and showed both the feasibility of this cell source and good survival (50%) at 3 years after transplant.[73]

TREATMENT STRATEGY FOR ACUTE LYMPHOBLASTIC LEUKEMIA

As discussed in this article, analysis of molecular genetic and clinical data treatment responses and changes in the approach to treatment have resulted in more refined recommendations on the timing of transplantation for the treatment of patients with ALL. Despite the MRC-ECOG results, most studies indicate that allogeneic transplantation in patients with high-risk disease in first remission provides a better chance of DFS. For patients who are younger than 50 years without other high-risk features, better control of disease can be achieved by early allogeneic transplantation, as reported in the MRC-ECOG trial, but this has not had a convincing impact on physicians' decisions and advice for patients with ALL. This is further complicated by the difficulty of achieving a second remission. For patients who relapse, transplantation is the only treatment with the potential for cure, especially if a second remission can be achieved. Therefore, it is important to perform HLA typing at the time of diagnosis to determine what the transplant possibilities might be either from related donors or through the unrelated donor registries, especially for patients with high-risk features such as high WBC count, older age, slow rate of achieving remission, or failure to achieve a remission. In addition, this information would be useful in planning for treatment in patients who suffer a relapse after achieving a remission. Clearly, identification of the Philadelphia chromosome early after diagnosis gives patients an additional beneficial therapeutic option with the inclusion of tyrosine kinase inhibitors as part of the induction, consolidation, and maintenance regimen. Trials are ongoing that will compare the outcome of this modern approach to ALL along with a more modern approach to ALL following transplantation. **Fig. 8** provides a suggested practical algorithm for the use of transplant in patients with ALL. MRD evaluations at certain time points after treatment could refine this strategy significantly by transplanting patients who truly are at risk before overt relapse.[74]

FUTURE CONSIDERATIONS

For many years, there were few, if any, innovations in the treatment of ALL in the adult, especially in the development of new agents. However, over the last few years, several agents, including monoclonal antibodies to CD20, CD52, and CD22, and new drugs for T cell ALL such as nelarabine and imatinib, dasatinib, and nilotinib for the treatment of Ph+ ALL may improve the treatment outcome for patients with ALL, and trials are being developed to include these agents and use MRD evaluation to assess their impact as an early end point.

The most important contribution may come from studies defining which patients are most likely to benefit from transplantation early in the course of their disease. Thus, the monitoring of MRD may have a predictive value for relapse, as a reflection of sensitivity to chemotherapy. This would be an important development for all patients. Those patients, even those with higher risk disease, who achieve a CR with lack of detection of MRD, may be spared the risk of transplantation, whereas other lower risk patients who have not achieved an adequate depth of remission would be better served by early transplantation, even if there were no overt high-risk features at the time of diagnosis. Thus, introduction of MRD monitoring over the course of treatment might provide a new strategy for how to advise patients about the timing of transplantation. This represents an unmet need for all adult patients with ALL.

In addition, transplantation regimens will be developed to address the needs of patients with high-risk disease that could include radioimmunotherapy targeted to the CD45 antigen. Studies are also being conducted to determine the efficacy of using antigen-specific T cells to augment a graft versus tumor effect. These cells can be derived from normal donors and could be transduced to recognize the CD19 antigen present in nearly all patients with pre-B ALL. Given the results of chemotherapy treatment of older patients with ALL, studies of reduced intensity conditioning should be pursued for such patients to explore the potential therapeutic role of GVL in this high-risk patient population.

REFERENCES

1. Rowe JM, Buck G, Burnett AK, et al. Induction therapy for adults with acute lymphoblastic leukemia: results of more than 1500 patients from the international ALL trial: MRC UKALL XII/ECOG E2993. Blood 2005;106:3760–7.
2. Larson RA, Dodge RK, Burns CP, et al. A five—drug remission induction regimen with intensive consolidation for adults with acute lymphoblastic leukemia: Cancer and Leukemia Group B study 8811. Blood 1995;85:2025–37.
3. Hoelzer D, Thiel H, Loffler H, et al. Prognostic factors in a multicenter study for treatment of acute lymhoblastic leukemia in adults. Blood 1988;71:123–31.
4. Rovera G, Wasserman R, Yamada M. Detection of minimal residual disease in childhood leukemia with the polymerase reaction. N Engl J Med 1991;324:774–81.
5. Cave H, van der Werff ten Bosch J, Suciu S, et al. Clinical significance of minimal residual disease in childhood acute lymphoblastic leukemia. N Engl J Med 1998; 339:591–8.
6. Mortuza FY, Papaioannou M, Moreira IM, et al. Minimal residual disease tests provide an independent predictor of clinical outcome in adult acute lymphoblastic leukemia. J Clin Oncol 2002;20:1094–104.
7. Bruggemann M, Raff T, Flohr T, et al. Clinical significance of minimal residual disease quantification in adult patients with standard-risk acute lymphoblastic leukemia. Blood 2006;107:1116–23.
8. Thomas X, Boiron JM, Huguet F, et al. Outcome of treatment in adults with acute lymphoblastic leukemia: analysis of the LALA-94 trial. J Clin Oncol 2004;22: 4075–86.
9. Rowe JM, Buck G, Burnett AK, et al. Induction therapy for adults with acute lymphoblastic leukemia: results of more than 1500 patients from the international ALL trial: MRC UKALL XII/ECOG E2993. Curr Oncol Rep 2006;8:413–4.
10. Attal M, Blaise D, Marit G, et al. Consolidation treatment of adult acute lymphoblastic leukemia: a prospective, randomized trial comparing allogeneic versus autologous bone marrow transplantation and testing the impact of recombinant interleukin-2 after autologous bone marrow transplantation. Blood 1995;86: 1619–28.
11. Doney K, Fisher LD, Appelbaum FR, et al. Treatment of adult acute lymphoblastic leukemia with allogeneic bone marrow transplantation: multivariate analysis of factors affecting acute graft-versus-host disease, relapse, and relapse-free survival. Bone Marrow Transplant 1991;7:453–9.
12. Blume KG, Forman SJ, Snyder DS, et al. Allogeneic bone marrow transplantation for acute lymphoblastic leukemia during first complete remission. Transplantation 1987;43:389–92.
13. Vernant JP, Marit G, Maraninchi D, et al. Allogeneic bone marrow transplantation in adults with acute lymphoblastic leukemia in first complete remission. J Clin Oncol 1988;6:227–31.
14. Chao NJ, Forman SJ, Schmidt GM, et al. Allogeneic bone marrow transplantation for high-risk acute lymphoblastic leukemia during first complete remission. Blood 1991;78:1923–7.

15. Sebban C, Lepage E, Vernant JP, et al. Allogeneic bone marrow transplantation in adult acute lymphoblastic leukemia in first complete remission: a comparative study. J Clin Oncol 1994;12:2580–7.

16. Vey N, Blaise D, Stoppa AM, et al. Bone marrow transplantation in 63 adult patients with acute lymphoblastic leukemia in first complete remission. Bone Marrow Transplant 1994;14:383–8.

17. Jamieson CH, Amylon MD, Wong RM, et al. Allogeneic hematopoietic cell transplantation for patients with high-risk acute lymphoblastic leukemia in first or second complete remission using fractionated total-body irradiation and high-dose etoposide: a 15-year experience. Exp Hematol 2003;31:981–6.

18. Goldstone AH, Richards SM, Lazarus HM, et al. In adults with standard-risk acute lymphoblastic leukemia, the greatest benefit is achieved from a matched sibling allogeneic transplantation in first complete remission, and an autologous transplantation is less effective than conventional consolidation/maintenance chemotherapy in all patients: final results of the international ALL trial (MRC UKALL XII/ECOG E2993). Blood 2008;111:1827–33.

19. Snyder DS. Allogeneic stem cell transplantation for Philadelphia chromosome-positive acute lymphoblastic leukemia. Biol Blood Marrow Transplant 2000;6: 597–603.

20. Dombret H, Gabert J, Boiron JM, et al. Outcome of treatment in adults with Philadelphia chromosome-positive acute lymphoblastic leukemia – results of the prospective multicenter LALA-94 trial. Blood 2002;100:2357–66.

21. Laport GG, Alvarnas JC, Palmer JM, et al. Long-term remission of Philadelphia chromosome-positive acute lymphoblastic leukemia after allogeneic hematopoietic cell transplantation from matched sibling donors: a 20-year experience with the fractionated total body irradiation-etoposide regimen. Blood 2008;112: 903–9.

22. Lee S, Kim YJ, Min CK, et al. The effect of first-line imatinib therapy on the outcome of allogeneic stem cell transplantation in adults with newly diagnosed Philadelphia chromosome-positive acute lymphoblastic leukemia. Blood 2005; 105:3449–57.

23. Radich J, Gehly G, Lee A, et al. Detection of bcr-abl transcripts in Philadelphia chromosome-positive acute lymphoblastic leukemia after marrow transplantation. Blood 1997;89:2602–9.

24. Carpenter PA, Snyder DS, Flowers ME, et al. Prophylactic administration of imatinib after hematopoietic cell transplantation for high-risk Philadelphia chromosome-positive leukemia. Blood 2007;109:2791–3.

25. Hiddemann W, Kreutzmann H, Straif K, et al. High-dose cytosine arabinoside in combination with mitoxantrone for the treatment of refractory acute myeloid leukemia and lymphoblastic leukemia. Semin Oncol 1987;14:73–7.

26. Cohen MH, Johnson JR, Massie T, et al. Approval summary: Nelarabine for the treatment of T-cell lymphoblastic leukemia/lymphoma. Clin Cancer Res. 2006; 12:5329–35.

27. Specchia G, Pastore D, Carluccio P, et al. FLAG-IDA in the treatment of refractory/relapsed adult acute lymphoblastic leukemia. Ann Hematol 2005;84:792–5.

28. Tavernier E, Boiron JM, Huguet F, et al. Outcome of treatment after first relapse in adults with acute lymphoblastic leukemia initially treated by the LALA-94 trial. Leukemia 2007;21:1907–14.

29. Fielding AK, Richards SM, Chopra R, et al. Outcome of 609 adults after relapse of acute lymphoblastic leukemia (ALL); an MRC UKALL12/ECOG 2993 study. Blood 2007;109:944–50.

30. Doney K, Hägglund H, Leisenring W, et al. Predictive factors for outcome of allogeneic hematopoietic cell transplantation for adult acute lymphoblastic leukemia. Biol Blood Marrow Transplant 2003;9:472–81.
31. Bachanova V, Weisdorf D. Unrelated donor allogeneic transplantation for adult acute lymphoblastic leukemia: a review. Bone Marrow Transplant 2008;41(5): 455–64.
32. Cornelissen JJ, Carston M, Kollman C, et al. Unrelated marrow transplantation for adult patients with poor-risk acute lymphoblastic leukemia: strong graft-versus-leukemia effect and risk factors determining outcome. Blood 2001;97: 1572–7.
33. Chim CS, Lie AK, Liang R, et al. Long-term results of allogeneic bone marrow transplantation for 108 adult patients with acute lymphoblastic leukemia: favorable outcome with BMT at first remission and HLA-matched unrelated donor. Bone Marrow Transplant 2007;40:339–47.
34. Dahlke J, Kroger N, Zabelina T, et al. Comparable results in patients with acute lymphoblastic leukemia after related and unrelated stem cell transplantation. Bone Marrow Transplant 2006;37:155–63.
35. Kiehl MG, Kraut L, Schwerdtfeger R, et al. Outcome of allogeneic hematopoietic stem-cell transplantation in adult patients with acute lymphoblastic leukemia: no difference in related compared with unrelated transplant in first complete remission. J Clin Oncol 2004;22:2816–25.
36. Horowitz MM, Gale RP, Sondel PM, et al. Graft-versus-leukemia reactions after bone marrow transplantation. Blood 1990;75:555–62.
37. Appelbaum FR. Graft versus leukemia (GVL) in the therapy of acute lymphoblastic leukemia (ALL). Leukemia 1997;11:S15–7.
38. Passweg JR, Tiberghien P, Cahn JY, et al. Graft-versus-leukemia effects in T lineage and B lineage acute lymphoblastic leukemia. Bone Marrow Transplant 1998;21:153–8.
39. Espérou H, Boiron JM, Cayuela JM, et al. A potential graft-versus-leukemia effect after allogeneic hematopoietic stem cell transplantation for patients with Philadelphia chromosome-positive acute lymphoblastic leukemia: results from the French Bone Marrow Transplantation Society. Bone Marrow Transplant 2003;31:909–18.
40. Lee S, Cho BS, Kim SY, et al. Allogeneic stem cell transplantation in first complete remission enhances graft-versus-leukemia effect in adults with acute lymphoblastic leukemia: antileukemic activity of chronic graft-versus-host disease. Biol Blood Marrow Transplant 2007;13:1083–94.
41. Appelbaum FR. Hematopoietic cell transplantation as immunotherapy. Nature 2001;411:385–9.
42. Mutis T, Verdijk R, Schrama E, et al. Feasibility of immunotherapy of relapsed leukemia with *ex vivo*-generated cytotoxic T lymphocytes specific for hematopoietic system-restricted minor histocompatibility antigens. Blood 1999;94:4374–6.
43. Warren EH, Greenberg PD, Riddell SR. Cytotoxic T-lymphocyte-defined human minor histocompatibility antigens with a restricted tissue distribution. Blood 1998;91:2197–207.
44. Tran CA, Burton L, Russom D, et al. Manufacturing of large numbers of patient-specific T cells for adoptive immunotherapy: an approach to improving product safety, composition, and production capacity. J Immunother 2007;30:644–54.
45. Berger C, Jensen MC, Lansdorp PM, et al. Adoptive transfer of effector CD +8 T cells derived from central memory cells establishes persistent T cell memory in primates. J Clin Invest 2008;118:294–305.

46. Cooper LJ, Topp MS, Serrano LM, et al. T-cell clones can be rendered specific for CD19: toward the selective augmentation of the graft-versus-B-lineage leukemia effect. Blood 2003;101:1637–44.

47. Valcarcel D, Martino R, Sureda A, et al. Conventional versus reduced-intensity conditioning regimen for allogeneic stem cell transplantation in patients with hematological malignancies. Eur J Haematol 2005;74:144–51.

48. Arnold R, Massenkeil G, Bornhäuser M, et al. Nonmyeloablative stem cell transplantation in adults with high-risk ALL may be effective in early but not in advanced disease. Leukemia 2002;16:2423–8.

49. Gutierrez-Aguirre CH, Gomez-Almaguer D, Cantu-Rodriguez OG, et al. Non-myeloablative stem cell transplantation in patients with relapsed acute lymphoblastic leukemia: results of a multicenter study. Bone Marrow Transplant 2007;40(6): 535–9.

50. Stein A, O'Donnell M, Snyder D, et al. Reduced-intensity stem cell transplantation for high-risk acute lymphoblastic leukemia, Submitted for publication.

51. Mohty M, Labopin M, Tabrizzi R, et al. Reduced intensity conditioning allogeneic stem cell transplantation for adult patients with acute lymphoblastic leukemia: a retrospective study from the European Group for Blood and Marrow Transplantation. Haematologica 2008;93:303–6.

52. Coccia PF, Strandjord SE, Warkentin PI, et al. High-dose cytosine arabinoside and fractionated total-body irradiation: an improved preparative regimen for bone marrow transplantation of children with acute lymphoblastic leukemia in remission. Blood 1988;71:888–93.

53. Champlin R, Jacobs A, Gale RP, et al. High-dose cytarabine in consolidation chemotherapy or with bone marrow transplantation for patients with acute leukemia: preliminary results. Semin Oncol 1985;12:190–5.

54. Santos GW, Tutschka PJ, Brookmeyer R, et al. Marrow transplantation for acute nonlymphocytic leukemia after treatment with busulfan and cyclophosphamide. N Engl J Med 1983;309:1347–53.

55. Tutschka PJ, Copelan EA, Klein JP. Bone marrow transplantation for leukemia following a new busulfan and cyclophosphamide regimen. Blood 1987;70: 1382–8.

56. Davies SM, Ramsay NKC, Klein JP, et al. Comparison of preparative regimens in transplants for children with acute lymphoblastic leukemia. J Clin Oncol 2000;18: 340–7.

57. Russell JA, Savoie ML, Balogh A, et al. Allogeneic transplantation for adult acute leukemia in first and second remission with a novel regimen incorporating daily intravenous busulfan, fludarabine, 400 CGY total-body irradiation and thymoglobulin. Biol Blood Marrow Transplant 2007;13:814–21.

58. Blume KG, Forman SJ, O'Donnell MR, et al. Total body irradiation and high-dose etoposide: a new preparatory regimen for bone marrow transplantation in patients with advanced hematologic malignancies. Blood 1987;69: 1015–20.

59. Blume KG, Kopecky KJ, Henslee-Downey JP, et al. A prospective randomized comparison of total body irradiation-etoposide versus busulfan cyclophosphamide as preparatory regimens for bone marrow transplantation in patients with leukemia who were not in first remission: a South-West Oncology Group study. Blood 1993;81:2187–93.

60. Marks DI, Forman SJ, Blume KG, et al. A comparison of cyclophosphamide and total body irradiation with etoposide and total body irradiation as conditioning regimens for patients undergoing sibling allografting for acute lymphoblastic

leukemia in first or second complete remission. Biol Blood Marrow Transplant 2006;12:438–53.

61. Matthews DC, Appelbaum FR, Eary JF, et al. Phase I study of ^{131}I-anti-CD45 antibody plus cyclophosphamide and total body irradiation for advanced acute leukemia and myelodysplastic syndrome. Blood 1999;94:1237–47.

62. Wong JY, Liu A, Schultheiss T, et al. Targeted total marrow irradiation using three-dimensional image-guided tomographic intensity-modulated radiation therapy: an alternative to standard total body irradiation. Biol Blood Marrow Transplant 2006;12:306–15.

63. Collins RH, Shpilberg O, Drobyski WR, et al. Donor leukocyte infusions in 140 patients with relapsed malignancy after allogeneic bone marrow transplantation. J Clin Oncol 1997;15:433–44.

64. Kolb HJ, Schattenberg A, Goldman JM, et al. Graft-versus-leukemia effect of donor lymphocyte transfusions in marrow grafted patients. European Group for Blood and Marrow Transplantation Working Party Chronic Leukemia. Blood 1995;86:2041–50.

65. Wassman B, Pfeifer H, Scheuring U, et al. Therapy with imatinib mesylate (Glivec) preceding allogeneic stem cell transplantation (SCT) in relapsed or refractory Philadelphia-positive acute lymphoblastic leukemia (Ph+ ALL). Leukemia 2002; 16:2358–65.

66. Gorin NC. Autologous stem cell transplantation in acute lymphocytic leukemia. Stem Cells 2002;20:3–10.

67. Fiere D, Lepage E, Sebban C, et al. Adult acute lymphoblastic leukemia: a multicentric randomized trial testing bone marrow transplantation as postremission therapy. J Clin Oncol 1993;11:1990–2001.

68. Willemze R, Labar B. Post-remission treatment for adult patients with acute lymphoblastic leukemia in first remission: is there a role for autologous stem cell transplantation? Seminar Hematol 2007;44:267–73.

69. Bishop MR, Logan BR, Gandham S, et al. Long-term outcomes of adults with acute lymphoblastic leukemia after autologous or unrelated donor bone marrow transplantation: a comparative analysis by the National Marrow Donor Program and Center for International Blood and Marrow Transplant Research. Bone Marrow Transplant 2008;41(7):635–42.

70. Ringdén O, Labopin M, Bacigalupo A, et al. Transplantation of peripheral blood stem cells as compared with bone marrow from HLA-identical siblings in adult patients with acute myeloid leukemia and acute lymphoblastic leukemia. J Clin Oncol 2002;20:4655–64.

71. Garderet L, Labopin M, Gorin NC, et al. Patients with acute lymphoblastic leukaemia allografted with a matched unrelated donor may have a lower survival with a peripheral blood stem cell graft compared to bone marrow. Bone Marrow Transplant 2003;31:23–9.

72. Ooi J, Iseki T, Takahashi S, et al. A clinical comparison of unrelated cord blood transplantation and unrelated bone marrow transplantation for adult patients with acute leukaemia in complete remission. Br J Haematol 2002;118:140–3.

73. Bachanova V, Verneris MR, DeFor T, et al. Prolonged survival in adults with acute lymphoblastic leukemia after reduced-intensity conditioning with cord blood or sibling donor transplantation. Blood 2009;113:2902–5.

74. Forman SJ. Hematopoietic cell transplantation for acute lymphoblastic leukemia in adults. In: Appelbaum FR, Forman SJ, Negrin RS, Blume KG, editors. Thomas' hematopoietic cell transplantation. 4th edition. Chichester, West Sussex, UK: Wiley-Blackwell; 2008. p. 791–805.

Acute Lymphoblastic Leukemia in Adolescents and Young Adults

Josep-Maria Ribera, MD, PhD*, Albert Oriol, MD

KEYWORDS

- Acute lymphoblastic • Leukemia • Adolescents
- Young adults • Treatment

The development of effective therapy for children with acute lymphoblastic leukemia (ALL) is one of the greatest successes of clinical oncology, with long-term survival achieved in more than 80% of children 1 to 10 years old.[1,2] However, cure rates for adults with ALL remain relatively low, at only 40% to 50%.[3,4] Age is a continuous prognostic variable in ALL, with no single age at which prognosis deteriorates markedly. Within childhood ALL populations, older children have shown inferior outcomes, whereas younger adults have shown superior outcomes among adult ALL patients. The type of treatment (pediatric-based versus adult-based) for adolescents and young adults (AYA) has recently been a matter of debate. In this article the biology and treatment of ALL in AYA is reviewed.

CLINICAL AND BIOLOGIC CHARACTERISTICS IN ADOLESCENTS AND YOUNG ADULTS

The incidence of ALL decreases with age, ranging from 9 to 10 cases/100,000 persons per year in childhood (representing 30% of all cancers) to 1 to 2 cases/100,000 persons per year in adults. In adolescents the incidence is 3 cases/100,000 persons per year, and represents 6% of all cancers at that age.[5] Differences between adolescents and other age categories include disease biology and host factors.

Several clinical and biologic characteristics of ALL are age dependent. In this sense, T-ALL is more frequent in AYA (25%) than in children (10%–15%) or in older adults.[6] However, the most important differences lie in cytogenetic and molecular characteristics. Regarding structural changes, the most outstanding feature is the progressive

This work was supported in part by grants RD06/0020/1056 from RETICS, PI051490 from Fondo de Investigaciones Sanitarias, and FIJC P/EF-08 from Jose Carreras Leukemia Foundation.
Clinical Hematology Department, Institut Català d'Oncologia, Hospital Universitari Germans Trias i Pujol, Badalona, Universitat Autonoma de Barcelona, C/Canyet s/n, 08916 Badalona, Spain
* Corresponding author.
E-mail address: jribera@iconcologia.net (J-M. Ribera)

Hematol Oncol Clin N Am 23 (2009) 1033–1042
doi:10.1016/j.hoc.2009.07.002
0889-8588/09/$ – see front matter © 2009 Elsevier Inc. All rights reserved.

increase in the frequency of t(9;22) (q34;q11) or *BCR-ABL* fusion gene, the frequency of which ranges from less than 3% in children under 18 years to 6% at ages 18 to 25 and to 15% to 20% at ages 25 to 35 years.[7] Another rearrangement with decreasing frequency with age is *TEL-AML1*,[8] which has been associated with a good treatment outcome with current pediatric regimens. Intrachromosomal amplification of chromosome 21 (iAMP21), previously known as amplification of *RUNX1*, is especially frequent in older children and adolescents with a common/pre-B immunophenotype. The reason for the poor prognosis of this subgroup of patients is unknown.[9] On the other hand, B-cell precursor ALL with rearrangements involving the immunoglobulin heavy chain (*IGH*) locus is a newly defined patient subgroup with a high number of partner genes interacting with the *IGH* locus, and typically involves older children and young adults, although the prognosis seems to be good.[9] On the contrary, translocation t(1;19) is the only rearrangement that occurs in most age groups at approximately the same rate. Regarding the numerical abnormalities, it is of note that the frequency of high hyperdiploidy (>50 chromosomes) also decreases with age (25%–30% in children vs 20% in adolescents and less than 10% in young adults), whereas there are no differences in the frequency of hypodiploid ALL. Finally, ALL in AYA comprises the largest group with unspecified chromosomal abnormalities, indicating the potential for the discovery of novel rearrangements.[9] In summary, with increasing age there is a progressive increase in the frequency of subsets of ALL patients with genetic abnormalities associated with poor prognosis, and these changes have already become evident in AYA patients. In addition to the phenotypic and cytogenetic differences, several studies have also reported differences in ALL cell sensitivity to corticosteroids and chemotherapy in vitro.

Regarding host factors, several may contribute to worse outcomes for older patients with ALL. These factors include differences in the metabolism of chemotherapeutic agents, depleted marrow reserve, and increased extramedullary toxicity. All these issues increase the frequency of life-threatening infections, organ failure, and treatment delays and dose reductions in planned chemotherapy.[10]

PEDIATRIC-BASED VERSUS ADULT-BASED TREATMENTS
Retrospective Studies

Several retrospective reports have shown that adolescents (15–20 years) and AYA treated by adult oncologists or hematologists with adult ALL protocols have poorer outcomes than similarly aged patients treated by pediatricians with pediatric protocols, despite having the same biologic disease.[11–18] The cutoff point of age for treatment of patients in pediatric or adult hemato-oncology units varies among different countries, but usually ranges between 15 and 18 years for the lower age group and up to 25 years for the upper age group.

The first study in which such different outcomes were reported was performed in France.[12] A comparison of AYA aged 15 to 20 years treated with the pediatric-based protocol FRALLE-93 (n = 77) with patients of the same age and comparable clinical and biologic characteristics of ALL who received the adult-based protocol LALA-94 (n = 100) showed a complete remission (CR) rate of 94% versus 83%. After a median follow-up of 3.5 years, the event-free survival (EFS) probabilities were 67% versus 41% at 5 years. Multivariate analysis showed an independent influence of the protocol on the outcome. The differences in the drugs employed, and especially in the dose intensity, could explain the better results of the FRALLE-93 protocol. In this protocol the cumulated dose of prednisone was five-fold higher, the vinca alkaloids 3-fold higher, and the asparaginase 20-fold higher than in the LALA-94 study. In addition, in the FRALLE-93 study asparaginase was initiated during induction, whereas in the LALA-94 trial it was administered only during early consolidation. Moreover, the time interval between CR and postremission therapy was 2 days in FRALL-93 versus 7 days in the LALA-94 study.

The North American Cancer and Acute Leukemia Group B (CALGB) and the Children's Cancer Group (CCG) performed a retrospective comparison of presenting features, planned treatment, CR rate, and outcome of 321 AYA aged 16 to 20 years who were treated in consecutive trials in either the CCG or the CALGB from 1988 to 2001.[11] CR rates were identical, being 90% for both the CALGB and CCG AYA. The CCG AYA had a 63% EFS and 67% overall survival (OS) at 7 years in contrast to the CALGB AYA, in which the 7-year EFS was only 34% and the OS was 46%. Whereas the CALGB AYA aged 16 to 17 years achieved similar outcomes to all the CCG AYA with a 7-year EFS of 55%, the EFS for 18- to 20-year-old CALGB patients was only 29%. Comparison of the regimens showed that the CCG AYA received earlier and more intensive central nervous system prophylaxis and higher cumulative doses of non-myelosuppressive agents. There were no differences in outcomes in those who reached maintenance therapy on time compared with those who were delayed.

A similar Dutch study in patients aged 15 to 21 years yielded similar results,[13] with a 5-year EFS of 69% for comparable patients treated with the more dose-intensive pediatric protocol DCOG versus 34% for those treated with adult protocols ALL-5 and ALL-18 from the HOVON group. Likewise, comparative retrospective studies from Italy also showed a poorer prognosis for patients aged 14 to 18 years treated with adult-type protocols.[14] In turn, a Swedish study compared patients aged 10 to 40 years treated with the pediatric trial NOPHO-92 (n = 144) versus a similar group of patients included in the Swedish Adult ALL group (n = 99).[15] A significantly higher CR rate (99% versus 90%) and EFS were observed in patients treated with the pediatric protocol, the type of treatment being an independent prognostic variable on multivariate analysis. However, it is of note that adults aged 26 to 40 years had a significantly poorer prognosis than AYA (15 to 25 years). Another study from Denmark yielded similar results.[16] In a retrospective study from the British Medical Research Council (MRC) performed only in adolescents (15 to 17 years) included in the ALL97/revised99 (pediatric, n = 61) or UKALLXII/E2993 (adult, n = 67) trials between 1997 and 2002,[17] the EFS (65% versus 49%) was higher and the rate of death in remission was lower in the former group of patients. Other studies from different countries[18] have shown similar results (**Table 1**).

Only one population-based study from Finland showed that the outcome of AYA with ALL treated with pediatric or adult protocols was comparable.[19] One hundred and twenty-eight patients (10 to 16 years) were treated with the pediatric Nordic (NOPHO) protocols and 97 patients (17 to 25 years) with Finnish Leukemia Group National protocols. All patients were centrally referred and treated in five academic centers. The 5-year EFS was 67% for the pediatric treatment group and 60% for the adult treatment group. There were no significant differences in the cumulative doses of corticosteroids, vincristine, and asparaginase between pediatric and adult protocols, whereas pediatric protocols used a higher cumulative dose of methotrexate and lower doses of anthracyclines than adult protocols. Epipodophyllotoxins and mitoxantrone were not included in the pediatric protocols. The investigators attributed the similar results to the similarity of the pediatric and adult protocols and to the centralized care of the patients in five academic centers, ensuring good compliance and adherence to the protocols even though two distinct age groups were evaluated.

In summary, the 5- to 6-year EFS rate for AYA treated with pediatric regimens ranges from 65% to 70% versus 35% to 50% for adult regimens in almost all

Table 1
Retrospective comparative studies in adolescents and young adults with acute lymphoblastic leukemia treated with pediatric-based versus adult-based protocols

Country	Protocol	Age	N	CR (%)	EFS (%)
USA[11]	CCG(P)	16–20	197	90	63
	CALGB(A)		124	90	34
France[12]	FRALLE93(P)	15–20	77	94	67
	LALA94 (A)		100	83	41
Netherlands[13]	DCOG (P)	15–18	47	98	69
	HOVON (A)		44	91	34
Italy[14]	AIEOP (P)	14–18	150	94	80
	GIMEMA (A)		95	89	71
Sweden[15]	NOPHO-92(P)	10–40	144	99	65
	Adult (A)		99	90	48
UK[17]	ALL97 (P)	15–17	61	98	65
	UKALLXII(A)		67	94	49
Mexico[18]	LALIN (P)	15–25	20	90	70
	LALA (A)		20	80	40
Finland[19]	NOPHO (P)	10–25	128	96	67
	ALL (A)		97	97	60

Abbreviations: A, adult based; CR, complete remission; EFS, event-free survival; N, number of patients; P, pediatric-based.

retrospective comparative studies. However, it is of note that these studies have focused on patients aged 15 to 21 years, but few have evaluated the results in young adults up to 30 years or older, in which the frequency of patients with adverse prognostic factors is progressively increasing.

The reasons for the better results of pediatric protocols are multiple.[20–23] The first and probably the most important reason is the dose intensity and the dose density of the nonmyelosuppressive chemotherapeutic agents, which are the mainstay of most pediatric protocols. This mainstay is especially relevant for drugs such as vincristine (usually capped to 2 mg in adult protocols), glucocorticoids, asparaginase, and methotrexate. In contrast, pediatric-based protocols include lower doses of alkylating agents, high-dose cytarabine, and anthracyclines than adult trials. The second reason is the model of protocol design. Most of the pediatric protocols include delayed intensifications and an extended maintenance chemotherapy phase, the former being omitted in many adult trials. In addition, the use of allogeneic stem cell transplantation (SCT) as part of first-line therapy (associated with a transplant-related mortality [TRM] of 20%), is restricted to patients with very high-risk features in pediatric trials,[24] whereas it is more widely used in adult trials, even in standard-risk patients in first CR.[25] The third reason is the tolerability to essential drugs such as asparaginase, steroids, and vincristine, which is poorer in AYA compared with children. The incidence of chemotherapy-related complications: diabetes mellitus, pancreatitis, and osteonecrosis are also more frequent in the former group, although in fact the differences in toxicity between these two subgroups are not very important. On the other hand, the adherence to treatment is usually higher in pediatric-derived than in adult-derived studies, probably due both to a better tolerability of pediatric protocols and a stricter control of time points of chemotherapy delivery in pediatric than in adult hematology units. The effect of other features such as team experience, supportive care, or patterns of referral is more difficult to assess.[26] However, in the United States and Canada most children and adolescents with ALL treated with pediatric protocols are managed in institutions and academic centers participating in national-sponsored clinical trials, whereas most AYA treated with adult protocols are managed throughout study groups by community-based medical oncologists. Kantarjian and O'Brien[27] recently have pointed out that the insurance policies in the United States may explain part of the outcome differences in AYA with ALL treated in adult versus pediatric regimens, suggesting that AYA included in adult regimens are more likely to be emancipated and therefore not covered by their parents' insurance. Their potentially poor insurance coverage could explain the higher dropout rates observed during consolidation and maintenance in adult trials in the United States.

United States adult and pediatric cooperative groups are embarking on a prospective trial to address some of these questions in a unified manner. Newly diagnosed patients 16 to 30 years old are being enrolled in an intergroup study (CALGB and Children's Oncology Group [COG]) in which the ability to administer safely and in a timely manner the same therapy used by the COG study for adolescents and high-risk children will be examined.[23]

Prospective Studies

Ongoing or fully published prospective studies that examined the outcome of AYA patients are shown in **Table 2**. Barry and colleagues[28] reported the outcome of adolescents treated in the Dana Farber Cancer Institute (DFCI) ALL Consortium Protocols conducted between 1991 and 2000. A total of 844 patients aged 1 to 18 years with newly diagnosed ALL were enrolled into two consecutive DFCI-ALL Consortium Protocols. Outcomes were compared in three age groups: children aged 1 to 10 years (n = 685), young adolescents aged 10 to 15 years (n = 108), and older adolescents aged 15 to 18 years (n = 51). With a median follow-up of 6.5 years, the 5-year EFS for those aged 1 to 10 years was 85%, compared with 77% for those aged 10 to 15 years and 78% for those aged 15 to 18 years. There was no difference in the rate of treatment-related complications between the 10- to 15-year and 15- to 18-year age groups. This 5-year EFS of 78% is superior to published outcomes for similarly aged patients treated with other pediatric and adult ALL regimens.

Some studies have evaluated or are currently evaluating the feasibility and results of the pediatric-based protocols administered to adults up to 30 or even up to 50 or 60 years. The Spanish PETHEMA group compared the results of the pediatric protocol ALL96 in adolescents (15–18 years, n = 35) and young adults (18–30 years, n = 46)

Table 2
Prospective studies in adolescents and young adults with acute lymphoblastic leukemia treated with pediatric-based or inspired protocols

Country	Protocol	Age	N	CR (%)	EFS (%)
USA[28]	DFCI 91-01, 95-01	15–18[a]	51[a]	94	78
Spain[29]	PETHEMA ALL-96	15–18	35	94	60
		19–30	46	100	63
France[30]	GRAALL-2003	15–45	172	95	58
USA[31]	DFCI	18–50	74	82	72.5[b]
Canada[32]	Modified DFCI	17–71	68	85	65[c]

[a] Results restricted to adolescents.
[b] Estimated at 2 years.
[c] Overall survival.

with standard-risk (SR) ALL.[29] Both groups were comparable for the main clinical and biologic characteristics of ALL. The CR rate was 98% and after a median follow-up of 4.2 years, 6-year EFS and OS were 61% and 69%, with no differences between AYA. No significant differences were observed in the timing of treatment delivery, although the hematologic toxicity in consolidation and reinforcement cycles was higher in young adults than in adolescents. These results suggest that pediatric protocols can be effectively and safely employed in adult patients with SR ALL, at least up to the age of 30 years.

The French GRAALL group has recently reported the results of the pediatric-inspired GRAALL-2003 study including 215 patients aged 15 to 60 years.[30] In this study there was an 8.6-fold, 3.7-fold, and 16-fold increase in cumulative doses of prednisone, vincristine, and asparaginase, respectively, compared with the previous adult-based LALA-94 protocol, although the GRAALL-2003 trial retained some adult options, such as allogeneic SCT for patients with high-risk ALL. The CR rate was 93.5%, and at 42 months the EFS and OS rates were 55% and 60%, respectively. The CR rate, EFS, and OS compared favorably with the previous LALA-94 experience. It is of note, however, that in patients over 45 years there was a higher cumulative incidence of chemotherapy-related deaths (23% vs 5%) and deaths in first CR (22% vs 5%), although the incidence of relapse remained stable (30 vs 32%). The results of this study suggest that pediatric-based therapy is feasible in young adults with ALL at least until the age of 45 years, in whom the outcome clearly improves.

Based on the promising results obtained in adolescents with ALL, the DFCI Combined Adult/Pediatric ALL Consortium has applied a pediatric protocol for adults aged 18 to 50 years.[31] Specifically, the investigators used an extended course of asparaginase for 30 weeks. The preliminary results in 74 patients have shown a CR rate of 82% with promising 2-year EFS and OS probabilities of 72.5% and 73.2%, respectively. This study proved that extended asparaginase treatment was feasible in adults and the drug-related toxicity was manageable, although the incidence of pancreatitis (13%) and thrombosis/embolism (19%) was a matter of concern. In turn, the Princess Margaret Hospital used a modified DFCI pediatric protocol in 68 adult patients (17–71 years), with a CR rate of 85%, and 3-year OS and disease-free survival (DFS) of 65% and 77%, respectively.[32] Finally, the University of South California group[33] used an augmented Berlin-Frankfurt-Muenster (BFM) pediatric regimen with 8 doses of pegylated asparaginase to treat adults with ALL aged 19 to 57 years (median 33), with a 3-year projected EFS of 65%. Toxicity attributable to asparaginase was frequent but manageable. However, patients older than 30 years appeared to have more asparaginase, vincristine, and steroid-related complications compared with children or adolescents.

The results from these prospective studies demonstrate the feasibility and tolerability of pediatric-based regimens in AYA with SR ALL, and the survival benefit may extend to patients from age 30 to 50 years. If these results can be confirmed with longer follow-up, they will have an impact on the clinical management of AYA patients in the future. In addition, the use of less toxic formulations of several major drugs such as pegylated asparaginase may further increase the adherence, and result in further improvements in treatment outcome [34-36] of AYA patients.

ROLE OF HEMATOPOIETIC STEM CELL TRANSPLANTATION IN ACUTE LYMPHOBLASTIC LEUKEMIA IN ADOLESCENTS AND YOUNG ADULTS

In children and adolescents, allogeneic SCT in first CR is only performed in cases with very high-risk ALL features.[37,38] In 2003 the German BFM Study Group initiated a prospective, international, multicenter trial on allogeneic SCT in children and adolescents with high-risk ALL. In this ongoing trial the main goals are the harmonization and standardization of the SCT procedure, and to answer the question as to whether SCT from an HLA-genoidentical sibling donor is equivalent to SCT from a matched unrelated donor. One-year TRM has been low (5%) in both groups of patients, and the results in adolescents with high-risk ALL are pending. In adult-based protocols, the practice of allogeneic SCT to all patients in first CR is still a matter of debate. The MRC UKALL XII/ECOG E2993 trial has shown superior results of allogeneic SCT over chemotherapy or autologous SCT in adults with SR ALL (5-year OS 62% vs 52%; $P = .02$).[25] This result has raised the question as to whether allogeneic SCT should be performed in young adults with SR ALL. In this sense, two aspects should be taken into account. First, the chemotherapy schedule of the MRC/ECOG trial was not pediatric based, and the results of current pediatric-based chemotherapy schedules are clearly superior to those of the chemotherapy arm reported in the MRC/ECOG trial. It is of note that the results of pediatric trials from the DFCI ALL Consortium[28] and from other groups have demonstrated that the outcome of adolescents has improved, with a 5-year EFS as high as 78%, being similar to that of older children. Second, in the SCT setting, age older than 14 years significantly correlates with higher TRM and lower DFS, especially for unrelated donor SCT. At present the decision to perform an allogeneic SCT in AYA with ALL in first CR remains open, and prospective comparative studies of SCT versus modern trials of pediatric-based chemotherapy are needed to clarify this issue. However, given the improved results of modern pediatric-based protocols in AYA, such studies are unlikely to be performed.

In addition to pediatric-based therapy, some variables must currently be taken into account for decision making. Among these variables minimal residual disease (MRD) is currently one of the most relevant prognostic factors in childhood ALL,[39] and some prospective data suggest that the detection of high levels of MRD at the time of CR, or the persistence of MRD after consolidation chemotherapy in adults with SR ALL, may predict increased risk of disease recurrence.[40–42] Sequential measurements of MRD in AYA treated with pediatric-based schedules will probably provide great help in selecting the minority of patients who should be treated with high-risk ALL approaches, including allogeneic SCT in first CR.

WHERE SHOULD ADOLESCENTS WITH ACUTE LYMPHOBLASTIC LEUKEMIA BE TREATED?

Until recently, outcomes for AYA patients had not improved significantly. One of the potential explanations for this has been the fragmentation of care between pediatric and adult hematologists. The paucity of prospective trials to examine differences in treatment outcomes of AYA enrolled on pediatric versus adult protocols have led to the hope that uniform treatment trials administered by pediatric and adult hematologists could improve the ability to recruit as many patients as possible, and would promote progress in the research on the treatment of ALL in AYA.[10,23] Redefining age limits according to risk-based strategies, as well as encouraging multicenter cooperation and minimizing competing protocols, should be taken into consideration to improve the outcome of this age category. These patients should ideally be treated in adolescent-specific hematology/oncology units, but these units are not numerous except in the United Kingdom.[43] A more feasible approach, perhaps, is the creation of research treatment teams with experience in the management of AYA ALL who collaborate to develop cooperative studies, ideally at an international level. The DFCI Combined Adult/Pediatric ALL Consortium and the aforementioned prospective trial comprising United States adult (CALGB, SWOG, ECOG) and pediatric (COG) cooperative groups constitute interesting initiatives directed to that goal. In addition to the chemotherapy schedules, psychosocial issues have major relevance and may actually contribute to optimal adherence to protocol, emotional support, and better outcomes. Improving psychosocial support during therapy, preventing treatment-related sequelae, and increasing the knowledge and practice of healthy lifestyle habits represent further challenges, especially for teams involved in the treatment of adolescents.[10] Finally, molecular, genomic, and proteomic evaluation of patients included in these studies will shed further light on the causes of the decrease in survival seen as the patients progress from childhood to adolescence and young adulthood.

REFERENCES

1. Pui CH, Robison LL, Look AT. Acute lymphoblastic leukaemia. Lancet 2008; 371(9617):1030–43.
2. Pulte D, Gondos A, Brenner H. Trends in 5-and 10-year survival after diagnosis with childhood hematologic malignancies in the United States 1990–2004. J Natl Cancer Inst 2008;100(18):1271–3.
3. Gokbuget N, Hoelzer D. Treatment of adult acute lymphoblastic leukemia. Semin Hematol 2009;46(1):64–75.
4. Larson R, Stock W. Progress in the treatment of adults with acute lymphoblastic leukemia. Curr Opin Hematol 2008;15(4):400–7.
5. Ries LAL, Melbert D, Krapcho M, et al. Cancer statistics review, 1975–2005, National Cancer Institute. Bethesda, MD, http://seer.cancer.gov/csr/1975_2005/. Accessed 2008.
6. Pullen J, Shuster JJ, Link M, et al. Significance of commonly used prognostic factors differs for children with T cell acute lymphocytic leukemia (ALL), as compared to those with B-precursor ALL. A Pediatric Oncology Group (POG) study. Leukemia 1999;13(11):1696–707.
7. Secker-Walker LM, Craig JM, Hawkins JM, et al. Philadelphia positive acute lymphoblastic leukemia in adults: age distribution, BCR breakpoint and prognostic significance. Leukemia 1991;5(3):196–9.
8. Aguiar RC, Sohal J, van Rhee F, et al. TEL-AML1 fusion in acute lymphoblastic leukaemia of adults. M.R.C. Adult Leukaemia Working Party. Br J Haematol 1996;95(4):673–7.
9. Harrison CJ. Cytogenentics in paediatric and adolescents acute lymphoblastic leukaemia. Br J Haematol 2009;144(2):147–56.
10. Dini G, Banov L, Dini S. Were should adolescents with ALL be treated? Bone Marrow Transplant 2008;42(Suppl 2):S35–9.
11. Stock W, La M, Sanford B, et al. What determines the outcomes for adolescents and young adults with acute lymphoblastic leukemia treated on cooperative protocols? A comparison of Children's Cancer Group and Cancer and Leukemia Group B studies. Blood 2008;112(5):1646–74.
12. Boissel N, Auclerc M-F, Lheritier V, et al. Should adolescents with acute lymphoblastic leukemia be treated as old children or young adults? Comparison of the French FRALLE-93 and LALA-94 trials. J Clin Oncol 2003;21(5):774–80.
13. de Bont JM, van der Holt B, Dekker AW, et al. Significant difference in outcome for adolescents with acute lymphoblastic leukemia treated on pediatric vs adult protocols in the Netherlands. Leukemia 2004;18(12):2032–5.
14. Testi AM, Valsecchi MG, Conter V, et al. Difference in outcome of adolescents with acute lymphoblastic leukemia (ALL) enrolled in pediatric (AIEOP) and adult (GIMEMA) protocols [abstract]. Blood 2004;104:1954.

15. Hallbook H, Gustafsson G, Smedmyr B, et al, Swedish Adult Acute Lymphocytic Leukemia Group, Swedish Childhood Leukemia Group. Treatment outcome in young adults and children >10 years of age with acute lymphoblastic leukemia in Sweden: a comparison between a pediatric protocol and an adult protocol. Cancer 2006;107(7):1551–61.
16. Schroder H, Kjeldahl M, Boesen AM, et al. Acute lymphoblastic leukemia in adolescents between 10 and 19 years of age in Denmark. Dan Med Bull 2006; 53(1):76–9.
17. Ramanujachar R, Richards S, Hann I, et al. Adolescents with acute lymphoblastic leukaemia: outcome on UK national paediatric (ALL97) and adult (UKALLXII/ E2993) trials. Pediatr Blood Cancer 2007;48(6):254–61.
18. Lopez-Hernandez MA, Alvarado-Ibarra M, Jiménez-Alvarado RM, et al. Adolescents with de novo acute lymphoblastic leukemia: efficacy and safety of a pediatric vs. adult treatment protocol. Gac Med Mex 2008;144(6):485–9.
19. Usvasalo A, Räty R, Knuutila S, et al. Acute lymphoblastic leukemia in adolescents and young adults in Finland. Haematologica 2008;93(8):1161–8.
20. Schiffer CA. Differences in outcome in adolescents with acute lymphoblastic leukemia: a consequence of better regimens? Better doctors? Both? J Clin Oncol 2003;21(5):760–1.
21. Sallan SE. Myths and lessons from the adult/pediatric interface in acute lymphoblastic leukemia. Hematology Am Soc Hematol Educ Program 2006;128–32.
22. Webb DKH. Management of adolescents with acute lymphoblastic leukemia: implications for adult therapy. Hematology Education. The Education Programme for the 13th Congress of the European Hematology Association 2008;2:71–5.
23. Seibel N. Treatment of acute lymphoblastic leukemia in children and adolescents: peaks and pitfalls. Hematology Am Soc Hematol Educ Program 2008;374–80.
24. Peters C, Schrander A, Schrappe M, et al. Allogeneic hematopoietic stem cell transplantation in children with acute lymphoblastic leukemia: the BFM/IBF-MEBMT concepts. Bone Marrow Transplant 2005;35(Suppl 1):S9–11.
25. Goldstone AH, Richards SM, Lazarus HM, et al. In adults with standard-risk acute lymphoblastic leukemia, the greatest benefit is achieved from a matched sibling allogeneic transplantation in first complete remission, and an autologous transplantation is less effective than conventional consolidation/maintenance chemotherapy in all patients: final results of the International ALL Trial (MRC UKALL XII/ECOG E2993). Blood 2008;111(4):1827–33.
26. Burke ME, Albriton K, Marina N. Challenges in the recruitment of adolescents and young adults to cancer clinical trials. Cancer 2007;110(11):2385–93.
27. Kantarjian HM, O'Brien S. Insurance policies in the United States may explain part of the outcome differences of adolescents and young adults with acute lymphoblastic leukemia treated on adult versus pediatric regimens [letter]. Blood 2009;113(8):1861.
28. Barry E, DeAngelo DJ, Neuberg D, et al. Favorable outcome for adolescents with acute lymphoblastic leukemia treated on Dana Farber Cancer Institute ALL Consortium protocols. J Clin Oncol 2007;25(7):813–9.
29. Ribera JM, Oriol A, Sanz MA, et al. Comparison of the results of the treatment of adolescents and young adults with standard-risk acute lymphoblastic leukemia with the pediatric-based protocol PETHEMA ALL-96. J Clin Oncol 2008;26(11):1843–9.
30. Huguet F, Raffoux E, Thomas X, et al. Pediatric inspired therapy in adults with Philadelphia chromosome-negative acute lymphoblastic leukemia: the GRAALL/2003 study. J Clin Oncol 2009;27(1):911–8.

31. DeAngelo DJ, Silverman LB, Couban S, et al. A multicenter phase II study using a dose intensified pediatric regimen in adults with untreated acute lymphoblastic leukaemia [abstract]. Blood 2006;108:526.

32. Storring JM, Brandwein J, Gupta V, et al. Treatment of adult acute lymphoblastic leukaemia (ALL) with a modified DFCI pediatric regimen. The Princess Margaret experience [abstract]. Blood 2006;108:316.

33. Srivastava P, Watkins K, Mark L, et al. Treatment of adults with newly diagnosed acute lymphoblastic leukemia with multiple doses of intravenous pegylated asparaginase in an intensified pediatric regimen [abstract]. Haematologica 2008;93(s1):366.

34. Appel IM, Kazemier KM, Boos J, et al. Pharmacokinetic, pharmacodynamic and intracellular effects of PEG-asparaginase in newly diagnosed childhood acute lymphoblastic leukemia: results from a single agent window study. Leukemia 2008;22(9):1665–79.

35. Wetzler M, Sanford BL, Kurtzberg J, et al. Effective asparagine depletion with pegylated asparaginase results in improved outcomes in adult acute lympho-blastic leukemia: Cancer and Leukemia Group B Study. Blood 2007;109(10): 4164–7.

36. Zeidan A, Wang ES, Wetzler M. Pegasparaginase: where do we stand? Expert Opin Biol Ther 2009;9(1):111–9.

37. Balduzzi A, Valsecchi MG, Uderzo C, et al. Chemotherapy versus allogeneic transplantation for very-high-risk childhood acute lymphoblastic leukaemia in first complete remission: comparison by genetic randomisation in an international prospective study. Lancet 2005;366(9486):635–42.

38. Ribera JM, Ortega JJ, Oriol A, et al. Comparison of intensive chemotherapy, allo-geneic, or autologous stem-cell transplantation as postremission treatment for children with very high risk acute lymphoblastic leukemia: PETHEMA ALL-93 Trial. Clin Oncol 2007;25(1):16–24.

39. Campana D. Minimal residual disease in acute lymphoblastic leukemia. Semin Hematol 2009;46(1):100–6.

40. Raff T, Gokbuget N, Luschen S, et al. Molecular relapse in adult standard-risk ALL patients detected by prospective MRD monitoring during and after maintenance treatment: data from the GMALL 06/99 and 07/03 trials. Blood 2007;109(3): 910–5.

41. Bruggemann M, Raff T, Flohr T, et al. Clinical significance of minimal residual disease quantification in adult patients with standard-risk acute lymphoblastic leukaemia. Blood 2006;107(3):116–23.

42. Bassan R, Spinelli O, Oldani E, et al. Improved risk classification for risk-specific therapy based on the molecular study of MRD in adult ALL. Blood 2009;113(18): 4153–62.

43. Reynolds BC, Windebank KP, Leonard RC, et al. A comparison of self-reported satisfaction between adolescents treated in a 'teenage' unit with those treated in adult or paediatric units. Pediatr Blood Cancer 2005;44(3):259–63.

Philadelphia Chromosome-Positive Acute Lymphoblastic Leukemia

Farhad Ravandi, MD[a],*, Partow Kebriaei, MD[b]

KEYWORDS

- Acute lymphoblastic leukemia • Philadelphia chromosome
- BCR-ABL • Tyrosine kinase inhibition
- Allogeneic stem cell transplant

BIOLOGY

The Philadelphia (Ph) chromosome, a short chromosome 22, results from the reciprocal translocation between chromosomes 9 and 22 that fuses the breakpoint cluster region (BCR) gene on chromosome 22 to the Ableson (ABL) gene on chromosome 9.[1,2] The protein product of the fusion gene, BCR-ABL, has enhanced tyrosine kinase activity leading to the constitutive activation of several downstream pro-proliferative and pro-survival signaling pathways, and hence to leukemogenesis.[3] The Ph chromosome is the most frequent cytogenetic abnormality in adult patients with acute lymphoblastic leukemia (ALL), occurring in approximately 20% to 30% of adults but only in about 5% of children with this disease.[4] The incidence rises with age, and it occurs in approximately 50% of patients older than 50 years.[5]

Depending on the location of the breakpoint within the BCR gene, two major varieties of the oncogenic protein of differing sizes have been recognized. The smaller P190[bcr-abl] protein is found in over two-thirds of patients with Ph+ ALL and the larger p210[bcr-abl] protein, which is typical of chronic myeloid leukemia (CML) but is also encountered in about one-third of Ph+ ALL patients.[6] In experimental models, the p190[bcr-abl] protein has a higher tyrosine kinase activity and is more efficient in stimulating the growth of lymphoid cells.[6,7] However, using traditional chemotherapy regimens, clinical outcomes in patients carrying either of the two proteins have been generally similar.[6,8]

[a] Department of Leukemia, The University of Texas M D Anderson Cancer Center, 1515 Holcombe Boulevard, Unit 428, Houston, TX 77030, USA
[b] Department of Stem Cell Transplantation and Cellular Therapy, The University of Texas M D Anderson Cancer Center, 1515 Holcombe Boulevard, Unit 428, Houston, TX 77030, USA
* Corresponding author.
E-mail address: fravandi@mdanderson.org (F. Ravandi).

Hematol Oncol Clin N Am 23 (2009) 1043–1063
doi:10.1016/j.hoc.2009.07.007
0889-8588/09/$ – see front matter © 2009 Elsevier Inc. All rights reserved.
hemonc.theclinics.com

TREATMENT OF ADULTS AND CHILDREN WITH PH+ ACUTE LYMPHOBLASTIC LEUKEMIA
Historical Perspectives

Before the introduction of imatinib, the outcome of patients with Ph+ ALL was poor. Although complete remission (CR) could be achieved in the majority of patients (60%–90%), the median CR duration was considerably shorter than that seen in patients with Ph-negative disease, leading to very few long-term survivors (**Table 1**). This discrepancy was to some degree age dependent, with better survival reported in children with Ph+ ALL, particularly for those with a good initial response to glucocorticoid therapy.[9,10] On the other end of the age spectrum, specifically those older than 50 to 60 years, the outcome was particularly dismal with high treatment-related mortality, low CR rates, and short disease-free survival (DFS) and overall survival (OS).[5,11,12]

The relatively uniform dismal prognosis in adult patients with Ph+ ALL using conventional chemotherapy regimens meant that few predictors of outcome had been identified. However, it is notable that even with such suboptimal regimens, the degree of reduction of *BCR-ABL* transcripts after induction and consolidation was found to be a powerful predictor of disease response and survival.[13] This finding may indicate the potential role for monitoring *BCR-ABL* transcript levels when using regimens containing tyrosine kinase inhibitors (TKIs).

Allogeneic stem cell transplantation (allo SCT) in first CR from a suitable donor has been the standard strategy in adult Ph+ ALL patients, given their poor outcome with chemotherapy alone. Several recent reports have better defined the feasibility and outcome of this strategy in the pre-imatinib era. The introduction of imatinib and other TKIs has improved the likelihood of identifying a donor, as these agents provide durable responses in patients thereby allowing for the conduct of the appropriate donor searches.

Management of patients with relapse after prior chemotherapy or transplant has been even more challenging, with the main focus to induce a second CR and proceed with allo SCT.[14] Second-generation TKIs are becoming particularly useful in this setting, as they have produced second CRs even in this group of patients with generally dire prognosis.

Table 1
Selected chemotherapy trials in Ph+ ALL

Study	Ph+, N (%)	CR%	Median EFS/CRD (Months)	Median OS (Months)
Bloomfield et al[100]	29 (17)	46	7	11
Gotz et al[101]	25	76	NA	8
Larsen et al[102]	30 (27)	70	7	11
GFCH[103]	127 (29)	59	5	NA
Secker-Walker et al[104]	40 (11)	83	13	11
Wetzler et al[105]	67 (29)	79	11	16
Faderl et al[106]	67 (13)	55, 90[a]	8, 10.8[a]	11.3, 16.5[a]
Dombret et al[31]	154	67	–	19% at 3 years[b]
Arico et al[9]	326	82	28% at 5 years[b]	40% at 5 years[b]
Schrappe et al[10]	61 (1)	75	38% at 5 years[b]	49% at 5 years[b]

Abbreviations: GFCH, Groupe Francais de Cytogenetique Hematologique; CR, complete remission; EFS, event-free survival; CRD, complete remission duration; OS, overall survival.
[a] Results for the VAD and hyper-CVAD regimens quoted, respectively.
[b] Estimated survival at X years.

Imatinib and Imatinib-Containing Regimens

Imatinib in younger Ph+ acute lymphoblastic leukemia patients

With the introduction of effective TKIs, the treatment of Ph+ ALL patients is undergoing a revolutionary transformation, with improved outcomes not only for patients who are eligible for and are able to receive allo SCT but also for those who are not candidates for or are unable to undergo such treatment. In fact, for the first time, the role of transplantation in first CR has been questioned, with early follow-up of several studies demonstrating comparable outcomes for patients receiving imatinib-containing regimens with and without a transplant in first CR.[15-17]

Imatinib mesylate (Gleevec, Novartis Pharmaceuticals, Basel, Switzerland) binds the inactive moiety of the bcr-abl kinase, partially blocking its adenosine triphosphate (ATP) binding site, thereby preventing a conformational switch to the active tyrosine kinase (**Fig. 1A**). Significant clinical activity and favorable toxicity profile of imatinib in Ph+ ALL was evident in the initial phase 1 and 2 trials of the drug.[18-20] In the phase 2 study in patients with Ph+ ALL, imatinib induced CRs and complete marrow responses (marrow-CRs) in 29% of patients, which were sustained for at least 4 weeks in 6%.[19] However, the median estimated time to progression and OS were short, 2.2 and 4.9 months, respectively.[19] In a follow-up study, the extent of reduction in the *BCR-ABL* transcript levels in peripheral blood (PB) and bone marrow (BM), analyzed by quantitative polymerase chain reaction (Q-PCR), in the treated patients was predictive of response and median time to progression.[21] Other predictors of response such as pretreatment white blood cell count (WBC), presence of circulating blasts before treatment, duration of prior CR, and presence of a double Ph chromosome or up to two additional *BCR-ABL* fusion signals have also been reported.[22] The probability of achieving complete hematological response (CHR) and response duration was higher in patients with a baseline WBC less than 10×10^9/L, no circulating blasts pretreatment, a prior CR of at least 6 months, and no *BCR-ABL* amplification.[22] Of interest, presence of additional chromosomal aberrations or the size of the protein (p190 vs p210) did not affect the clinical outcome.

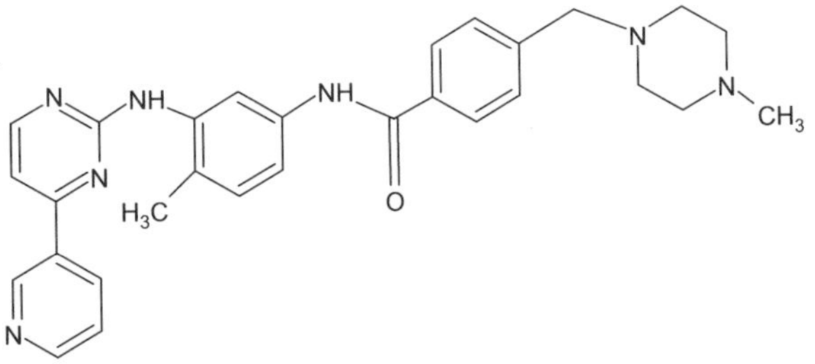

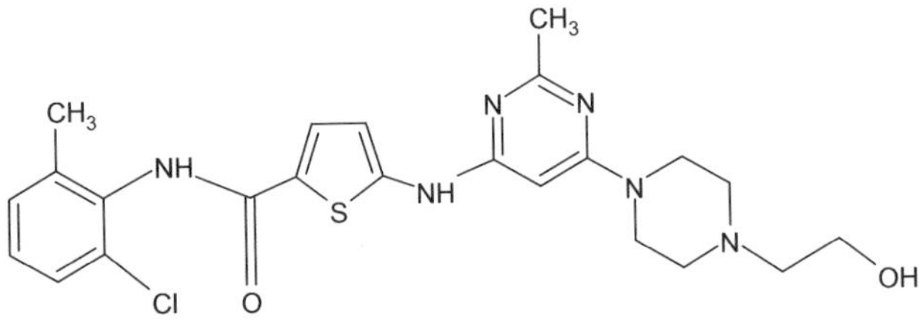

Fig. 1. (*A*) Imatinib. (*B*) Dasatinib.

Therefore, from these early studies it was clear that few, if any, patients can achieve durable responses with single-agent imatinib. At the same time, in vitro studies demonstrated synergistic or additive effects in Ph+ cell lines when imatinib was administered in combination with various chemotherapy agents, suggesting a potential role for these combinations in patients.[23–25] Several investigators explored the efficacy of imatinib in combination with chemotherapy for frontline treatment of Ph+ ALL patients, although initially the optimal schedule was debated, and concurrent as well as sequential schedules were investigated (**Table 2**).

In the first clinical trial reporting the combination of imatinib with chemotherapy, imatinib 400 mg was administered daily for the first 14 days of each of the eight cycles of the hyper-CVAD regimen (fractionated cyclophosphamide, vincristine, doxorubicin, and dexamethasone, alternating with high-dose cytarabine and methotrexate).[15] This phase was followed by a maintenance phase whereby imatinib 600 mg was given continuously together with monthly vincristine and prednisone for 12 months.[15] A CR rate of 96% with a 2-year DFS of 85% was reported. Half of the initial cohort of 20 patients underwent allo SCT. These results were significantly superior to historical data using chemotherapy alone. Furthermore, molecular complete responses, as analyzed by Q-PCR, were reported in 60% of the patients. Of importance is that there was no unexpected toxicity related to the addition of imatinib to the regimen.

The same investigators have modified the regimen, with the final regimen including imatinib 600 mg on days 1 to 14 of induction, then 600 mg continuously with courses 2 to 8, followed by escalation to 800 mg as tolerated during 24 months of maintenance therapy with monthly vincristine and prednisone. Maintenance was interrupted by two intensification courses of hyper-CVAD and imatinib, and after its completion imatinib was administered indefinitely. Allo SCT was performed in first CR as feasible. In a follow-up report in 54 patients with untreated or minimally treated disease, a CR

Table 2
Clinical trials incorporating imatinib into frontline chemotherapy for Ph+ ALL

Study	N	Median Age (Range)	Imatinib and Chemo Schedule	CR %	Relapse %	EFS % (Years)	Survival % (Years)
Thomas et al[15,26]	45	51 (17–84)	Concurrent	93	22	68 (3)[a]	55 (3)
Yanada et al[16,28]	80	48 (15–63)	Concurrent	96	26	51 (2)	58 (20)
Lee et al[27]	20	37 (15–67)	Concurrent	95	32	62 (2)	59 (2)
Lee et al[42,43]	29	36 (18–55)	Alternating	79	4	78 (3)	78 (3)
Wassmann et al[29]	45	41 (19–63)	Concurrent	a	a	61 (2)	43 (2)
	47	46 (21–65)	Alternating	a	a	52 (2)	36 (2)
de Labarthe et al[30]	45	45 (16–59)	Concurrent	96	19	51 (1.5)	65 (1.5)
Delannoy et al[33]	30	66 (58–78)	Alternating	72	60	58 (1)	66 (1)
Vignetti et al[32]	30	69 (61–83)	+Prednisone	100	48	48 (1)	74 (1)
Ottmann et al[34]	28	68 (54–79)	Chemo→Concurrent	96	41	29 (1.5)	35 (1.5)
	27	–	Imatinib→Concurrent	50	54	57 (1.5)	41 (1.5)

Abbreviations: CR, complete remission; EFS, event-free survival.
[a] CR duration reported.

rate of 93% was reported for those with active disease.[26] Sixteen patients (33%) underwent allo SCT in first CR within a median of 5 months from start of therapy (range, 1–13). In the untreated group, 14 patients with a median age of 37 years underwent SCT in first CR whereas 33 patients with a median age of 53 years did not. The 3-year OS rates were similar (66% vs 49% with or without allo SCT, respectively, $P = .36$). The 3-year CR duration rate was 84% for patients who achieved molecular CR (2 of 16 had allo SCT) compared with 64% for those who did not (14 of 35 had allo SCT), $P = .1$; OS rates were similar regardless of molecular CR status. With a median follow-up of 52 months (range, 19–83+), 22% of the patients relapsed within a median of 15 months from the start of therapy (range, 8–42), including two after allo SCT without imatinib maintenance.[26]

Other investigators have reported the results of studies incorporating imatinib into ALL chemotherapy regimens (**Table 2**). In general, trials designed for younger patients have added imatinib for varying lengths and doses to standard regimens, whereas the emphasis in the older population has been to minimize poorly tolerated cytotoxic chemotherapy. The initial debates focusing on the optimal schedule, concurrent versus sequential imatinib, have been largely settled by several reports of good tolerability and improved efficacy of the concurrent treatment.

Lee and colleagues[27] reported on 20 patients with a median age of 37 years (range, 15–67 years) with newly diagnosed Ph+ ALL who received an induction regimen of daunorubicin, vincristine, prednisone, and L-asparaginase together with imatinib 600 mg daily on days 1 to 14. Imatinib 400 mg daily was also administered in the first 14 days of each course of consolidation. After the first 12 patients, imatinib was administered continuously in both induction and consolidation cycles. Nineteen (95%) patients achieved CR and 15 underwent allo SCT in first CR.[27] Median CR duration and median survival were significantly longer compared with a historical cohort of 18 patients treated with the same regimen but without imatinib.[27] The reported toxicities of the regimen included reversible hyperbilirubinemia in four patients.

The Japan Adult Leukemia Study Group (JALSG) reported on a concurrent induction regimen of imatinib, cyclophosphamide, daunorubicin, vincristine, and prednisolone.[16,28] Consolidation therapy consisted of odd courses of high-dose cytarabine and methotrexate, alternating with single-agent imatinib 600 mg daily for 28 days. Patients then received 2 years of maintenance with imatinib, vincristine, and prednisone. In the more recent report of 80 patients (median age 48 years, range, 15–63) a CR rate of 96% was reported.[16] A PCR-negative status was reported in 71% of patients at least at one point during their follow-up. Among the 57 patients who achieved PCR negativity, 17 patients had molecular relapse. Of them, seven patients had hematological relapse, six underwent allo SCT, and four were in continuous CR without allo SCT. Allo SCT was conducted in 49 patients including 39 who underwent allo SCT in first CR. The 1-year event-free survival (EFS) and OS were estimated to be 60% and 76%, respectively, which were significantly better than historical controls treated without imatinib ($P<.0001$ for both). The probability of survival at 1 year was 73% and 85% for those who received or did not receive allo SCT, respectively.

To establish the best strategy of incorporating imatinib into ALL chemotherapy, The German Multicenter Acute Lymphoblastic Leukemia (GMALL) trial evaluated 92 patients (median age 46 years, range 21–65 years) in two schedules.[29] Imatinib was administered alternating with chemotherapy cycles in the first cohort of patients; then it was administered concurrently with chemotherapy throughout the second induction phase, consolidation, and up to allo SCT in the second cohort. Before consolidation, PCR negativity rates of 52% and 19% were reported in the concurrent and alternating cohorts, respectively. A poor hematological response to the first induction cycle of chemotherapy was compensated by subsequent concurrent administration of imatinib with chemotherapy.[29] In each cohort, 77% of patients underwent allo SCT, and toxicity was acceptable for both schedules. The investigators concluded that the concurrent regimen had a greater antileukemic efficacy. However, this greater activity did not translate to improvements in EFS and OS.[29]

In the Group for Research on Adult Acute Lymphoblastic Leukemia (GRAAPH) 2003 study, imatinib was started with cytarabine and mitoxantrone (HAM) consolidation in good early responders (corticosteroid and chemosensitive ALL), or earlier during the induction course in combination with dexamethasone and vincristine in poor early responders (corticosteroid or chemoresistant ALL). Imatinib was then continuously administered until allo SCT.[30] Overall CR and Q-PCR negativity rates were 96% and 29%, respectively. The CR rate was significantly higher compared with the previous report from the pre-imatinib era by the same group (96% vs 71%, $P<.001$), and the DFS and OS were significantly longer ($P = .02$ and 0.05, respectively).[30,31] Furthermore, patients younger than 55 years were eligible for allo SCT and all 22 with a donor underwent SCT. Early results of a study by the Children's Oncology Group in which imatinib at 340 mg/m^2 was administered for an increasing number of days in combination with an intensive chemotherapy backbone seem to confirm the benefit of the addition of imatinib, even in the pediatric population, and irrespective of the availability of a donor.[17]

Therefore, it is clear that the addition of imatinib to the initial therapy for patients with Ph+ ALL has significantly improved their outcome. Despite relatively short follow-up and variations in the design and schedule of treatment, higher response rates, improved feasibility of allo SCT. and improved EFS and OS rates were observed in all trials.

Imatinib in elderly Ph+ acute lymphoblastic leukemia patients

The question of the more imatinib and less chemotherapy approach has been of particular interest in the elderly population, who are less tolerant of the intensive chemotherapy regimens used in ALL, are less likely to be candidates for allo SCT, and comprise a significant portion of patients with this disease.[12] Several trials have examined various approaches in this population (**Table 2**).

In the Gruppo Italiano Malattie Ematologiche dell'Adulto (GIMEMA) study, 30 patients with Ph+ ALL, 60 years and older, were treated with imatinib 800 mg as well as prednisone 40 mg/m^2 daily from days 1 to 45.[32] Twenty-nine were assessable for response and all (100%) achieved CR. Molecular CR was achieved only in 1 of the 27 evaluable patients.[32] The median CR duration and survival were 8 months and 20 months, respectively.[32] Fourteen patients relapsed after a median of 4 months (range, 3–28 months). Two patients died in CR and 13 were alive in continuous remission after a median of 10 months (range, 1–32 months).[32] In a study by Group for Research on Adult Acute Lymphocytic Leukemia (GRAALL), patients 55 years or older were treated with chemotherapy-based induction after a pre-phase of steroids.[33] This phase was followed by a consolidation phase of steroids and imatinib, and 10 maintenance blocks of alternating chemotherapy, including two imatinib-containing blocks. Among the 30 patients treated, a CR rate of 72% was reported, with additional patients achieving CR after salvage imatinib.[33] The outcome was significantly better than in historical patients treated by the same group, with 1-year OS of 66% versus 43% ($P = .005$), and 1-year relapse-free survival of 58% versus 11% ($P = .0003$).

Ottmann and colleagues[34] conducted a randomized trial of imatinib monotherapy versus standard induction therapy in 55 patients with a median age of 67 years (range, 54–79 years). The CR rate was 96% in the imatinib-treated arm versus 50% in the patients receiving induction chemotherapy ($P = .0001$). Severe adverse events were significantly more frequent during induction with chemotherapy. Patients in either treatment arm then received imatinib 600 mg daily in combination with all successive cycles of chemotherapy, which were administered irrespective of response to induction. The estimated OS for all patients was 42% at 2 years, with no significant difference between the 2 arms.[34] The molecular CR rates did not differ with either approach but PCR negativity occurred earlier in the imatinib induction arm. Median DFS was significantly longer in the patients achieving PCR-negative status (18.3 months vs 7.2 months, $P = .002$).

Role of Allogeneic Stem Cell Transplantation Before and After Imatinib Era

Pre-imatinib era

With the incorporation of imatinib and other TKIs in the treatment of Ph+ ALL, the role of allo SCT is undergoing transformation. In the past, it was the only strategy that had a significant curative potential. However, it was limited in its application by the availability of suitable donors, and by its diminished feasibility and effectiveness in older patients, those with comorbid conditions, and those with active leukemia at the time of transplantation. The outcome after allo SCT in the pre-imatinib era has been better characterized by several recent reports. Laport and colleagues[35] reported the outcomes for the largest series to date of uniformly treated Ph+ ALL patients. From 1985 to 2005, 79 patients with Ph+ ALL, with a median age of 36 years, received a matched sibling transplant following total body irradiation (TBI) and etoposide-based conditioning, and cyclosporine-based graft versus host disease (GVHD) prophylaxis. For patients transplanted in first CR, the 10-year OS and cumulative incidence of non-relapse mortality (NRM) were 54% and 31%, respectively. Acute GVHD, grades 2 to 4, was noted in 35% of patients, with 13% of patients developing chronic extensive GVHD. Of note, patients transplanted with PB stem cells were twice as likely to develop chronic GVHD compared with patients who received BM stem cells, confirming results of other randomized studies assessing the impact of stem cell source on transplant outcome.[36,37] The median time to relapse was 12 months (range, 1–27 months), and all deaths due to NRM occurred within 3 years of allo SCT.[35]

The results of single-center studies have been corroborated in large, multicenter studies designed to prospectively assess the role of allo SCT in adult ALL patients. In the largest trial to date, 267 Ph+ ALL patients were treated between 1993 and 2004 as part of the MRC UKALL XII/ECOG E2993 study.[38] Patients with Ph+ disease who were younger than 55 years and had achieved CR were assigned to a matched sibling or matched unrelated donor (MUD). Patients without a donor or with a performance status that prohibited allo SCT were eligible for randomization to continued chemotherapy versus autologous SCT; very few patients were actually randomized, with the majority of patients receiving continued chemotherapy.[38] The conditioning regimen for the allo SCT consisted of TBI and etoposide, and a cyclosporine-based GVHD prophylaxis regimen was recommended; imatinib was not used in the patients reported in this series. Twenty-eight percent of patients received a matched-related or unrelated donor allo SCT in first CR. At 5 years, OS was 44% following sibling SCT, 36% following MUD SCT, and 19% following chemotherapy, with treatment-related mortality (TRM) of 27% following sibling SCT and 39% following MUD SCT.[38] After adjusting for differences in age and WBC at presentation in the two groups and after excluding chemotherapy-treated patients who relapsed or died before the median time to allo SCT, only relapse-free survival remained significantly better in the allo SCT group; the TRM rate became significantly lower for the chemotherapy group, and OS became nonsignificantly worse in the allo SCT group, underscoring the need to carefully weigh the benefit of disease control with the TRM associated with allo SCT. An intention-to-treat analysis, using the availability of a matched sibling donor, showed no significant difference in survival between the two groups (34% with and 25% without a donor).[38]

The results of this trial are consistent with the conclusions of two earlier studies, the LALA-87 and LALA-94 trials, which were designed to prospectively evaluate the role of allo SCT in first CR.[31,39] Analyzed on an intention-to-treat basis, the LALA-87 trial showed a statistically significant advantage for allo SCT versus chemotherapy for patients with high-risk ALL, including Ph+ patients, with 10-year survival rates of 44% and 11%, respectively.[39] In the follow-up LALA-94 trial, the advantage of allo SCT over chemotherapy in Ph+ ALL patients was confirmed (estimated survival at 3 years 37% vs 12%, $P = .02$).[31] Furthermore, the advantage of a molecular response before SCT was demonstrated, with 3-year survival estimated at 54% for the group achieving a negative PCR versus 19% for those remaining BCR-ABL positive.[31] This result is in agreement with studies in the pediatric population in which the level of residual disease before allo SCT correlates with outcome after SCT.[40,41]

Post-imatinib era

The incorporation of imatinib into standard ALL therapy has improved the ability to undergo allo SCT in first CR, resulting in improved OS rates of 43% to 78% at 1 to 3 years of follow-up.[15,16,29,30] As discussed previously, even before imatinib, patients in molecular remission at time of allo SCT had a longer DFS.[31] As a result, interim monotherapy with imatinib has been used to reduce the disease burden prior to allo SCT.[42,43] In a study by Lee and colleagues,[42,43] interim cycles of imatinib between induction and consolidation, and between consolidation and allo SCT significantly improved the DFS and OS compared with a historical group of patients treated with the same chemotherapy regimen but without imatinib. The patients' BCR-ABL/ABL ratios declined by a median of 0.77 and 0.34 logs after each of the two cycles of imatinib.[42,43] As a result, a significantly higher proportion of patients proceeded to allo SCT in first CR. Therefore, such interim imatinib therapy not only improves the likelihood of allo SCT to be conducted in Ph+ ALL patients but also allows it to occur in a more favorable status.[44] Of note, thus far the early results of studies incorporating imatinib into pretransplant therapy have not demonstrated a clear survival difference between patients who receive an allo SCT for consolidation compared with those who do not.[15,16,29,30] Thus, whether consolidation with allo SCT in first CR will remain the standard of care for Ph+ ALL will depend on the durability of the remissions achieved with chemotherapy plus imatinib regimens.

Radich and colleagues[45] had shown that Ph+ ALL patients who remained PCR-positive after allo SCT had a significantly higher incidence of relapse than PCR-negative patients. Therefore, use of imatinib in the posttransplant setting to eradicate minimal residual disease (MRD) has been investigated by several groups.[46–48] In the study by Wassmann and colleagues,[47] 27 Ph+ ALL patients received imatinib 400 mg daily on detection of MRD after SCT. The dose could be escalated to 600 mg and 800 mg in patients remaining PCR-positive. BCR-ABL transcripts were undetectable in 14 (52%) of the patients, after a median of 1.5 months of imatinib therapy (range, 0.9–3.7 months). Failure to achieve a molecular remission within 6 weeks of starting imatinib predicted relapse, occurring in 12 of 13 (92%) patients at a median of 3 months. DFS in patients with molecular CR at 12 and 24 months was 91% and 54% compared with only 8% in patients remaining MRD-positive after 12 months.[47] These data suggested the benefit of prophylactic administration of imatinib in the post allo SCT setting.[48] Imatinib could be administered safely from the time of engraftment at a dose intensity comparable to that used in primary therapy. Similar strategies combining interferon and imatinib to maintain remission have also been investigated.[49,50]

As evident in the MRC UKALL XII/ECOG 2993 study, TRM overcomes any survival advantage for transplant in older patients. Because the incidence of ALL, particularly the Ph+ subtype, increases in adults older than 50 years, transplant approaches with reduced TRM such as nonmyeloablative regimens are needed. Martino and colleagues[51] reported the largest series of nonmyeloablative SCT in ALL. These investigators reported a TRM of 23%, OS of 31%, and disease progression of 49% at 2 years among 27 patients with a median age of 55 years. A higher relapse rate was observed for patients transplanted with overt disease compared with those transplanted in CR (60% vs 33%, respectively). These data suggest that this strategy is feasible in older patients in CR, but must be validated in multicenter, prospective studies.

Beyond first remission, allo SCT is curative in only a small fraction of ALL patients, with long-term OS ranging between 5% and 43%, the primary cause of failure being relapse (>50%).[38,52-55] In a study of 60 adult patients with advanced ALL (primary refractory n = 8, first relapse n = 52), including 14 patients with Ph+ disease, those who did not undergo reinduction chemotherapy after relapse had a better outcome, with 5-year OS 47% versus 18%.[55] The investigators suggested that patients who did not undergo salvage chemotherapy before SCT sustained less TRM, leading ultimately to a better outcome.[55] In the subset of patients who relapsed in the MRC ECOG/UKALL study, patients who were able to receive a matched sibling transplant had the best survival at 5 years (23%).[56] Factors predicting a better outcome were young age (OS 12% for patients <20 years old versus 3% for patients >50 years old) and long duration of first remission (OS 11% for CR1 >2 years versus 5% for CR1 <2 years).[56]

With current induction regimens, only 5% to 10% of newly diagnosed Ph+ ALL adults fail to achieve remission with initial induction chemotherapy, and additional attempts at induction chemotherapy may be unsuccessful. Several studies suggest that patients with a human leukocyte antigen (HLA)-identical sibling can benefit if they proceed directly to allo SCT without undergoing a second attempt at induction therapy.[57,58] In the largest study, 38 patients with ALL failing to achieve remission received HLA-identical sibling transplants without reinduction.[57] Approximately 35% of these patients with refractory disease achieved long-term DFS. A second study with 22 patients (5 with ALL) with refractory disease had a similar survival of 38% following HLA-matched sibling transplants.[58] Other studies suggest lower survival rates of 20% or less for these refractory patients.[57,59] Nevertheless, allogeneic transplant should be considered for patients with relapsed/refractory disease who otherwise have a dismal chance of long-term survival.

In conclusion, transplant offered superior disease control compared with chemotherapy in the pre-TKI era, and allo SCT with a matched sibling or unrelated donor was recommended for all patients in first CR. The addition of TKIs to standard ALL therapy seems to improve disease control, albeit with relatively short follow-up. Allo SCT in first CR remains standard, but older or frail patients may be monitored closely with Q-PCR and transplanted at time of increasing BCR-ABL transcript levels. Alternatively, nonmyeloablative transplants with an expected lower TRM may be considered. Allo SCT with matched sibling or unrelated donors should be recommended for all patients with primary refractory or relapsed disease. Furthermore, alternative donor transplants should be considered in these patients, despite their significant TRM and relapse rates of up to 40%. Small patient numbers and heterogeneity in remission status limit conclusions regarding the use of umbilical cord blood transplants. An estimated 20% to 50% of patients transplanted in remission can achieve long-term disease control; relapse and engraftment remain significant issues.[60]

Resistance to Imatinib

Both acquired and intrinsic resistance to imatinib has been described in Ph+ ALL patients. Acquired imatinib resistance may be due to *BCR-ABL*–dependent mechanisms such as bcr-abl overexpression or mutations in the kinase domains (KD) (**Table 3**).[61,62] Resistance may also arise through *BCR-ABL*–independent mechanisms such as pharmacokinetic factors reducing the availability of imatinib within Ph+ cells, or through activation of alternative signaling pathways such as the Src-kinase related pathways.[63–67]

Although several KD mutations have limited consequence, those that interfere with imatinib binding to the bcr-abl protein have been identified as a major mechanism of acquired resistance in patients with CML.[61,62,68] These include (1) mutations that directly impede contact between imatinib and bcr-abl, such as T315I and F317L, and (2) mutations in the ATP-binding P-loop or in the activation loop, which alter the spatial conformation of the protein.[61,62,69,70] Data on the frequency and spectrum of these mutations in Ph+ ALL is more limited. Two early studies in patients with advanced Ph+ lymphoid leukemias identified 5 different KD mutations in 14 of 17 patients with acquired imatinib resistance.[71,72] In one report E255K/V mutations were noted in 67% of patients, but this was not confirmed by the other study.[71,72] However, in these studies KD mutations occurring before initiation of therapy with imatinib that could potentially account for primary resistance were not identified. More recently the same investigators, using a more sensitive cloning and sequencing strategy, were able to demonstrate the presence of low-level KD mutations in imatinib-naïve patients.[73] In a follow-up study in a larger cohort of elderly patients enrolled into the GMALL randomized study,[34] approximately 40% of patients with imatinib-naïve with no or minimal prior exposure to chemotherapy harbored a small leukemic clone (allele frequency of 2%, range 0.1%–2%) with these mutations.[74] The frequency of the mutant allele at the time of diagnosis was always below the level of detection by direct cDNA sequencing, and ATP-binding P-loop mutations were the dominant type, accounting for 83% of the mutations with the other 17% being T315I. It is remarkable

Table 3
Reported potential mechanisms of resistance to imatinib

Mechanisms related to cellular uptake and retention of imatinib
  Increased MDR1 expression[107]
  Reduced hOCT1 mediated influx[67,108]
  Increased binding to α1-acid glycoprotein-1[109]

BCR-ABL dependent mechanisms
  BCR-ABL overexpression[61]
  BCR-ABL kinase domain mutations[61,62]

BCR-ABL independent mechanisms
  Activation of alternate signaling pathways such as Src[65]
  Clonal evolution[110]

Miscellaneous
  Noncompliance
  Stem cell quiescence[111]

that preexistence of mutations including T315I did not adversely affect the CR rate or the achievement of molecular CR when compared with patients who only had unmutated *BCR-ABL* at diagnosis.[74] This finding raises the hypothesis that these clones were eradicated by chemotherapy.

Only the presence of T315I at diagnoses was associated with a more rapid relapse; however, nearly all of the patients with a detectable mutation at diagnosis relapsed as opposed to only 50% of patients with unmutated BCR-ABL. Among the patients who relapsed, 84% harbored mutations, with the most frequent site of mutations being P-loop (58%) and T315I (19%). Comparing the mutations at diagnosis and relapse, only 1 of 11 patients with detectable mutation at diagnosis had a switch. On the other hand, 67% of patients with no mutation at baseline were found to have a dominant mutant clone at relapse.[74] Jones and colleagues[75] have also recently reported the presence of KD mutations in most patients with relapsed disease following imatinib therapy. KD mutations were detected in 88% of patients who had received either imatinib (n = 11) or dasatinib (n = 1), and in 86% of patients who had had two or more prior TKIs compared with none of the patients who never received TKIs.[75] A limited spectrum of mutations, mostly Y253H, T315I, and F317L, were noted, which were not present before treatment with TKIs in those with available samples. Other investigators have also reported a high frequency of mutations at relapse, suggesting a pivotal role for the *BCR-ABL* KD mutations in acquired imatinib resistance in Ph+ ALL patients.[75,76] Whether such acquired imatinib resistance is a result of outgrowth of small clones with mutant KD existing before the initiation of imatinib, or the effect of selection leading to the emergence of mutations after the initiation of and continuous exposure to TKIs, requires further studies.[74,75]

A new mechanism of resistance involves the expression of spliced isoforms of Ikaros (*IKZF1*).[77] Ikzf1 functions as a critical regulator of normal lymphocyte development and is involved in the rapid development of leukemia in mice expressing non-DNA binding isoforms.[78] The Ik6 isoform, lacking all 4 N-terminal zinc fingers responsible for DNA binding, was detected in 43 of 47 (91%) Ph+ ALL patients resistant to imatinib or dasatinib.[77] In addition, the expression level of Ik6 correlated with the *BCR-ABL* transcript level. Restoring Ikzf1 function would be of great benefit in this condition.

Finally, stromal support was proposed as an additional mechanism of resistance to TKIs.[79] Cells with low expression of *BCR-ABL* were able to grow in the presence of stroma. The stromal effect did not require cell-cell contact and the stromal-cell derived factor 1α, the ligand to the chemokine receptor 4 (CXCR4), could substitute for the presence of the stromal cells. Interfering with the stroma-lymphoblast interaction, possibly by the CXCR4 inhibitor plerixafor (AMD3100), could be of benefit in eradicating Ph+ ALL cells.

Second-Generation Tyrosine Kinase Inhibitors

The development of resistance and intolerance to imatinib in Ph+ leukemia patients has fuelled the search for alternative, second-generation inhibitors capable of overcoming the resistance.[80–82] Dasatinib is a dual Src and Abl kinase inhibitor that binds both active and inactive moieties of the bcr-abl protein, and is approximately 325 times more potent against the kinase in preclinical studies (**Fig. 1**B).[80] The inhibition of other kinases, particularly Src, may be important in overcoming imatinib resistance, particularly in patients with lymphoid leukemias in whom Src-kinase activity may be important in the pathogenesis of the disease.[83] Dasatinib is active in vitro against all imatinib-resistant BCR-ABL mutants with the notable exception of T315I.[80] It has demonstrated significant activity in phase I and II studies in Ph+ leukemia patients who were resistant to or intolerant of imatinib. Cortes and colleagues[84] reported the results of a phase II trial in which patients with blast phase of CML who had failed imatinib were treated with dasatinib 70 mg orally twice daily. Among 42 patients with lymphoid blast phase, 31% achieved a major hematological response (HR) and 50% a major cytogenetic response, mostly CRs. Response rates were similar in patients with or without imatinib-resistant BCR-ABL mutations. Ottmann and colleagues[85] conducted a phase 2 study of dasatinib in 36 Ph+ ALL patients after failing imatinib. The median age of the patients was 46 years (range, 15–85 years). Major HR was achieved in 15 (42%) of patients and cytogenetic CR in 21 (58%). Six patients had a baseline T315I mutation and none responded, but response rates were similar in patients with other mutations compared with those with no mutations.[85] More recent data have suggested that administering dasatinib once daily in CML or Ph+ ALL patients produces similar responses and is associated with a better toxicity profile, including a lower incidence of grade III and IV myelosuppression or pleural effusions.[86] In another report it was suggested that this regimen was effective in achieving CR in patients who had relapsed from prior, mostly imatinib-based therapy.[87]

Based on the significant activity of dasatinib against BCR-ABL, and impressive data in patients with relapsed disease, the authors have conducted a phase 2 study of combining the hyper-CVAD regimen with dasatinib, administered at 50 mg orally twice daily for the first 14 days of each of the eight induction/consolidation chemotherapy cycles, as frontline therapy.[88] Patients would then receive dasatinib continuously and indefinitely, with monthly cycles of prednisone and vincristine for the first 2 years. A lower dasatinib dose was chosen to avoid excessive myelosuppression when combined with intensive chemotherapy. Preliminary data have been recently reported demonstrating the feasibility of this regimen in relapsed and previously untreated patients.[88] Among 28 patients with newly diagnosed disease (median age 52 years, range 21–79 years), 26 (93%) achieved CR after one course of treatment; 20 of 26 (81%) achieved a cytogenetic CR after 1 cycle, and 19 (68%) achieved a major molecular response including 14 (50%) with molecular CR. With a median follow-up of 10 months (range, 2–21 months), 21 were alive and 18 alive in CR, 2 died at induction and 3 died in CR; 5 patients had relapsed with a median CR duration of 47 weeks in the relapsing patients; 2 relapsing patients died.[88] Of note, BCR-ABL mutations were identified in 4 of the 5 relapsing patients (including 3 with T315I and 1 with F359V).[88]

Early reports of ongoing studies have suggested improved outcomes in older patients using dasatinib-based regimens for newly diagnosed patients. In a study by the European Working Group on adult ALL (EWALL), patients older than 55 years received an induction schedule of vincristine and dexamethasone repeated weekly for 4 weeks, followed by consolidation methotrexate and asparaginase alternating with cytarabine for a total of 6 cycles.[89] Dasatinib was administered at 140 mg daily during the induction and at 100 mg/day sequentially during the consolidation and maintenance courses. A CR rate of 95% was reported in the first 22 patients treated. Only 1 relapse and 3 deaths in CR were reported at a median follow-up of 3.6 months.[89] In the GIMEMA LAL 1205 study, dasatinib 70 mg twice daily was administered for 12 weeks, in combination with prednisone and intrathecal chemotherapy, to treat adult patients with newly diagnosed Ph+ ALL.[90] Among the first 48 patients (median age, 54 years; range, 24–76 years) 34 were evaluable for response, and a CR rate of 100% was reported with no deaths attributable to treatment.[90] With a median follow-up of 11 months, survival at 10 months was 81%. Nine patients had relapsed, with five showing a T315I, one an E255K, and two without mutations. Details of consolidation treatment were not provided.[90]

Existence of BCR-ABL mutations that may induce resistance to dasatinib is of significant concern.[91] Mutations in the gatekeeper region of BCR-ABL, in particular T315I, confer resistance to dasatinib (as well as imatinib and other available TKIs). Crystal studies have demonstrated that the aromatic ring in the side chain of phenyl-alanine 317 directly interacts with the pyrimidine and thiazole rings of dasatinib.[92] Furthermore, in the in vitro saturation mutagenesis, several amino acid substitutions affecting residue 317 have been reported to induce dasatinib resistance, including both the imatinib-resistant F317L and other variants like F317V, F317I, and F317S. In cellular assays, the F317L has been shown to induce an approximately 10-fold increase of dasatinib IC_{50} with respect to wild-type BCR-ABL.[93] As with imatinib-based therapy, at present it is not clear whether these mutants exist pretherapy and dasatinib treatment induces their overgrowth, or if their development is a direct result of treatment with the TKIs. Other second-generation TKIs, including nilotinib and bo-sutinib as well other investigational agents have been evaluated in phase 1 and 2 trials. Of potential interest are agents with activity against the T315I mutants.

Central Nervous System Disease

Central nervous system (CNS) involvement is common in ALL, with up to 6% of patients having evidence of involvement at diagnosis and without adequate pro-phylaxis, Up to 30% of patients will develop CNS disease during treatment and follow-up.[94,95] However, with routine CNS-directed treatment, this risk has subsided to less than 10%. Several recent studies have reported a relatively high incidence of isolated CNS relapse in Ph+ acute leukemia patients, with generally unfavorable outcomes.[96,97] In the study by Leis and colleagues,[97] 5 of 24 (21%) Ph+ acute leukemia (ALL or CML lymphoid blast phase) patients who were treated with imatinib and without intensive chemotherapy or specific CNS prophylaxis developed CNS disease despite achieving a CR. Simultaneous plasma and cerebrospinal fluid (CSF) imatinib levels were measured in four subsequent patients, and imatinib levels were noted to be two logs lower in the CSF than in plasma, with the CSF levels being below the level required for bcr-abl inhibition. Another report confirmed an almost 100-fold lower imatinib level in the CSF compared with plasma in a patient with relapsed Ph+ ALL and concurrent CNS disease.[98] These studies suggest that imatinib poorly penetrates the blood-brain barrier, and underscore the need for adequate CNS-directed therapy in patients receiving imatinib-based therapy. At least in part, this may be because imatinib is a substrate for the drug efflux P-glycoprotein with the latter's high expression in the CNS.

Imatinib and dasatinib have been compared in a preclinical mouse model of intra-cranial Ph+ leukemia for their ability to penetrate the blood-brain barrier.[99] Dasatinib has antileukemic activity in the multidrug-resistant K562/ADM, with a high expression of P-glycoprotein, and as such may have a better penetrance of the blood-brain barrier.[99] In the mouse model, dasatinib led to the regression of CNS disease and improved survival, whereas imatinib was unable to inhibit the intracranial tumor growth. Furthermore, clinical responses to dasatinib in patients with imatinib-resistant disease involving the CNS have been reported, with responses being durable in some patients.[99] Furthermore, KD mutational analysis on the blasts from the CSF of two patients who experienced a CNS relapse while receiving dasatinib demonstrated the presence of dasatinib-resistant mutations, suggesting a selection pressure further indicating its CNS penetration.[99] Prospective studies evaluating the dasatinib CSF

Table 4	
Selected new agents being evaluated in Ph+ leukemias	
Drug	**Mechanism of Action**
Bosutinib	Bcr-Abl and Src-kinase inhibitor
Homoharringtonine	Inhibition of protein synthesis, induction of differentiation and apoptosis
PHA739358	Bcr-Abl and Aurora kinase A, B, and C inhibitor
AP24534	Bcr-Abl, FLT3, and FGF1-R inhibitor
DCC2036	Bcr-Abl inhibitor (binds the "switch pocket")
XL228	Bcr-Abl, Src and IGF1-R inhibitor

levels and its ability to decrease the incidence of CNS relapse are necessary to confirm these data.

Future Challenges in Ph+ Acute Lymphoblastic Leukemia

The introduction of effective TKIs in the treatment of Ph+ ALL has introduced several avenues of research in a disease that was hitherto difficult to treat. In the younger patients, the standard therapy should include combination of chemotherapy with one of the TKIs, likely imatinib but potentially dasatinib, with further maturation of emerging data. In the older patients who are less able to tolerate intensive chemo-therapy regimens, rationally designed combinations including dasatinib, in addition to the careful monitoring for response, MRD, and toxicity to decide on the continuation of treatment may further improve the outcome. The emergence or resurgence of KD mutations, particularly those resistant to the available TKIs (such as T315I), is a signif-icant concern that requires careful design of potential strategies to circumvent it. Several new TKIs are in development, with potential efficacy against clones resistant to first- and second-generation TKIs, including T315I mutants (**Table 4**). The role of allo SCT will likely continue to be refined, incorporating TKI-based strategies before and after allo SCT to maximize the benefits from all of the therapeutic armamentarium against this disease.

REFERENCES

1. Nowell PC, Hungerford DA. Chromosome studies on normal and leukemic human leukocytes. J Natl Cancer Inst 1960;25:85–109.
2. Rowley JD. Letter: a new consistent chromosomal abnormality in chronic myelogenous leukaemia identified by quinacrine fluorescence and Giemsa staining. Nature 1973;243:290–3.
3. Daley GQ, Van Etten RA, Baltimore D. Induction of chronic myelogenous leukemia in mice by the P210bcr/abl gene of the Philadelphia chromosome. Science 1990;247:824–30.
4. Schlieben S, Borkhardt A, Reinisch I, et al. Incidence and clinical outcome of children with BCR/ABL-positive acute lymphoblastic leukemia (ALL). A prospec-tive RT-PCR study based on 673 patients enrolled in the German pediatric multi-center therapy trials ALL-BFM-90 and CoALL-05-92. Leukemia 1996;10:957–63.
5. Hoelzer D. Advances in the management of Ph-positive ALL. Clin Adv Hematol Oncol 2006;4:804–5.

6. Kantarjian HM, Talpaz M, Dhingra K, et al. Significance of the P210 versus P190 molecular abnormalities in adults with Philadelphia chromosome-positive acute leukemia. Blood 1991;78:2411–8.

7. Li S, Ilaria RL Jr, Million RP, et al. The P190, P210, and P230 forms of the BCR/ABL oncogene induce a similar chronic myeloid leukemia-like syndrome in mice but have different lymphoid leukemogenic activity. J Exp Med 1999;189: 1399–412.

8. Gleissner B, Gokbuget N, Bartram CR, et al. Leading prognostic relevance of the BCR-ABL translocation in adult acute B-lineage lymphoblastic leukemia: a prospective study of the German Multicenter Trial Group and confirmed polymerase chain reaction analysis. Blood 2002;99:1536–43.

9. Arico M, Valsecchi MG, Camitta B, et al. Outcome of treatment in children with Philadelphia chromosome-positive acute lymphoblastic leukemia. N Engl J Med 2000;342:998–1006.

10. Schrappe M, Arico M, Harbott J, et al. Philadelphia chromosome-positive (Ph+) childhood acute lymphoblastic leukemia: good initial steroid response allows early prediction of a favorable treatment outcome. Blood 1998;92:2730–41.

11. Radich JP. Philadelphia chromosome-positive acute lymphocytic leukemia. Hematol Oncol Clin North Am 2001;15:21–36.

12. Larson RA. Management of acute lymphoblastic leukemia in older patients. Semin Hematol 2006;43:126–33.

13. Pane F, Cimino G, Izzo B, et al. Significant reduction of the hybrid BCR/ABL transcripts after induction and consolidation therapy is a powerful predictor of treatment response in adult Philadelphia-positive acute lymphoblastic leukemia. Leukemia 2005;19:628–35.

14. Garcia-Manero G, Thomas DA. Salvage therapy for refractory or relapsed acute lymphocytic leukemia. Hematol Oncol Clin North Am 2001;15:163–205.

15. Thomas DA, Faderl S, Cortes J, et al. Treatment of Philadelphia chromosome-positive acute lymphocytic leukemia with hyper-CVAD and imatinib mesylate. Blood 2004;103:4396–407.

16. Yanada M, Takeuchi J, Sugiura I, et al. High complete remission rate and promising outcome by combination of imatinib and chemotherapy for newly diagnosed BCR-ABL-positive acute lymphoblastic leukemia: a phase II study by the Japan Adult Leukemia Study Group. J Clin Oncol 2006;24:460–6.

17. Schultz KR, Bowman WP, Slayton W, et al. Improved early event free survival (EFS) in children with Philadelphia chromosome-positive (Ph+) acute lymphoblastic leukemia (ALL) with intensive Imatinib in combination with high dose chemotherapy: Children's Oncology Group (COG) Study AALL0031. Blood 2007;110 [Abstract #4].

18. Druker BJ, Sawyers CL, Kantarjian H, et al. Activity of a specific inhibitor of the BCR-ABL tyrosine kinase in the blast crisis of chronic myeloid leukemia and acute lymphoblastic leukemia with the Philadelphia chromosome. N Engl J Med 2001;344:1038–42.

19. Ottmann OG, Druker BJ, Sawyers CL, et al. A phase 2 study of imatinib in patients with relapsed or refractory Philadelphia chromosome-positive acute lymphoid leukemias. Blood 2002;100:1965–71.

20. Champagne MA, Capdeville R, Krailo M, et al. Imatinib mesylate (STI571) for treatment of children with Philadelphia chromosome-positive leukemia: results from a Children's Oncology Group phase 1 study. Blood 2004;104:2655–60.

21. Scheuring UJ, Pfeifer H, Wassmann B, et al. Early minimal residual disease (MRD) analysis during treatment of Philadelphia chromosome/Bcr-Abl-positive

acute lymphoblastic leukemia with the Abl-tyrosine kinase inhibitor imatinib (STI571). Blood 2003;101:85–90.

22. Wassmann B, Pfeifer H, Scheuring UJ, et al. Early prediction of response in patients with relapsed or refractory Philadelphia chromosome-positive acute lymphoblastic leukemia (Ph+ ALL) treated with imatinib. Blood 2004;103: 1495–8.

23. Thiesing JT, Ohno-Jones S, Kolibaba KS, et al. Efficacy of STI571, an abl tyrosine kinase inhibitor, in conjunction with other antileukemic agents against bcr-abl-positive cells. Blood 2000;96:3195–9.

24. Kano Y, Akutsu M, Tsunoda S, et al. In vitro cytotoxic effects of a tyrosine kinase inhibitor STI571 in combination with commonly used antileukemic agents. Blood 2001;97:1999–2007.

25. Topaly J, Zeller WJ, Fruehauf S. Synergistic activity of the new ABL-specific tyrosine kinase inhibitor STI571 and chemotherapeutic drugs on BCR-ABL-positive chronic myelogenous leukemia cells. Leukemia 2001;15:342–7.

26. Thomas DA, Kantarjian HM, Cortes J, et al. Outcome after frontline therapy with the hyper-CVAD and imatinib mesylate regimen for adults with de novo or minimally treated Philadelphia Chromosome (Ph) positive acute lymphoblastic leukemia (ALL). Blood 2008;112 [Abstract #2931].

27. Lee KH, Lee JH, Choi SJ, et al. Clinical effect of imatinib added to intensive combination chemotherapy for newly diagnosed Philadelphia chromosome-positive acute lymphoblastic leukemia. Leukemia 2005;19:1509–16.

28. Towatari M, Yanada M, Usui N, et al. Combination of intensive chemotherapy and imatinib can rapidly induce high-quality complete remission for a majority of patients with newly diagnosed BCR-ABL-positive acute lymphoblastic leukemia. Blood 2004;104:3507–12.

29. Wassmann B, Pfeifer H, Goekbuget N, et al. Alternating versus concurrent schedules of imatinib and chemotherapy as front-line therapy for Philadelphia-positive acute lymphoblastic leukemia (Ph+ ALL). Blood 2006;108:1469–77.

30. de Labarthe A, Rousselot P, Huguet-Rigal F, et al. Imatinib combined with induction or consolidation chemotherapy in patients with de novo Philadelphia chromosome-positive acute lymphoblastic leukemia: results of the GRAAPH-2003 study. Blood 2007;109:1408–13.

31. Dombret H, Gabert J, Boiron JM, et al. Outcome of treatment in adults with Philadelphia chromosome-positive acute lymphoblastic leukemia—results of the prospective multicenter LALA-94 trial. Blood 2002;100:2357–66.

32. Vignetti M, Fazi P, Cimino G, et al. Imatinib plus steroids induces complete remissions and prolonged survival in elderly Philadelphia chromosome-positive patients with acute lymphoblastic leukemia without additional chemotherapy: results of the Gruppo Italiano Malattie Ematologiche dell'Adulto (GIMEMA) LAL0201-B protocol. Blood 2007;109:3676–8.

33. Delannoy A, Delabesse E, Lheritier V, et al. Imatinib and methylprednisolone alternated with chemotherapy improve the outcome of elderly patients with Philadelphia-positive acute lymphoblastic leukemia: results of the GRAALL AFR09 study. Leukemia 2006;20:1526–32.

34. Ottmann OG, Wassmann B, Pfeifer H, et al. Imatinib compared with chemotherapy as front-line treatment of elderly patients with Philadelphia chromosome-positive acute lymphoblastic leukemia (Ph+ ALL). Cancer 2007;109: 2068–76.

35. Laport GG, Alvarnas JC, Palmer JM, et al. Long-term remission of Philadelphia chromosome-positive acute lymphoblastic leukemia after allogeneic

hematopoietic cell transplantation from matched sibling donors: a 20-year experience with the fractionated total body irradiation-etoposide regimen. Blood 2008;112:903–9.

36. Champlin RE, Schmitz N, Horowitz MM, et al. Blood stem cells compared with bone marrow as a source of hematopoietic cells for allogeneic transplantation. IBMTR Histocompatibility and Stem Cell Sources Working Committee and the European Group for Blood and Marrow Transplantation (EBMT). Blood 2000; 95:3702–9.

37. Schmitz N, Beksac M, Hasenclever D, et al. Transplantation of mobilized peripheral blood cells to HLA-identical siblings with standard-risk leukemia. Blood 2002;100:761–7.

38. Fielding AK, Rowe JM, Richards SM, et al. Prospective outcome data on 267 unselected adult patients with Philadelphia-chromosome positive acute lymphoblastic leukaemia confirms superiority of allogeneic transplant over chemotherapy in the pre-imatinib era: Results from the international ALL trial MRC UKALLXII/ECOG2993. Blood 2009;113:4489–96.

39. Thiebaut A, Vernant JP, Degos L, et al. Adult acute lymphocytic leukemia study testing chemotherapy and autologous and allogeneic transplantation. A follow-up report of the French protocol LALA 87. Hematol Oncol Clin North Am 2000;14: 1353–66, x.

40. Krejci O, van der Velden VH, Bader P, et al. Level of minimal residual disease prior to haematopoietic stem cell transplantation predicts prognosis in paediatric patients with acute lymphoblastic leukaemia: a report of the Pre-BMT MRD Study Group. Bone Marrow Transplant 2003;32:849–51.

41. Goulden N, Bader P, Van Der Velden V, et al. Minimal residual disease prior to stem cell transplant for childhood acute lymphoblastic leukaemia. Br J Haematol 2003;122:24–9.

42. Lee S, Kim DW, Kim YJ, et al. Minimal residual disease-based role of imatinib as a first-line interim therapy prior to allogeneic stem cell transplantation in Philadelphia chromosome-positive acute lymphoblastic leukemia. Blood 2003;102: 3068–70.

43. Lee S, Kim YJ, Min CK, et al. The effect of first-line imatinib interim therapy on the outcome of allogeneic stem cell transplantation in adults with newly diagnosed Philadelphia chromosome-positive acute lymphoblastic leukemia. Blood 2005; 105:3449–57.

44. Shimoni A, Kroger N, Zander AR, et al. Imatinib mesylate (STI571) in preparation for allogeneic hematopoietic stem cell transplantation and donor lymphocyte infusions in patients with Philadelphia-positive acute leukemias. Leukemia 2003;17:290–7.

45. Radich J, Gehly G, Lee A, et al. Detection of bcr-abl transcripts in Philadelphia chromosome-positive acute lymphoblastic leukemia after marrow transplantation. Blood 1997;89:2602–9.

46. Anderlini P, Sheth S, Hicks K, et al. Re: Imatinib mesylate administration in the first 100 days after stem cell transplantation. Biol Blood Marrow Transplant 2004;10:883–4.

47. Wassmann B, Pfeifer H, Stadler M, et al. Early molecular response to posttransplantation imatinib determines outcome in MRD+ Philadelphia-positive acute lymphoblastic leukemia (Ph+ ALL). Blood 2005;106:458–63.

48. Carpenter PA, Snyder DS, Flowers ME, et al. Prophylactic administration of imatinib after hematopoietic cell transplantation for high-risk Philadelphia chromosome-positive leukemia. Blood 2007;109:2791–3.

49. Visani G, Isidori A, Malagola M, et al. Efficacy of imatinib mesylate (STI571) in conjunction with alpha-interferon: long-term quantitative molecular remission in relapsed P-190(BCR-ABL)-positive acute lymphoblastic leukemia. Leukemia 2002;16:2159–60.

50. Wassmann B, Scheuring U, Pfeifer H, et al. Efficacy and safety of imatinib mesylate (Glivec) in combination with interferon-alpha (IFN-alpha) in Philadelphia chromosome-positive acute lymphoblastic leukemia (Ph+ ALL). Leukemia 2003;17:1919–24.

51. Martino R, Giralt S, Caballero MD, et al. Allogeneic hematopoietic stem cell transplantation with reduced-intensity conditioning in acute lymphoblastic leukemia: a feasibility study. Haematologica 2003;88:555–60.

52. Sullivan KM, Weiden PL, Storb R, et al. Influence of acute and chronic graft-versus-host disease on relapse and survival after bone marrow transplantation from HLA-identical siblings as treatment of acute and chronic leukemia. Blood 1989;73:1720–8.

53. Doney K, Fisher LD, Appelbaum FR, et al. Treatment of adult acute lymphoblastic leukemia with allogeneic bone marrow transplantation. Multivariate analysis of factors affecting acute graft-versus-host disease, relapse, and relapse-free survival. Bone Marrow Transplant 1991;7:453–9.

54. Cornelissen JJ, Carston M, Kollman C, et al. Unrelated marrow transplantation for adult patients with poor-risk acute lymphoblastic leukemia: strong graft-versus-leukemia effect and risk factors determining outcome. Blood 2001;97:1572–7.

55. Terwey TH, Massenkeil G, Tamm I, et al. Allogeneic SCT in refractory or relapsed adult ALL is effective without prior reinduction chemotherapy. Bone Marrow Transplant 2008;42:791–8.

56. Fielding AK, Richards SM, Chopra R, et al. Outcome of 609 adults after relapse of acute lymphoblastic leukemia (ALL); an MRC UKALL12/ECOG 2993 study. Blood 2007;109:944–50.

57. Biggs JC, Horowitz MM, Gale RP, et al. Bone marrow transplants may cure patients with acute leukemia never achieving remission with chemotherapy. Blood 1992;80:1090–3.

58. Forman SJ, Schmidt GM, Nademanee AP, et al. Allogeneic bone marrow transplantation as therapy for primary induction failure for patients with acute leukemia. J Clin Oncol 1991;9:1570–4.

59. Grigg AP, Szer J, Beresford J, et al. Factors affecting the outcome of allogeneic bone marrow transplantation for adult patients with refractory or relapsed acute leukaemia. Br J Haematol 1999;107:409–18.

60. Marks DI, Aversa F, Lazarus HM. Alternative donor transplants for adult acute lymphoblastic leukaemia: a comparison of the three major options. Bone Marrow Transplant 2006;38:467–75.

61. Gorre ME, Mohammed M, Ellwood K, et al. Clinical resistance to STI-571 cancer therapy caused by BCR-ABL gene mutation or amplification. Science 2001;293: 876–80.

62. Shah NP, Nicoll JM, Nagar B, et al. Multiple BCR-ABL kinase domain mutations confer polyclonal resistance to the tyrosine kinase inhibitor imatinib (STI571) in chronic phase and blast crisis chronic myeloid leukemia. Cancer Cell 2002;2:117–25.

63. Burger H, van Tol H, Boersma AW, et al. Imatinib mesylate (STI571) is a substrate for the breast cancer resistance protein (BCRP)/ABCG2 drug pump. Blood 2004;104:2940–2.

64. Thomas J, Wang L, Clark RE, et al. Active transport of imatinib into and out of cells: implications for drug resistance. Blood 2004;104:3739–45.

65. Donato NJ, Wu JY, Stapley J, et al. BCR-ABL independence and LYN kinase overexpression in chronic myelogenous leukemia cells selected for resistance to STI571. Blood 2003;101:690–8.

66. White DL, Saunders VA, Dang P, et al. OCT-1-mediated influx is a key determinant of the intracellular uptake of imatinib but not nilotinib (AMN107): reduced OCT-1 activity is the cause of low in vitro sensitivity to imatinib. Blood 2006; 108:697–704.

67. White DL, Saunders VA, Dang P, et al. Most CML patients who have a suboptimal response to imatinib have low OCT-1 activity: higher doses of imatinib may overcome the negative impact of low OCT-1 activity. Blood 2007;110: 4064–72.

68. Corbin AS, La Rosee P, Stoffregen EP, et al. Several Bcr-Abl kinase domain mutants associated with imatinib mesylate resistance remain sensitive to imatinib. Blood 2003;101:4611–4.

69. Hochhaus A, Kreil S, Corbin AS, et al. Molecular and chromosomal mechanisms of resistance to imatinib (STI571) therapy. Leukemia 2002;16:2190–6.

70. Jabbour E, Kantarjian H, Jones D, et al. Frequency and clinical significance of BCR-ABL mutations in patients with chronic myeloid leukemia treated with imatinib mesylate. Leukemia 2006;20:1767–73.

71. Hofmann WK, Jones LC, Lemp NA, et al. Ph(+) acute lymphoblastic leukemia resistant to the tyrosine kinase inhibitor STI571 has a unique BCR-ABL gene mutation. Blood 2002;99:1860–2.

72. von Bubnoff N, Schneller F, Peschel C, et al. BCR-ABL gene mutations in relation to clinical resistance of Philadelphia-chromosome-positive leukaemia to STI571: a prospective study. Lancet 2002;359:487–91.

73. Hofmann WK, Komor M, Wassmann B, et al. Presence of the BCR-ABL mutation Glu255Lys prior to STI571 (imatinib) treatment in patients with Ph+ acute lymphoblastic leukemia. Blood 2003;102:659–61.

74. Pfeifer H, Wassmann B, Pavlova A, et al. Kinase domain mutations of BCR-ABL frequently precede imatinib-based therapy and give rise to relapse in patients with de novo Philadelphia-positive acute lymphoblastic leukemia (Ph+ ALL). Blood 2007;110:727–34.

75. Jones D, Thomas D, Yin CC, et al. Kinase domain point mutations in Philadelphia chromosome-positive acute lymphoblastic leukemia emerge after therapy with BCR-ABL kinase inhibitors. Cancer 2008;113:985–94.

76. Soverini S, Colarossi S, Gnani A, et al. Contribution of ABL kinase domain mutations to imatinib resistance in different subsets of Philadelphia-positive patients: by the GIMEMA Working Party on Chronic Myeloid Leukemia. Clin Cancer Res 2006;12:7374–9.

77. Iacobucci I, Lonetti A, Messa F, et al. Expression of spliced oncogenic Ikaros isoforms in Philadelphia-positive acute lymphoblastic leukemia patients treated with tyrosine kinase inhibitors: implications for a new mechanism of resistance. Blood 2008;112:3847–55.

78. Cobb BS, Smale ST. Ikaros-family proteins: in search of molecular functions during lymphocyte development. Curr Top Microbiol Immunol 2005;290:29–47.

79. Mishra S, Zhang B, Cunnick JM, et al. Resistance to imatinib of bcr/abl p190 lymphoblastic leukemia cells. Cancer Res 2006;66:5387–93.

80. Shah NP, Tran C, Lee FY, et al. Overriding imatinib resistance with a novel ABL kinase inhibitor. Science 2004;305:399–401.

81. Talpaz M, Shah NP, Kantarjian H, et al. Dasatinib in imatinib-resistant Philadelphia chromosome-positive leukemias. N Engl J Med 2006;354:2531–41.

82. Kantarjian H, Giles F, Wunderle L, et al. Nilotinib in imatinib-resistant CML and Philadelphia chromosome-positive ALL. N Engl J Med 2006;354:2542–51.

83. Brown VI, Seif AE, Reid GS, et al. Novel molecular and cellular therapeutic targets in acute lymphoblastic leukemia and lymphoproliferative disease. Immunol Res 2008;42:84–105.

84. Cortes J, Rousselot P, Kim DW, et al. Dasatinib induces complete hematologic and cytogenetic responses in patients with imatinib-resistant or -intolerant chronic myeloid leukemia in blast crisis. Blood 2007;109:3207–13.

85. Ottmann O, Dombret H, Martinelli G, et al. Dasatinib induces rapid hematologic and cytogenetic responses in adult patients with Philadelphia chromosome positive acute lymphoblastic leukemia with resistance or intolerance to imatinib: interim results of a phase 2 study. Blood 2007;110:2309–15.

86. Larson RA, Ottmann OG, Shah NP, et al. Dasatinib 140 mg once daily (QD) has equivalent efficacy and improved safety compared with 70 mg twice daily (BID) in patients with imatinib-resistant or -Intolerant Philadelphia chromosome-positive acute lymphoblastic leukemia (Ph+ ALL): 2-year data from CA180-035. Blood 2008;112 [Abstract #2926].

87. Jabbour E, O'Brien S, Thomas D, et al. Combination of the hyperCVAD regimen with dasatinib is effective in patients with relapsed Philadelphia chromosome (Ph) positive acute lymphoblastic leukemia (ALL) and lymphoid blast phase chronic myeloid leukemia (CML-LB). Blood 2008;112 [Abstract #2919].

88. Ravandi F, Thomas D, Kantarjian H, et al. Phase II study of combination of hyperCVAD with dasatinib in frontline therapy of patients with Philadelphia chromosome (Ph) positive acute lymphoblastic leukemia (ALL). Blood 2008;112 [Abstract #2921].

89. Rousselot P, Cayuela J-M, Recher C, et al. Dasatinib (Sprycel®) and chemotherapy for first-line treatment in elderly patients with de novo Philadelphia positive ALL: Results of the first 22 patients Included in the EWALL-Ph-01 trial (on behalf of the European Working Group on Adult ALL (EWALL)). Blood 2008; 112 [Abstract #2920].

90. Foà R, Vitale A, Guarini A, et al. Line treatment of adult Ph+ acute lymphoblastic leukemia (ALL) patients. Final results of the GIMEMA LAL1205 study [abstract]. Blood 2008;112.

91. Soverini S, Martinelli G, Colarossi S, et al. Presence or the emergence of a F317L BCR-ABL mutation may be associated with resistance to dasatinib in Philadelphia chromosome-positive leukemia. J Clin Oncol 2006;24:e51–2.

92. Tokarski JS, Newitt JA, Chang CY, et al. The structure of Dasatinib (BMS-354825) bound to activated ABL kinase domain elucidates its inhibitory activity against imatinib-resistant ABL mutants. Cancer Res 2006;66:5790–7.

93. O'Hare T, Walters DK, Stoffregen EP, et al. In vitro activity of Bcr-Abl inhibitors AMN107 and BMS-354825 against clinically relevant imatinib-resistant Abl kinase domain mutants. Cancer Res 2005;65:4500–5.

94. Cortes J. Central nervous system involvement in adult acute lymphocytic leukemia. Hematol Oncol Clin North Am 2001;15:145–62.

95. Lazarus HM, Richards SM, Chopra R, et al. Central nervous system involvement in adult lymphoblastic leukemia at diagnosis: results from the international ALL trial MRC UKALL XII/ECOG E2993. Blood 2006;108:465–72.

96. Pfeifer H, Wassmann B, Hofmann WK, et al. Risk and prognosis of central nervous system leukemia in patients with Philadelphia chromosome-positive acute leukemias treated with imatinib mesylate. Clin Cancer Res 2003;9: 4674–81.

97. Leis JF, Stepan DE, Curtin PT, et al. Central nervous system failure in patients with chronic myelogenous leukemia lymphoid blast crisis and Philadelphia chromosome positive acute lymphoblastic leukemia treated with imatinib (STI-571). Leuk Lymphoma 2004;45:695–8.

98. Takayama N, Sato N, O'Brien SG, et al. Imatinib mesylate has limited activity against the central nervous system involvement of Philadelphia chromosome-positive acute lymphoblastic leukaemia due to poor penetration into cerebrospinal fluid. Br J Haematol 2002;119:106–8.

99. Porkka K, Koskenvesa P, Lundan T, et al. Dasatinib crosses the blood-brain barrier and is an efficient therapy for central nervous system Philadelphia chromosome-positive leukemia. Blood 2008;112:1005–12.

100. Bloomfield CD, Goldman AI, Alimena G, et al. Chromosomal abnormalities identify high-risk and low-risk patients with acute lymphoblastic leukemia. Blood 1986;67:415–20.

101. Gotz G, Weh HJ, Walter TA, et al. Clinical and prognostic significance of the Philadelphia chromosome in adult patients with acute lymphoblastic leukemia. Ann Hematol 1992;64:97–100.

102. Larson RA, Dodge RK, Burns CP, et al. A five-drug remission induction regimen with intensive consolidation for adults with acute lymphoblastic leukemia: cancer and leukemia group B study 8811. Blood 1995;85:2025–37.

103. Cytogenetic abnormalities in adult acute lymphoblastic leukemia: correlations with hematologic findings outcome. A collaborative study of the Groupe Francais de Cytogenetique Hematologique. Blood 1996;87:3135–42.

104. Secker-Walker LM, Prentice HG, Durrant J, et al. Cytogenetics adds independent prognostic information in adults with acute lymphoblastic leukaemia on MRC trial UKALL XA. MRC Adult Leukaemia Working Party. Br J Haematol 1997;96:601–10.

105. Wetzler M, Dodge RK, Mrozek K, et al. Prospective karyotype analysis in adult acute lymphoblastic leukemia: the cancer and leukemia Group B experience. Blood 1999;93:3983–93.

106. Faderl S, Kantarjian HM, Thomas DA, et al. Outcome of Philadelphia chromosome-positive adult acute lymphoblastic leukemia. Leuk Lymphoma 2000;36:263–73.

107. Mahon FX, Belloc F, Lagarde V, et al. MDR1 gene overexpression confers resistance to imatinib mesylate in leukemia cell line models. Blood 2003;101:2368–73.

108. Crossman LC, Druker BJ, Deininger MW, et al. hOCT 1 and resistance to imatinib. Blood 2005;106:1133–4, author reply 1134.

109. Gambacorti-Passerini C, Barni R, le Coutre P, et al. Role of alpha1 acid glycoprotein in the in vivo resistance of human BCR-ABL(+) leukemic cells to the abl inhibitor STI571. J Natl Cancer Inst 2000;92:1641–50.

110. Wendel HG, de Stanchina E, Cepero E, et al. Loss of p53 impedes the antileukemic response to BCR-ABL inhibition. Proc Natl Acad Sci U S A 2006;103:7444–9.

111. Graham SM, Jorgensen HG, Allan E, et al. Primitive, quiescent, Philadelphia-positive stem cells from patients with chronic myeloid leukemia are insensitive to STI571 in vitro. Blood 2002;99:319–25.

Long-term Outcomes in Survivors of Childhood Acute Lymphoblastic Leukemia

Paul C. Nathan, MD, MSc[a,b,*], Karen Wasilewski-Masker, MSc, MD[c,d], Laura A. Janzen, PhD[e]

KEYWORDS

- Acute lymphoblastic leukemia • Childhood
- Cancer survivor • Late effects • Cranial radiation

One-quarter of children newly diagnosed with cancer have acute lymphoblastic leukemia (ALL),[1] and more than 80% of those will become long-term survivors.[2,3] Consequently, survivors of childhood ALL are the largest portion of the over 325,000 survivors of childhood cancer who are alive in the United States. Many long-term survivors of childhood cancer will develop chronic physical[4,5] or psychosocial[6] problems as a result of their cancer or its therapy. Fortunately, most ALL survivors are at a lower than average risk of developing a late effect of therapy when compared with survivors of other pediatric cancers. However, children who were treated for ALL in the 1970s and 1980s are almost four times more likely than their siblings to develop a severe or life-threatening chronic medical condition.[7] By the time they reach 25 years from diagnosis, 65% report one or more chronic physical conditions, and 21% report a severe or life-threatening condition or have died of such a complication. Long-term outcomes of children treated more recently are not as well documented because of the shorter follow-up time.

Late effects in survivors of ALL are less commonly the result of the leukemia itself, but rather a consequence of therapy. Much of the evolution of ALL therapy over the

[a] Division of Hematology/Oncology, Department of Paediatrics, The Hospital for Sick Children, 555 University Avenue, Toronto, ON, M5G 1X8, Canada
[b] Management and Evaluation, The University of Toronto, Toronto, Ontario, Canada
[c] Aflac Cancer Center and Blood Disorders Service, Childhood Cancer Program, 5455 Merdian Mark Road, Suite 400, Atlanta, GA 30342, USA
[d] Emory University School of Medicine, Atlanta, GA, USA
[e] Department of Psychology, The Hospital for Sick Children, 555 University Avenue, Toronto, ON, M5G 1X8, Canada
* Corresponding author.
E-mail address: paul.nathan@sickkids.ca (P.C. Nathan).

Hematol Oncol Clin N Am 23 (2009) 1065–1082
doi:10.1016/j.hoc.2009.07.003
0889-8588/09/$ – see front matter © 2009 Elsevier Inc. All rights reserved.

hemonc.theclinics.com

past 4 decades has been targeted at maintaining or improving survival while minimizing long-term sequelae. Cranial radiation therapy (CRT) has been implicated as the most important risk factor for the development of physical, neurocognitive, and psychosocial morbidity. The inclusion of CRT in ALL treatment protocols in the late 1960s resulted in a major improvement in survival by reducing the risk of central nervous system (CNS) relapse. Early CNS-directed therapy consisted of 24 Gray (Gy) of craniospinal radiation, but this had significant detrimental effects on neurocognitive[8,9] and neuroendocrine[10] function. To reduce the risk of these late effects, subsequent protocols eliminated radiation to the spine, decreased the CRT dose to 18 Gy or 12 Gy, or replaced CRT with intrathecal and/or systemic drugs such as high-dose methotrexate.[11,12] Currently, CRT has been eliminated for all but the less than 20% of patients at highest risk for CNS relapse, and the feasibility of eliminating CRT for all newly diagnosed ALL patients is being studied.[13] Of the numerous chemotherapy agents used for the treatment of ALL, only a few have been implicated as causing late effects. These include anthracyclines (eg, doxorubicin, daunorubicin), oxazaphosphorine alkylating agents (eg, cyclophosphamide), corticosteroids (eg, prednisone, dexamethasone) and high-dose methotrexate. Most patients treated with anthracyclines or oxazaphosphorines receive them at relatively low doses and the risk of late effects is correspondingly low. Emerging research has suggested that susceptibility to certain late effects of chemotherapy, such as neurocognitive dysfunction after methotrexate treatment and cardiac toxicity as a result of anthracycline exposure, may be mediated by polymorphisms in specific genes responsible for chemotherapy metabolism.[14,15] More recently, the use of allogeneic hematopoietic stem cell transplantation (HSCT) for those groups of patients at highest risk for relapse, or those who have recurrent disease, has created a new subset of ALL survivors at increased risk for long-term medical problems. However, despite the risks arising from exposure to CRT, HSCT, and certain chemotherapy agents, it is likely that most children who survive after current ALL therapies will live normal lives with minimal or no long-term morbidity. The purpose of this paper is to review the more common, serious late effects of ALL therapy and to discuss the treatment exposures and patient characteristics that predispose some survivors to their development.

NEUROCOGNITIVE OUTCOMES

Survivors of childhood ALL may experience long-term neurocognitive deficits that limit their academic attainment, vocational options, and social success. Although current chemotherapy-only treatment regimens are significantly less neurotoxic than their predecessors, which included CRT, a significant proportion of survivors experience a decline in cognitive functioning following treatment. These neurocognitive difficulties contribute to some long-term survivors' perception of poorer overall quality of life,[16] and may impede them in achieving their full potential. Survivors of ALL treated with CRT are at the highest risk for neurocognitive impairment. Cognitive outcomes are related to CRT dose, with early studies reporting losses of approximately 10 intelligence quotient (IQ) points following whole brain radiation with 24 Gy.[17] More contemporary CRT dosages of 12–18 Gy are less neurotoxic, yet children treated with 18 Gy demonstrate some intellectual decline following treatment, with an average decrease of nearly four IQ points per year over at least 6 years after diagnosis.[9] The effects of CRT on neurocognitive function are delayed, and may not be evident for several years following treatment.[18] Further, the effects are progressive, with poorer intellectual outcomes associated with increasing time since treatment.[19] Individual patient variables have been shown to moderate the effects of CRT on intellectual function such that younger age at radiation exposure and female gender are associated with lower long-term intelligence.[20,21] CRT-related declines in basic cognitive processes, such as attention, processing speed, and working memory are believed to underlie the declines seen on multidimensional intelligence tests,[22] whereas verbal and language-related abilities are typically spared.[23] Academic abilities in children treated with CRT are significantly lower relative to matched controls[24,25] and as a group, ALL survivors treated with CRT are more likely than their siblings to require special education services, and less likely to graduate from high school.[26]

Because of the marked cognitive and academic declines associated with CRT, chemotherapy-only protocols are now used for all but the highest risk patients. Although less severe than with CRT, CNS prophylaxis with chemotherapy-only is associated with mild, yet measurable cognitive decline. Approximately 20% to 30% of children who receive chemotherapy without CRT experience some degree of neurocognitive impairment.[27,28] Within the multi-agent chemotherapy regimens, high-dose systemic or intrathecal methotrexate (MTX), cytosine arabinoside (ARA-C), and corticosteroids are most often investigated as potential causes of neurocognitive deficits.

Longitudinal studies of children treated with chemotherapy who are assessed up to 6 years following the completion of treatment indicate that there are modest declines in intelligence, attention, reading, arithmetic, and visual-motor function; however, performance typically remains within the average range.[27–29] Cross-sectional studies of long-term survivors paint a similar picture of mild but measurable deficits in some areas of neurocognitive function. A recent meta-analysis of the neuropsychological sequelae of chemotherapy-only treatment included 13 studies and concluded that ALL survivors demonstrate significantly lower IQ, attention, visual-perception, mathematics and reading achievement, and verbal memory than controls.[30] Again, a gender effect was reported, with girls showing lower intellectual performance than boys. Despite relatively good neurocognitive outcomes for school-age children treated with current chemotherapy-only protocols for standard-risk ALL, there are particular subgroups of survivors who experience more significant cognitive impairments. Children treated for infant ALL, CNS positive disease and those who experience relapse display greater long-term neurocognitive impairment,[31,32] due primarily to their need for more aggressive treatments.

Because of these long-term neurocognitive deficits, ranging from mild to severe, regular and comprehensive neuropsychological evaluations of ALL survivors is highly recommended.[33] Educating patients and their families about typical cognitive effects following treatment and how to cope with these changes is part of the neuropsychological consultation. In addition, assessment of neurocognitive and academic function forms the basis of recommendations for educational programming and interventions. Repeat assessment is particularly helpful before expected changes in the demands placed on survivors, such as transition from elementary to high school, or high school to college. Interventions provided to ALL survivors, based on the neuropsychological assessment results, may include access to special education services, along with school-based accommodations and modifications to teaching strategies and assessment methods. In addition, cognitive rehabilitation programs that have been used with traumatic brain injury survivors are now being applied to ALL survivors, and aim to specifically mediate attention or executive functioning difficulties.[34,35] Because the attention and behavioral difficulties seen in long-term ALL survivors can mimic those characteristic of attention-deficit/hyperactivity disorder (ADHD), primarily the inattentive subtype, the use of stimulant medication in ALL survivors has been investigated. There is preliminary support for the use of methylphenidate to improve inattention and possibly social skills, but not necessarily other cognitive deficits or academic problems.[36,37] Going beyond treatment of existing deficits, efforts to minimize or prevent neurocognitive late effects in ALL survivors are underway, and include risk-adapted treatment protocols and the search for neuroprotective agents. If successful, the growing number of childhood ALL survivors would enjoy greater academic, vocational and social success, and increased overall quality of life.

NEUROLOGIC OUTCOMES

Beyond neuropsychological difficulties, survivors are also at risk for neurologic sequelae of their therapy, including stroke and peripheral neuropathies. Acute CNS events such as ischemic or hemorrhagic stroke can cause cerebral injury.[38] The chemotherapeutic agent, asparaginase, can alter the balance of coagulation factors resulting in thrombosis or less commonly, hemorrhage. Although most patients who experience asparaginase-induced CNS events have gross recovery of neurologic impairment, some may not.[39] Although rare, stroke can also occur in long-term survivors at a higher rate than is observed in the general population. The Childhood Cancer Survivor Study (CCSS) reported on the incidence of stroke in 4828 leukemia survivors (including ALL and acute myelogenous leukemia (AML)) who were at least 5 years from diagnosis.[40] A stroke was reported by 37 survivors, with an actuarial cumulative incidence of 0.73% at 25 years. The mean interval from ALL diagnosis to late-occurring stroke was approximately 10 years. Almost half of the survivors who had a stroke had a prior history of relapse, and those treated with greater than 30 Gy CRT were nearly 8 times more likely to suffer a stroke than those treated with chemotherapy alone. Risk factors for stroke in the general population, such as hypertension, diabetes mellitus, oral contraceptive use by women, and tobacco use did not modify the risk of stroke in this survivor cohort.

Treatment with vinca alkaloids (particularly vincristine) is associated with the development of peripheral neuropathies during therapy, and can be particularly severe in patients with Charcot-Marie-Tooth disease.[41,42] However, even survivors without Charcot-Marie-Tooth may have abnormal nerve conduction that persists after the completion of therapy, as shown by prolongation of motor evoked potentials at 5 years after the completion of therapy.[43] Although most survivors do not display physical signs of impaired nerve conduction after therapy ends, some may have persistent fine or gross motor difficulties.[43] The cause of persistent motor dysfunction in ALL survivors likely extends beyond vincristine-induced peripheral neuropathy and may include muscle weakness[44] and CNS damage that affects visual-motor integration.[45]

Finally, high-dose intravenous ARA-C is associated with acute neurotoxicity, including cerebellar dysfunction.[46] Children who experience acute toxicity are likely at increased risk of long-term sequelae, but because ARA-C use is confounded with methotrexate and dexamethasone use, there is no independent evidence to support this.

NEUROENDOCRINE OUTCOMES

CRT, used as either treatment or prophylaxis for CNS disease, is associated with an increased risk for neuroendocrine dysfunction as a result of damage to the hypothalamus. In general, these complications are dose dependent and have become less common with the trend toward decreasing the dose of CRT or avoiding it completely. Growth hormone (GH) deficiency and precocious puberty are the most common central endocrinopathies observed in ALL survivors. Survivors treated with conventional CRT doses do not usually develop other central endocrinopathies, such as central adrenal insufficiency, hyperprolactinemia, gonadotropin insufficiency, or central (secondary) hypothyroidism, as these are associated with doses of ≥ 40 Gy[47] and, with the exception of recurrent CNS disease, doses of this magnitude are rarely administered in the treatment of ALL. Primary hypothyroidism, however, can occur after cranial, craniospinal and total body irradiation (TBI) because of direct exposure of the thyroid gland to radiation, even at relatively low doses (≥ 10 Gy).[48]

GH deficiency is the most common endocrinopathy detected after CRT.[49] It is a likely complication with doses ≥ 24 Gy, but has been observed with doses as low as 18 Gy, or 10 Gy given as a single dose as part of TBI.[10,49] Although chemotherapy, specifically corticosteroids, can result in growth delay during treatment, this is normally followed by a period of catch-up growth after completion of therapy.[10,50] In addition to higher CRT dose, risk factors for GH deficiency and short stature include younger age at diagnosis and female gender.[10,49,51] In addition, exposure to craniospinal radiation and TBI further impairs growth because of direct effects on skeletal growth.[51,52] GH replacement therapy in ALL survivors is controversial. In an analysis from the CCSS cohort, there was no increased risk of leukemia recurrence in those treated with GH; however, there was an increase in second malignant neoplasms (SMNs).[53] Of 119 survivors of acute leukemia and non-Hodgkin lymphoma treated with GH, 6 (4 of whom had survived ALL) developed an SMN. Due to the small number of events in this study, further research is warranted to obtain an accurate estimate of risk.[54]

Precocious puberty is the development of physical signs of puberty before a normal age. The age that is considered normal varies by gender, race, and physical characteristics. Precocious puberty is a well-described late effect of CRT in doses of 18 to 24 Gy, and is more common in girls.[55–57] However, most female ALL survivors experience menarche at a normal age. In two large cohorts, the CCSS and the National Cancer Institute Children's Cancer Group Leukemia Follow-up Study, 92% of female ALL survivors reported a normal age of menarche compared with 97% and 96% of controls, respectively.[58,59]

Individual chemotherapy agents have not been found to affect the hypothalamus or pituitary gland, or to be associated with endocrine late effects.[49] In a report from the CCSS, young adult survivors of ALL were more than three times as likely as sibling controls to have a chronic endocrine condition; however, the risk in nonrelapsed, nonirradiated survivors was similar to that seen in the sibling control group.[7] Growth and puberty should be monitored closely in all survivors. Survivors treated with CRT, craniospinal radiation or TBI warrant even closer monitoring (at least every 6 months) for growth, pubertal development, and symptoms of hypothyroidism.[47] If a problem is suspected, patients should be referred to a pediatric endocrinologist for hormonal evaluation and consideration of therapy. Although survivors of ALL are at low risk for the development of central endocrinopathies (central adrenal insufficiency, hyperprolactinemia, gonadotropin insufficiency, secondary hypothyroidism) because of their relatively low-dose CRT exposure, they should be monitored clinically for symptoms of these disorders and tested as indicated.

OBESITY AND METABOLIC OUTCOMES

Many studies have demonstrated an increased risk of being overweight in childhood ALL survivors.[60–65] The largest of these, conducted by the CCSS, compared 1765 adult survivors of pediatric ALL with 2565 siblings.[66] Survivors who received greater than 20 Gy CRT were significantly more likely than their siblings to be overweight. Girls treated before the age of 4 years were at particular risk. A repeat assessment 8 years later revealed that all survivors treated with CRT (even at doses less than 20 Gy) had a more rapid increase in their body mass index (calculated as the weight in kilograms divided by height in meters squared) than their siblings over the follow-up period.[62] Overall, 61% of female survivors and 67% of male survivors were either overweight or obese. Possible mechanisms of CRT-induced obesity include the induction of GH deficiency[66] and insensitivity to leptin, an adipose-derived hormone that plays a key role in the regulation of energy intake and expenditure via its effect on the hypothalamus.[67] One polymorphism in the leptin receptor gene (Gln223Arg) has been demonstrated to significantly increase the risk of developing obesity among female survivors of ALL treated with $\geq$20 Gy CRT.[67]

The risk of obesity in ALL survivors who are not treated with CRT is controversial. In the CCSS study, survivors treated with chemotherapy alone were not at an increased risk of being overweight compared with their siblings.[62,66] However, other studies have demonstrated an increased prevalence of overweight in this group.[63,64,68] Treatment with corticosteroids has been linked to increased energy intake[69,70] and decreased physical activity,[70] both of which may lead to weight gain during therapy. Corticosteroids may cause physical inactivity secondary to myopathy[44,71] or damage to bones[72] or joints.[73] Vincristine-induced peripheral neuropathy may further limit activity.[43] Young children receiving ALL therapy seem to have an earlier adiposity rebound (when body mass index begins to increase after its nadir in childhood) than healthy controls, and this may further potentiate the development of overweight.[74] In addition, survivors of ALL have been shown to have reduced habitual physical activity[75,76] both during and after therapy, resulting in a decrease in total energy expenditure.

Independent of specific leukemia therapies, several factors may predispose children with ALL to becoming overweight. As therapy continues for up to 3 years, many children miss opportunities to participate in physical activity during times of hospitalization or periods of suppressed immunity. Often, teachers and parents restrict activity unnecessarily.[77] Risk factors for overweight that are common in the general population, including poor dietary choices, increased sedentary behavior (television, computers, video games), and decreased physical activity,[76,78] may contribute to the risk of overweight, although the interaction between these behavior patterns and the cancer therapy has not been studied adequately. However, even if survivors of ALL treated with chemotherapy alone are not at increased risk of overweight compared with the general population, the consequences of their being overweight are potentially more severe given their predisposition to cardiovascular and metabolic disease.

Beyond obesity, survivors of ALL treated with CRT seem to be at increased risk of developing the metabolic syndrome,[79-81] a clustering of three or more of obesity, hypertension, impaired glucose metabolism, and dyslipidemia.[82] This syndrome has been linked conclusively to an increased risk of coronary artery disease [83,84] and the development of type 2 diabetes in adults. A small study of both irradiated and nonirradiated adult survivors of childhood ALL demonstrated that 62% of patients manifested at least one of obesity, dyslipidemia, hypertension, or insulin resistance, with irradiated survivors being at a greater risk.[79] GH deficiency may play a central role in the development of abdominal obesity and the metabolic syndrome in these survivors. A comparison of 44 adults who had received CRT for childhood ALL to an equal number of age- and gender-matched controls demonstrated higher levels of plasma insulin, glucose, low density lipoprotein cholesterol, triglycerides, and leptin, and lower levels of high density lipoprotein cholesterol, along with increased body mass index in the survivor group.[85] Another study of 75 survivors (50 irradiated, 25 not irradiated) revealed that 17% of the survivors met the criteria for the metabolic syndrome.[86] Sixty percent of subjects treated with CRT, compared with 20% of those who were not, had two or more components of metabolic syndrome. Low GH levels were detected in 64% of subjects overall and 85% of those who had received CRT, suggesting a relationship between GH levels and metabolic dysfunction. Abdominal obesity, particularly visceral adiposity, seems to be a strong predictor of metabolic abnormalities such as insulin resistance, hypertension, and lipid abnormalities, and is an independent predictor of mortality.[87] CRT is a risk factor for the redistribution of fat resulting in increased abdominal obesity and particularly visceral adiposity in some survivors.[88] Given the risk and potential morbidity associated with becoming overweight after ALL treatment, prevention of overweight and other metabolic dysfunction should be emphasized, both during therapy and at follow-up. Patients with ALL tend to gain weight during therapy and in the first year after treatment,[60,89,90] suggesting that interventions are likely best implemented during therapy, rather than waiting until the conclusion of treatment. Implementing and testing such programs, preferably multidimensional programs that target diet, exercise, and sedentary behavior, should be a priority in future ALL trials.

BONE TOXICITIES

Osteonecrosis (avascular necrosis) and bone mineral density (BMD) deficits are both associated with treatment of ALL, specifically prolonged corticosteroid exposure. Osteonecrosis, a condition in which bone death occurs because of poor blood supply and marrow ischemia can manifest with debilitating pain and immobility. Corticosteroids are believed to cause direct damage by inducing apoptosis of osteoblasts and mature osteocytes, and indirectly by increasing the fat content of the marrow leading to fat embolization and vascular compression.[91,92] Asparaginase is associated with coagulation abnormalities, and may contribute to the development of osteonecrosis in a manner similar to thrombophilia, which is a known risk factor in the general population.[93,94] The overall incidence of osteonecrosis has been reported as 1.6% to 9.3% in various ALL protocols.[95–98] Higher incidence is associated with higher cumulative corticosteroid doses and older age ($\geq$10 years) at treatment.[97] Additional risk factors may include white race and the use of dexamethasone compared with prednisone.[97] Both genders are affected; however, the peak incidence occurs at an older age in boys (16–20 years) versus girls (15–19 years), likely because of their later onset of puberty.[97] Pain is the main symptom of osteonecrosis, although this may not be a good indicator of its presence or severity. Patients may also present with a joint effusion or isolated limp. Symptoms usually develop within 2 to 3 years of therapy, with most patients presenting during the maintenance phase of their therapy.[95–98] Weight-bearing joints are affected in 90% of patients, with the knees and hips being the most common joints; multiple joints are affected in more than 75% of patients.[95–101] Magnetic resonance imaging (MRI) is considered to be the best modality for evaluating osteonecrosis, and detection can precede symptoms.[94,100,101] However, the role of MRI in screening is still being established as not all patients with radiographic evidence of osteonecrosis will develop symptoms or progressive joint destruction.[102] Depending on the location, stage, age of the patient, and status of their cancer treatment, patients can be treated supportively with physical therapy, limitation of weight-bearing and pain management and/or surgically. Surgical interventions include core decompression, rotational osteotomy, vascularized bone graft and arthroplasty (joint replacement).[103] Newer treatments being investigated include the use of hyperbaric oxygen for treatment and statins for prevention.[103]

Decreased BMD is not associated with acute morbidity; however, its presence may increase long-term morbidity by increasing the risk of fracture at a younger-than-expected age in adulthood. Corticosteroids can cause a decrease in BMD by inhibiting osteoblast activity, increasing bone resorption, interfering with the GH/insulin-like growth factor 1 axis, reducing muscle strength, and disturbing calcium balance at the level of the gut and kidney.[104–106] Methotrexate is cytotoxic to the osteoblast and may act in synergy with corticosteroids.[107] Endocrinopathies, such as hypogonadism and GH deficiency, may also lead to low BMD. Whereas some treatment protocols have been associated with a risk of fracture during or shortly after therapy,[98,108] low BMD after the completion of therapy has not necessarily been associated with fracture risk. However, studies have shown that ALL survivors have a relatively low BMD compared with the general population.[72,109–111] Whereas most survivors will recover bone mass with increasing time off therapy, some demonstrate severe BMD deficits (Z-scores of more than 2.5 standard deviations [SD] less than the mean) years after therapy.[72,112,113] Failure to reach an optimal peak bone mass may increase the risk of osteoporosis and fracture as an older adult, although this is unproven. Current guidelines for patients treated with corticosteroids, methotrexate or HSCT recommend a baseline evaluation of BMD by dual x-ray absorptiometry or quantitative computed tomography at entry into long-term follow-up, typically 2 years after completion of therapy.[47] A severe BMD deficit is defined as a Z-score more than 2.5 SD less than the mean and low BMD as a Z-score value between 1 and 2.5 SD less than the mean. Because the World Health Organization definitions of osteopenia and osteoporosis apply only to postmenopausal women, it is not recommended that these terms be used in children and adolescents.[114] By detecting problems before attainment of peak BMD (typically in the third decade of life), diet and lifestyle can be adjusted. Treatment of BMD deficits in children includes weight-bearing exercise, adequate nutritional intake of calcium and vitamin D, supplementation of calcium and vitamin D if dietary intake is insufficient, and treatment of underlying conditions such as hypogonadism and GH deficiency.[115] Educating survivors to avoid smoking, alcohol, and excess caffeine intake is important as these factors can all worsen BMD deficits. Cancer survivors with a severe BMD deficit may benefit from consultation with an endocrinologist for evaluation of predisposing conditions and consideration of pharmacologic intervention with hormonal treatment, calcitonin, or bisphosphonates.[115]

OTHER SERIOUS PHYSICAL LATE EFFECTS OF THERAPY

Other serious late effects observed in some ALL survivors include cardiotoxicity, SMN and infertility. Cardiotoxicity is associated with exposure to anthracyclines and irradiation to the heart, particularly at a young age. With the exception of TBI given in the HSCT setting, and relatively small doses of thoracic spine radiation given as part of craniospinal irradiation, cardiac exposure to radiation in ALL patients is rare. Cumulative anthracycline doses vary widely between ALL protocols, and many protocols contain no anthracycline agent. Doses of ≥ 300 mg/m^2 of doxorubicin or daunorubicin are associated with the highest risk of cardiotoxicity, usually in the form of left ventricular dysfunction.[116–118] Due to additional cardiovascular risk factors such as obesity, physical inactivity, and the metabolic syndrome, ALL survivors, particularly those who receive ≥ 24 Gy of CRT, may be at an even further increased risk for cardiac events.[119] This risk increases with time, emphasizing the need for life-long surveillance. The Children's Oncology Group recommends a screening echocardiogram or MUGA at frequencies of every 1, 2, or 5 years, depending on age at exposure, cumulative anthracycline dose, and concomitant radiation exposure.[47]

SMN include AML and myelodysplastic syndrome (MDS) as a result of exposure to certain chemotherapy agents, and solid tumors as a result of radiation exposure. Although the risk of an SMN is much greater than that observed in the general population, the actual risk for an individual ALL survivor is low, especially in those with no history of radiation exposure.[7,120,121] The 15-year cumulative incidence of developing an SMN after ALL treatment has been estimated between 1.4% and 4.2%.[120–124] However, this risk estimate decreases to 1.2% in nonirradiated survivors.[121] Chemotherapy agents associated with secondary AML/MDS include anthracyclines, oxazaphosphorines, and epipodophyllotoxins.[47] These malignancies usually occur within 2 to 5 years of exposure, although some late occurrences (10–15 years from exposure) have been associated with oxazaphosphorines.[47] Not all ALL treatment protocols contain these classes of chemotherapy. SMN risk caused by radiation exposure increases with time and these neoplasms usually occur at least 10 to 15 years after exposure.[120] Although many of these malignancies are basal cell carcinomas and meningiomas, other carcinomas, brain tumors, sarcomas, and lymphomas have been reported.[120–124] Survivors should be counseled to practice general health maintenance such as using sunscreen, avoiding cancer-associated habits including smoking or excessive alcohol consumption, eating a healthful diet, exercising, and pursuing preventative health services. Survivors with high-risk exposures such as radiation may require more careful monitoring, including annual physical examinations with attention to radiation-exposed areas, and early screening for adult malignancies such as breast and colon cancer.[47]

Fertility is a concern for many cancer survivors once they enter their young adult years. Fortunately, most ALL survivors treated on current regimens for newly diagnosed patients are at relatively low risk for reduced fertility. Although gonadal toxicity can result from exposure to alkylating agents, such as cyclophosphamide, the cumulative doses commonly used in ALL regimens (1–2 g/m^2) are generally less than the threshold associated with permanent gonadal damage.[47,125,126] High-risk groups include patients who have received an HSCT with high-dose alkylating agent conditioning, TBI, or both. In addition, males with testicular disease are treated with testicular radiation resulting in infertility. Although doses of CRT used in ALL rarely reach the cumulative doses of ≥ 40 Gy associated with central gonadotropin insufficiency, craniospinal radiation can result in direct ovarian damage, even at modest doses.[127,128] It is recommended that all patients be followed closely with Tanner staging throughout puberty, and laboratory evaluation (eg, FSH, LH, estradiol, or testosterone) if concerns about pubertal delay arise.[47] Although the risk for gonadal toxicity is relatively low after up-front ALL therapy, some centers consider offering sperm banking to all pubertal males at the time of diagnosis, because those that develop recurrent disease may be rendered infertile by their relapse therapy. Although premature ovarian failure has been reported in survivors of some types of childhood cancer,[129,130] particularly those treated during puberty, it is unlikely to occur in females treated on standard ALL protocols. Further research is needed to quantify the risk of premature ovarian failure in survivors of relapse protocols and HSCT.

PROVIDING LIFE-LONG RISK-BASED CARE TO SURVIVORS OF ACUTE LYMPHOBLASTIC LEUKEMIA

In 2003, the National Research Council's Institute of Medicine (IOM) published a report entitled "Childhood cancer survivorship: improving care and quality of life."[131] This was 1 of 2 seminal reports addressing issues among cancer survivors, both of which included a series of recommendations aimed at ensuring life-long medical care for survivors of cancer on the premise that the risk for many serious health problems can be reduced by prevention or early detection.[131,132] The IOM concluded that all cancer survivors require a systematic plan for periodic screening, surveillance, and prevention that is adapted to the risks arising from their previous cancer and its therapy, and genetic predispositions, lifestyle behaviors, and co-morbid health conditions.[131,132] To guide the frequency and focus of medical visits, and the ordering of appropriate surveillance tests, comprehensive guidelines for the life-long care of childhood cancer survivors have been published in North America,[133] the United Kingdom[134] and Scotland,[135] among others. Many North American insti-tutions adhere to guidelines created by the Children's Oncology Group, entitled "Long-Term Follow-Up Guidelines for Survivors of Childhood, Adolescent, and Young Adult Cancers"[133] (available at www.survivorshipguidelines.org). Because there is considerable heterogeneity in the treatment protocols used for each type of cancer, the specific recommendations are based on each survivor's treatment exposures rather than their diagnosis. Thus, it is crucial that ALL survivors have knowledge of their prior therapies, including radiation field and dose, the names of the chemotherapy agents that they received, and the cumulative doses of those agents for which there is a relationship between dose and risk of late effects (eg, an-thracyclines, oxazaphosphorines). Ideally, all survivors should be provided with a survivor care plan before discharge from a pediatric center that documents their exposures, any late effects that have developed before discharge, and a detailed plan for their ongoing medical care, including the frequency of medical appointments and the recommended timing of specific surveillance tests, such as echocardio-grams or neurocognitive testing.[136] Unfortunately, there are numerous barriers to the successful transition of survivors from pediatric to adult care. These barriers include limitations in survivors' knowledge about their exposure-related risks and their need for follow-up, psychological and developmental factors that influence survivors' maturity and readiness to assume responsibility for their own health care, a lack of adult health care providers with the knowledge, experience, or willing-ness to care for these patients, and the absence of health insurance for some survi-vors.[137] Preparation for transition needs to occur early to "facilitate the continuous, medically and developmentally appropriate implementation of risk-based guidelines for the monitoring and management of late effects of childhood cancer and its treat-ment; and to support the normal maturational processes involved with growing from childhood to adulthood."[137]

SUMMARY

Most children diagnosed with ALL in the current era will become long-term survivors, and many of these survivors can be expected to suffer minimal or no morbidity as a result of their cancer therapy. However, some therapeutic exposures, including CRT, HSCT, and certain chemotherapy agents, will place some ALL survivors at a risk for the development of serious late effects from their therapy. Such late effects include neurocognitive and neurologic dysfunction, endocrine and metabolic abnor-malities, bone toxicity, SMNs, and cardiac damage. Thus, all ALL survivors require periodic, life-long medical care that is adapted to the specific risks arising from their specific treatment exposures, along with counseling about ways to live a healthy lifestyle.

ACKNOWLEDGMENTS

The authors are grateful to Mark Greenberg, Kevin Oeffinger, and Lillian Meacham for their invaluable help in reviewing this manuscript.

REFERENCES

1. Ries LAG, Smith MA, Gurney JG, et al, editors Cancer incidence and survival among children and adolescents: United States SEER program 1975-1995. (NIH publication no. 99-4649). Bethesda (MD): National Cancer Institute, SEER Program; 1999.
2. Moghrabi A, Levy DE, Asselin B, et al. Results of the Dana Farber Cancer Institute ALL Consortium Protocol 95-01 for children with acute lymphoblastic leukemia. Blood 2007;109(3):896–904.
3. Schrappe M, Reiter A, Ludwig WD, et al. Improved outcome in childhood acute lymphoblastic leukemia despite reduced use of anthracyclines and cranial radiotherapy: results of trial ALL-BFM 90. German-Austrian Swiss ALL-BFM study group. Blood 2000;95(11):3310–22.
4. Oeffinger KC, Mertens AC, Sklar CA, et al. Chronic health conditions in adult survivors of childhood cancer. N Engl J Med 2006;355:1572–82.
5. Geenen MM, Cardous-Ubbink MC, Kremer LCM, et al. Medical assessment of adverse health outcomes in long-term survivors of childhood cancer. JAMA 2007;297(24):2705–15.
6. Langeveld NE, Ubbink MC, Last BF, et al. Educational achievement, employment and living situation in long-term young adult survivors of childhood cancer in the Netherlands. Psychooncology 2003;12(3):213–25.
7. Mody R, Li S, Dover DC, et al. Twenty-five-year follow-up among survivors of childhood acute lymphoblastic leukemia: a report from the childhood cancer survivor study. Blood 2008;111(12):5515–23.
8. Spiegler BJ, Kennedy K, Maze R, et al. Comparison of long-term neurocognitive outcomes in young children with acute lymphoblastic leukemia treated with cranial radiation or high-dose or very high-dose intravenous methotrexate. J Clin Oncol 2006;24(24):3858–64.
9. Jankovic M, Brouwers P, Valsecchi MG, et al. Association of 1800 cGy cranial irradiation with intellectual function in children with acute lymphoblastic leukaemia. ISPACC. International study group on psychosocial aspects of childhood cancer. Lancet 1994;344(8917):224–7.
10. Howard SC, Pui CH. Endocrine complications in pediatric patients with acute lymphoblastic leukemia. Blood Rev 2002;16(4):225–43.
11. Nesbit ME Jr, Sather HN, Robison LL, et al. Presymptomatic central nervous system therapy in previously untreated childhood acute lymphoblastic leukaemia: comparison of 1800 rad and 2400 rad. A report for Children's Cancer Study Group. Lancet 1981;1(8218):461–6.
12. Bleyer WA, Poplack D. Prophylaxis and treatment of leukemia in the central nervous system and other sanctuaries. Semin Oncol 1985;12(2):131–48.
13. Pui CH, Robison LL, Look AT. Acute lymphoblastic leukaemia. Lancet 2008; 371(9617):1030–43.
14. Krull KR, Brouwers P, Jain N, et al. Folate pathway genetic polymorphisms are related to attention disorders in childhood leukemia survivors. J Pediatr 2008; 152(1):101–5.
15. Blanco JG, Leisenring WM, Gonzalez-Covarrubias VM, et al. Genetic polymorphisms in the carbonyl reductase 3 gene CBR3 and the NAD(P)H:quinone

oxidoreductase 1 gene NQO1 in patients who developed anthracycline-related congestive heart failure after childhood cancer. Cancer 2008;112(12):2789–95.

16. Wu E, Robison LL, Jenney ME, et al. Assessment of health-related quality of life of adolescent cancer patients using the Minneapolis-Manchester quality of life adolescent questionnaire. Pediatr Blood Cancer 2007;48(7):678–86.

17. Cousens P, Waters B, Said J, et al. Cognitive effects of cranial irradiation in leukaemia: a survey and meta-analysis. J Child Psychol Psychiatry 1988; 29(6):839–52.

18. Rubenstein CL, Varni JW, Katz ER. Cognitive functioning in long-term survivors of childhood leukemia: a prospective analysis. J Dev Behav Pediatr 1990;11(6):301–5.

19. Kato M, Azuma E, Ido M, et al. Ten-year survey of the intellectual deficits in children with acute lymphoblastic leukemia receiving chemoimmunotherapy. Med Pediatr Oncol 1993;21(6):435–40.

20. Bleyer WA, Fallavollita J, Robison L, et al. Influence of age, sex, and concurrent intrathecal methotrexate therapy on intellectual function after cranial irradiation during childhood: a report from the Children's Cancer Study Group. Pediatr Hematol Oncol 1990;7(4):329–38.

21. Waber DP, Urion DK, Tarbell NJ, et al. Late effects of central nervous system treatment of acute lymphoblastic leukemia in childhood are sex-dependent. Dev Med Child Neurol 1990;32(3):238–48.

22. Schatz J, Kramer JH, Ablin A, et al. Processing speed, working memory and IQ: a developmental model of cognitive deficits following cranial radiation therapy. Neuropsychology 2000;14(2):189–200.

23. Fletcher JM, Copeland DR. Neurobehavioral effects of central nervous system prophylactic treatment of cancer in children. J Clin Exp Neuropsychol 1988; 10(4):495–537.

24. Smibert E, Anderson V, Godber T, et al. Risk factors for intellectual and educational sequelae of cranial irradiation in childhood acute lymphoblastic leukaemia. Br J Cancer 1996;73(6):825–30.

25. Anderson V, Smibert E, Ekert H, et al. Intellectual, educational, and behavioural sequelae after cranial irradiation and chemotherapy. Arch Dis Child 1994;70(6): 476–83.

26. Mitby PA, Robison LL, Whitton JA, et al. Utilization of special education services and educational attainment among long-term survivors of childhood cancer: a report from the Childhood Cancer Survivor Study. Cancer 2003;97(4):1115–26.

27. Mulhern RK, Fairclough D, Ochs J. A prospective comparison of neuropsychologic performance of children surviving leukemia who received 18-Gy, 24-Gy, or no cranial irradiation. J Clin Oncol 1991;9(8):1348–56.

28. Copeland DR, Moore BD 3rd, Francis DJ, et al. Neuropsychologic effects of chemotherapy on children with cancer: a longitudinal study. J Clin Oncol 1996;14(10):2826–35.

29. Ochs J, Mulhern R, Fairclough D, et al. Comparison of neuropsychologic functioning and clinical indicators of neurotoxicity in long-term survivors of childhood leukemia given cranial radiation or parenteral methotrexate: a prospective study. J Clin Oncol 1991;9(1):145–51.

30. Peterson CC, Johnson CE, Ramirez LY, et al. A meta-analysis of the neuropsychological sequelae of chemotherapy-only treatment for pediatric acute lymphoblastic leukemia. Pediatr Blood Cancer 2008;51(1):99–104.

31. Silverman LB, McLean TW, Gelber RD, et al. Intensified therapy for infants with acute lymphoblastic leukemia: results from the Dana Farber Cancer Institute consortium. Cancer 1997;80(12):2285–95.

32. Mulhern RK, Ochs J, Fairclough D, et al. Intellectual and academic achievement status after CNS relapse: a retrospective analysis of 40 children treated for acute lymphoblastic leukemia. J Clin Oncol 1987;5(6): 933–40.

33. Nathan PC, Patel SK, Dilley K, et al. Guidelines for identification of, advocacy for, and intervention in neurocognitive problems in survivors of childhood cancer: a report from the Children's Oncology Group. Arch Pediatr Adolesc Med 2007;161(8):798–806.

34. Butler RW. Attentional processes and their remediation in childhood cancer. Med Pediatr Oncol 1998;(Suppl 1):75–8.

35. Butler RW, Copeland DR. Attentional processes and their remediation in children treated for cancer: a literature review and the development of a therapeutic approach. J Int Neuropsychol Soc 2002;8(1):115–24.

36. Thompson SJ, Leigh L, Christensen R, et al. Immediate neurocognitive effects of methylphenidate on learning-impaired survivors of childhood cancer. J Clin Oncol 2001;19(6):1802–8.

37. Mulhern RK, Khan RB, Kaplan S, et al. Short-term efficacy of methylphenidate: a randomized, double-blind, placebo-controlled trial among survivors of childhood cancer. J Clin Oncol 2004;22(23):4795–803.

38. Hogan AM, Kirkham FJ, Isaacs EB. Intelligence after stroke in childhood: review of the literature and suggestions for future research. J Child Neurol 2000;15(5): 325–32.

39. Ott N, Ramsay NK, Priest JR, et al. Sequelae of thrombotic or hemorrhagic complications following L-asparaginase therapy for childhood lymphoblastic leukemia. Am J Pediatr Hematol Oncol 1988;10(3):191–5.

40. Bowers DC, Liu Y, Leisenring W, et al. Late-occurring stroke among long-term survivors of childhood leukemia and brain tumors: a report from the childhood cancer survivor study. J Clin Oncol 2006;24(33):5277–82.

41. Chauvenet AR, Shashi V, Selsky C, et al. Vincristine-induced neuropathy as the initial presentation of Charcot-Marie-Tooth disease in acute lymphoblastic leukemia: a Pediatric Oncology Group study. J Pediatr Hematol Oncol 2003; 25(4):316–20.

42. Trobaugh-Lotrario AD, Smith AA, Odom LF. Vincristine neurotoxicity in the presence of hereditary neuropathy. Med Pediatr Oncol 2003;40(1):39–43.

43. Lehtinen SS, Huuskonen UE, Harila-Saari AH, et al. Motor nervous system impairment persists in long-term survivors of childhood acute lymphoblastic leukemia. Cancer 2002;94(9):2466–73.

44. Wright MJ, Halton JM, Martin RF, et al. Long-term gross motor performance following treatment for acute lymphoblastic leukemia. Med Pediatr Oncol 1998;31(2):86–90.

45. Hockenberry M, Krull K, Moore K, et al. Longitudinal evaluation of fine motor skills in children with leukemia. J Pediatr Hematol Oncol 2007; 29(8):535–9.

46. Nand S, Messmore HL Jr, Patel R, et al. Neurotoxicity associated with systemic high-dose cytosine arabinoside. J Clin Oncol 1986;4(4):571–5.

47. Mills J, Bonner A, Francis K. The development of constructivist grounded theory. International Journal of Qualitative Methods 2006;5(1):25–35.

48. DeGroot LJ. Effects of irradiation on the thyroid gland. Endocrinol Metab Clin North Am 1993;22(3):607–15.

49. Sklar CA, Constine LS. Chronic neuroendocrinological sequelae of radiation therapy. Int J Radiat Oncol Biol Phys 1995;31(5):1113–21.

50. Haddy TB, Mosher RB, Nunez SB, et al. Growth hormone deficiency after chemotherapy for acute lymphoblastic leukemia in children who have not received cranial radiation. Pediatr Blood Cancer 2006;46(2):258–61.

51. Chow EJ, Friedman DL, Yasui Y, et al. Decreased adult height in survivors of childhood acute lymphoblastic leukemia: a report from the childhood cancer survivor study. J Pediatr 2007;150(4):370–5, 75 e1.

52. Chemaitilly W, Sklar CA. Endocrine complications of hematopoietic stem cell transplantation. Endocrinol Metab Clin North Am 2007;36(4):983–98, ix.

53. Mertens AC, Yasui Y, Liu Y, et al. Pulmonary complications in survivors of childhood and adolescent cancer. A report from the Childhood Cancer Survivor Study. Cancer 2002;95(11):2431–41.

54. Ergun-Longmire B, Mertens AC, Mitby P, et al. Growth hormone treatment and risk of second neoplasms in the childhood cancer survivor. J Clin Endocrinol Metab 2006;91(9):3494–8.

55. Leiper AD, Stanhope R, Kitching P, et al. Precocious and premature puberty associated with treatment of acute lymphoblastic leukaemia. Arch Dis Child 1987;62(11):1107–12.

56. Ogilvy-Stuart AL, Clayton PE, Shalet SM. Cranial irradiation and early puberty. J Clin Endocrinol Metab 1994;78(6):1282–6.

57. Quigley C, Cowell C, Jimenez M, et al. Normal or early development of puberty despite gonadal damage in children treated for acute lymphoblastic leukemia. N Engl J Med 1989;321(3):143–51.

58. Chow EJ, Friedman DL, Yasui Y, et al. Timing of menarche among survivors of childhood acute lymphoblastic leukemia: a report from the childhood cancer survivor study. Pediatr Blood Cancer 2008;50(4):854–8.

59. Mills JL, Fears TR, Robison LL, et al. Menarche in a cohort of 188 long-term survivors of acute lymphoblastic leukemia. J Pediatr 1997;131(4):598–602.

60. Reilly JJ, Ventham JC, Newell J, et al. Risk factors for excess weight gain in children treated for acute lymphoblastic leukaemia. Int J Obes Relat Metab Disord 2000;24(11):1537–41.

61. Sklar CA, Mertens AC, Walter A, et al. Changes in body mass index and prevalence of overweight in survivors of childhood acute lymphoblastic leukemia: role of cranial irradiation. Med Pediatr Oncol 2000;35(2):91–5.

62. Garmey EG, Liu Q, Sklar CA, et al. Longitudinal changes in obesity and body mass index among adult survivors of childhood acute lymphoblastic leukemia: a report from the Childhood Cancer Survivor Study. J Clin Oncol 2008;26(28):4639–45.

63. Mayer EI, Reuter M, Dopfer RE, et al. Energy expenditure, energy intake and prevalence of obesity after therapy for acute lymphoblastic leukemia during childhood. Horm Res 2000;53(4):193–9.

64. Van Dongen-Melman JE, Hokken-Koelega AC, Hahlen K, et al. Obesity after successful treatment of acute lymphoblastic leukemia in childhood. Pediatr Res 1995;38(1):86–90.

65. Warner JT, Evans WD, Webb DK, et al. Body composition of long-term survivors of acute lymphoblastic leukaemia. Med Pediatr Oncol 2002;38(3):165–72.

66. Oeffinger KC, Mertens AC, Sklar CA, et al. Obesity in adult survivors of childhood acute lymphoblastic leukemia: a report from the childhood cancer survivor study. J Clin Oncol 2003;21(7):1359–65.

67. Ross JA, Oeffinger KC, Davies SM, et al. Genetic variation in the leptin receptor gene and obesity in survivors of childhood acute lymphoblastic leukemia: a report from the Childhood Cancer Survivor Study. J Clin Oncol 2004;22(17):3558–62.

68. Nathan PC, Jovcevska V, Ness KK, et al. The prevalence of overweight and obesity in pediatric survivors of cancer. J Pediatr 2006;149(4):518–25, e2.
69. Reilly JJ, Brougham M, Montgomery C, et al. Effect of glucocorticoid therapy on energy intake in children treated for acute lymphoblastic leukemia. J Clin Endocrinol Metab 2001;86(8):3742–5.
70. Jansen H, Postma A, Stolk RP, et al. Acute lymphoblastic leukemia and obesity: increased energy intake or decreased physical activity? Support Care Cancer 2009;17(1):103–6.
71. van Brussel M, Takken T, Lucia A, et al. Is physical fitness decreased in survivors of childhood leukemia? A systematic review. Leukemia 2005;19(1):13–7.
72. Kaste SC, Jones-Wallace D, Rose SR, et al. Bone mineral decrements in survivors of childhood acute lymphoblastic leukemia: frequency of occurrence and risk factors for their development. Leukemia 2001;15(5):728–34.
73. Kadan-Lottick NS, Dinu I, Wasilewski-Masker K, et al. Osteonecrosis in adult survivors of childhood cancer: a report from the Childhood Cancer Survivor Study. J Clin Oncol 2008;26(18):3038–45.
74. Reilly JJ, Kelly A, Ness P, et al. Premature adiposity rebound in children treated for acute lymphoblastic leukemia. J Clin Endocrinol Metab 2001;86(6):2775–8.
75. Reilly JJ, Ventham JC, Ralston JM, et al. Reduced energy expenditure in preobese children treated for acute lymphoblastic leukemia. Pediatr Res 1998;44(4):557–62.
76. Warner JT, Bell W, Webb DK, et al. Daily energy expenditure and physical activity in survivors of childhood malignancy. Pediatr Res 1998;43(5):607–13.
77. Aznar S, Webster AL, San Juan AF, et al. Physical activity during treatment in children with leukemia: a pilot study. Appl Physiol Nutr Metab 2006;31(4):407–13.
78. Jago R, Baranowski T, Baranowski JC, et al. BMI from 3–6 y of age is predicted by TV viewing and physical activity, not diet. Int J Obes (Lond) 2005;29(6):557–64.
79. Oeffinger KC, Buchanan GR, Eshelman DA, et al. Cardiovascular risk factors in young adult survivors of childhood acute lymphoblastic leukemia. J Pediatr Hematol Oncol 2001;23(7):424–30.
80. Talvensaari KK, Lanning M, Tapanainen P, et al. Long-term survivors of childhood cancer have an increased risk of manifesting the metabolic syndrome. J Clin Endocrinol Metab 1996;81(8):3051–5.
81. Taskinen M, Saarinen-Pihkala UM, Hovi L, et al. Impaired glucose tolerance and dyslipidaemia as late effects after bone-marrow transplantation in childhood. Lancet 2000;356:993–7.
82. Cook S. The metabolic syndrome: antecedent of adult cardiovascular disease in pediatrics. J Pediatr 2004;145:427–30.
83. Reaven GM. Banting lecture 1988. Role of insulin resistance in human disease. Diabetes 1988;37:1595–607.
84. Lakka H-M, Laaksonen DE, Lakka TA, et al. The metabolic syndrome and total and cardiovascular disease mortality in middle-aged men. JAMA 2002;288(21):2709–16.
85. Link K, Moell C, Garwicz S, et al. Growth hormone deficiency predicts cardiovascular risk in young adults treated for acute lymphoblastic leukemia in childhood. J Clin Endocrinol Metab 2004;89(10):5003–12.
86. Gurney JG, Ness KK, Sibley SD, et al. Metabolic syndrome and growth hormone deficiency in adult survivors of childhood acute lymphoblastic leukemia. Cancer 2006;107(6):1303–12.

87. Kuk JL, Katzmarzyk PT, Nichaman MZ, et al. Visceral fat is an independent predictor of all-cause mortality in men. Obesity (Silver Spring) 2006;14(2): 336–41.

88. Janiszewski PM, Oeffinger KC, Church TS, et al. Abdominal obesity, liver fat, and muscle composition in survivors of childhood acute lymphoblastic leukemia. J Clin Endocrinol Metab 2007;92(10):3816–21.

89. Halton JM, Atkinson SA, Barr RD. Growth and body composition in response to chemotherapy in children with acute lymphoblastic leukemia. Int J Cancer Suppl 1998;11:81–4.

90. Baillargeon J, Langevin AM, Lewis M, et al. Therapy-related changes in body size in Hispanic children with acute lymphoblastic leukemia. Cancer 2005; 103(8):1725–9.

91. Lafforgue P. Pathophysiology and natural history of avascular necrosis of bone. Joint Bone Spine 2006;73(5):500–7.

92. Mattano L. The skeletal remains: porosis and necrosis of bone in the marrow transplantation setting. Pediatr Transplant 2003;7(Suppl 3):71–5.

93. Hanada T, Horigome Y, Inudoh M, et al. Osteonecrosis of vertebrae in a child with acute lymphocytic leukaemia during L-asparaginase therapy. Eur J Pediatr 1989;149(3):162–71.

94. Watson RM, Roach NA, Dalinka MK. Avascular necrosis and bone marrow edema syndrome. Radiol Clin North Am 2004;42(1):207–19.

95. Arico M, Boccalatte MF, Silvestri D, et al. Osteonecrosis: an emerging complication of intensive chemotherapy for childhood acute lymphoblastic leukemia. Haematologica 2003;88(7):747–53.

96. Burger B, Beier R, Zimmermann M, et al. Osteonecrosis: a treatment related toxicity in childhood acute lymphoblastic leukemia (ALL) – experiences from trial ALL-BFM 95. Pediatr Blood Cancer 2005;44(3):220–5.

97. Mattano LA Jr, Sather HN, Trigg ME, et al. Osteonecrosis as a complication of treating acute lymphoblastic leukemia in children: a report from the Children's Cancer Group. J Clin Oncol 2000;18(18):3262–72.

98. Strauss AJ, Su JT, Dalton VM, et al. Bony morbidity in children treated for acute lymphoblastic leukemia. J Clin Oncol 2001;19(12):3066–72.

99. Enright H, Haake R, Weisdorf D. Avascular necrosis of bone: a common serious complication of allogeneic bone marrow transplantation. Am J Med 1990;89(6):733–8.

100. Koo KH, Kim R. Quantifying the extent of osteonecrosis of the femoral head. A new method using MRI. J Bone Joint Surg Br 1995;77(6):875–80.

101. Ojala AE, Paakko E, Lanning FP, et al. Osteonecrosis during the treatment of childhood acute lymphoblastic leukemia: a prospective MRI study. Med Pediatr Oncol 1999;32(1):11–7.

102. Ribeiro RC, Fletcher BD, Kennedy W, et al. Magnetic resonance imaging detection of avascular necrosis of the bone in children receiving intensive prednisone therapy for acute lymphoblastic leukemia or non-Hodgkin lymphoma. Leukemia 2001;15(6):891–7.

103. Jones LC, Hungerford DS. Osteonecrosis: etiology, diagnosis, and treatment. Curr Opin Rheumatol 2004;16(4):443–9.

104. Hochberg Z. Mechanisms of steroid impairment of growth. Horm Res 2002; 58(Suppl 1):33–8.

105. Leonard MB. Assessment of bone health in children and adolescents with cancer: promises and pitfalls of current techniques. Med Pediatr Oncol 2003; 41(3):198–207.

106. Pfeilschifter J, Diel IJ. Osteoporosis due to cancer treatment: pathogenesis and management. J Clin Oncol 2000;18(7):1570–93.
107. Davies JH, Evans BA, Jenney ME, et al. Skeletal morbidity in childhood acute lymphoblastic leukaemia. Clin Endocrinol (Oxf) 2005;63(1):1–9.
108. Halton JM, Atkinson SA, Fraher L, et al. Altered mineral metabolism and bone mass in children during treatment for acute lymphoblastic leukemia. J Bone Miner Res 1996;11(11):1774–83.
109. Hoorweg-Nijman JJ, Kardos G, Roos JC, et al. Bone mineral density and markers of bone turnover in young adult survivors of childhood lymphoblastic leukaemia. Clin Endocrinol (Oxf) 1999;50(2):237–44.
110. Kaste SC, Rai SN, Fleming K, et al. Changes in bone mineral density in survivors of childhood acute lymphoblastic leukemia. Pediatr Blood Cancer 2006;46(1): 77–87.
111. Warner JT, Evans WD, Webb DK, et al. Relative osteopenia after treatment for acute lymphoblastic leukemia. Pediatr Res 1999;45(4 Pt 1):544–51.
112. Henderson RC, Madsen CD. Bone mineral content and body composition in children and young adults with cystic fibrosis. Pediatr Pulmonol 1999;27(2): 80–4.
113. Hesseling PB, Hough SF, Nel ED, et al. Bone mineral density in long-term survivors of childhood cancer. Int J Cancer Suppl 1998;11:44–7.
114. Leslie WD, Adler RA, El-Hajj Fuleihan G, et al. Application of the 1994 WHO classification to populations other than postmenopausal Caucasian women: the 2005 ISCD official positions. J Clin Densitom 2006;9(1):22–30.
115. Wasilewski-Masker K, Kaste SC, Hudson MM, et al. Bone mineral density deficits in survivors of childhood cancer: long-term follow-up guidelines and review of the literature. Pediatrics 2008;121(3):e705–13.
116. Adams MJ, Lipshultz SE, Schwartz C, et al. Radiation-associated cardiovascular disease: manifestations and management. Semin Radiat Oncol 2003; 13(3):346–56.
117. Lipshultz SE, Lipsitz SR, Sallan SE, et al. Chronic progressive cardiac dysfunction years after doxorubicin therapy for childhood acute lymphoblastic leukemia. J Clin Oncol 2005;23(12):2629–36.
118. Nysom K, Holm K, Lipsitz SR, et al. Relationship between cumulative anthracycline dose and late cardiotoxicity in childhood acute lymphoblastic leukemia. J Clin Oncol 1998;16(2):545–50.
119. Oeffinger KC. Are survivors of acute lymphoblastic leukemia (ALL) at increased risk of cardiovascular disease? Pediatr Blood Cancer 2008;50(2 Suppl):462–7 [discussion: 468].
120. Hijiya N, Hudson MM, Lensing S, et al. Cumulative incidence of secondary neoplasms as a first event after childhood acute lymphoblastic leukemia. JAMA 2007;297(11):1207–15.
121. Loning L, Zimmermann M, Reiter A, et al. Secondary neoplasms subsequent to Berlin-Frankfurt-Munster therapy of acute lymphoblastic leukemia in childhood: significantly lower risk without cranial radiotherapy. Blood 2000;95(9):2770–5.
122. Bhatia S, Sather HN, Pabustan OB, et al. Low incidence of second neoplasms among children diagnosed with acute lymphoblastic leukemia after 1983. Blood 2002;99(12):4257–64.
123. Borgmann A, Zinn C, Hartmann R, et al. Secondary malignant neoplasms after intensive treatment of relapsed acute lymphoblastic leukaemia in childhood. Eur J Cancer 2008;44(2):257–68.

124. Neglia JP, Meadows AT, Robison LL, et al. Second neoplasms after acute lymphoblastic leukemia in childhood. N Engl J Med 1991;325(19):1330–6.

125. Meistrich ML, Wilson G, Brown BW, et al. Impact of cyclophosphamide on long-term reduction in sperm count in men treated with combination chemotherapy for Ewing and soft tissue sarcomas. Cancer 1992;70(11):2703–12.

126. Ridola V, Fawaz O, Aubier F, et al. Testicular function of survivors of childhood cancer: a comparative study between ifosfamide- and cyclophosphamide-based regimens. Eur J Cancer 2009;45(5):814–8.

127. Hamre MR, Robison LL, Nesbit ME, et al. Effects of radiation on ovarian function in long-term survivors of childhood acute lymphoblastic leukemia: a report from the Childrens Cancer Study Group. J Clin Oncol 1987;5(11):1759–65.

128. Howell S, Shalet S. Gonadal damage from chemotherapy and radiotherapy. Endocrinol Metab Clin North Am 1998;27(4):927–43.

129. Sklar C. Maintenance of ovarian function and risk of premature menopause related to cancer treatment. J Natl Cancer Inst Monogr 2005;(34):25–7.

130. Chiarelli AM, Marrett LD, Darlington G. Early menopause and infertility in females after treatment for childhood cancer diagnosed in 1964–1988 in Ontario, Canada. Am J Epidemiol 1999;150(3):245–54.

131. Hewitt M, Weiner SL, Simone JV. Childhood cancer survivorship: improving care and quality of life. Washington, DC: The National Academies Press; 2003.

132. Hewitt M, Greenfield S, Stovall E. From cancer patient to cancer survivor: lost in transition. Washington, DC: National Academies Press; 2005.

133. Hudson M, Landier W, Eshelman D, et al, editors. Long-term follow-up guidelines for survivors of childhood, adolescent, and young adult cancers. Acadia (CA): Children's Oncology Group; 2006.

134. Skinner R, Wallace WHB, Levitt GA, editors. Therapy based long term follow up: practice statement. 2nd edition. United Kingdom Children's Cancer Study Group; 2005.

135. Long term follow up of survivors of childhood cancer: a national clinical guideline. Scottish Collegiate Guidelines Network. Available at: http://www.sign.ac.uk/pdf/sign76.pdf. Accessed March 11, 2009.

136. Landier W, Wallace WH, Hudson MM. Long-term follow-up of pediatric cancer survivors: education, surveillance, and screening. Pediatr Blood Cancer 2006; 46(2):149–58.

137. Freyer DR, Brugieres L. Adolescent and young adult oncology: transition of care. Pediatr Blood Cancer 2008;50(5 Suppl):1116–9.

Role of Minimal Residual Disease Monitoring in Adult and Pediatric Acute Lymphoblastic Leukemia

Dario Campana, MD, PhD[a,b,c,*]

KEYWORDS

- Acute lymphoblastic leukemia • Minimal residual disease
- Flow cytometry • Polymerase chain reaction • Prognosis

The response to treatment in patients with leukemia traditionally has been assessed by counting cells in blood while attempting to identify residual leukemic blasts in blood and bone marrow by microscopic analysis. The latter task is challenging when leukemic cells are present in small numbers. This is particularly true in patients with acute lymphoblastic leukemia (ALL), because the morphology of ALL blast cells is often indistinguishable from that of lymphoid precursors (the progenitors of B-lymphocytes, often called hematogones by hemopathologists) and activated mature lymphocytes. The distinction between leukemic and normal cells is exceedingly difficult in bone marrow samples recovering after cessation of chemotherapy or after transplant, where the percentage of hematogones may surpass 10% of the total cellular population. Hence, the morphologic assessment of remission by morphology in patients with ALL can be imprecise, especially if samples are examined when normal hematopoiesis is reconstituting. With contemporary chemotherapy regimens, only a few patients with ALL have unusually high percentages of marrow leukemic lymphoblasts

This work was supported by grants CA60419 and CA21765 from the National Cancer Institute, and by the American Lebanese Syrian Associated Charities (ALSAC).
[a] Department of Oncology, St. Jude Children's Research Hospital, 262 Danny Thomas Place, Memphis TN 38105, USA
[b] Departments of Oncology and Pathology, St. Jude Children's Research Hospital, 262 Danny Thomas Place, Memphis TN 38105, USA
[c] University of Tennessee Health Science Center, 920 Madison Avenue, Memphis, TN 38163, USA
* Department of Oncology, St. Jude Children's Research Hospital, 262 Danny Thomas Place, Memphis TN 38105.
E-mail address: dario.campana@stjude.org

Hematol Oncol Clin N Am 23 (2009) 1083–1098
doi:10.1016/j.hoc.2009.07.010
0889-8588/09/$ – see front matter © 2009 Elsevier Inc. All rights reserved.

persisting during remission induction therapy.[1] Most patients achieve morphologic remission, and the amount of residual disease not detectable by morphology (ie, minimal residual disease [MRD]) has remained unknown until relatively recently.

Janossy and colleagues were among the first to examine the remission status of patients with ALL with a method more sensitive and specific than morphology. During the initial attempts to leukemia immunophenotype nearly 30 years ago, these investigators noticed that T-lineage ALL cells simultaneously expressed nuclear terminal deoxynucleotidyl transferase (TdT) and T-cell markers, whereas peripheral blood and bone marrow cells of healthy individuals did not.[2] Logically, they used this cell marker combination to investigate whether patients with T-lineage ALL in morphologic remission had measurable MRD and found cells with the immunophenotype of T-lineage ALL in the bone marrow of some patients.[3] The usefulness of immunologic markers to identify residual leukemic cells was corroborated and expanded by the development of monoclonal antibodies and clinical flow cytometers, which allowed the detection of MRD, not only in T-lineage ALL, but also in B-lineage ALL.[4–6] In parallel to these developments, other investigators took advantage of the development of the polymerase chain reaction (PCR) technique to amplify fusion transcripts in ALL cells[7,8] and to use antigen receptor genes as a PCR target to detect MRD.[9–12] This groundbreaking work was enriched by the subsequent research of numerous laboratories, resulting in methods for objective MRD detection whose sensitivity is much higher than that of morphology.[13,14]

In addition to developing and refining MRD assays, early studies had to define the value of MRD testing to assess response to treatment and predict relapse. Although the clinical significance of MRD is now clear, initial efforts to systematically study MRD in patients were met with some skepticism about the clinical value of MRD testing. This often stemmed from the belief, supported by animal studies and clinical observations,[15,16] that leukemia distribution might be extremely heterogeneous, rendering MRD testing uninformative in regards to residual leukemic burden and treatment response. Others thought that MRD studies might not provide any additional information over established clinicobiologic prognostic features of ALL. As discussed in this article, numerous studies now have demonstrated conclusively that MRD is a powerful prognostic indicator in childhood ALL, and there is mounting evidence that this is also the case in adult ALL patients. Therefore, an increasing number of treatment protocols use MRD measurements for ALL risk assignment.

MINIMAL RESIDUAL DISEASE ASSAYS
Targets for Flow Cytometric Studies

ALL cells express immunophenotypic features that can be used to distinguish them from normal hematopoietic cells, including hematogones and activated lymphocytes.[14] These leukemia-associated immunophenotypes can be grouped into three main categories. First, are immunophenotypes that are expressed during normal development but are limited to cells in certain tissues. This group is exemplified by the immunophenotypic features of T-lineage ALL cells, which are expressed only by a subset of thymocytes and never found outside the thymus. These leukemia-associated immunophenotypes are those that were used by Janossy and colleagues[3] in their early studies of MRD, and they now can be used effectively with flow cytometry to monitor MRD in T-lineage ALL, and also to detect disease dissemination in T-cell lymphoblastic lymphoma.[17]

The second group of leukemia-associated immunophenotypes is constituted by the expression of fusion proteins derived from chromosomal breakpoints, such as BCR-ABL1, ETV6-RUNX1, or TCF3-PBX1. This set of markers is attractive because of its leukemia specificity. Its use, however, has been limited by the lack of suitable anti-bodies for reliable flow cytometric analysis of these proteins. Within this category, one also can include the ectopic expression of proteins promoted by gene transloca-tions, such as expression of PBX1 in lymphoblasts (PBX1 expression normally is confined to nonlymphoid cells)[18] and the high molecular weight melanoma-associated antigen, the human homolog of the rat NG2, on the surface of 11q23-positive ALL.[19,20]

The third type of leukemia-associated immunophenotype is represented by markers normally expressed during lymphohematopoiesis but found in abnormal combinations in leukemic cells. These phenotypes at times are termed asynchronous or aber-rant.[4,21–23] They offer the most widely available option to monitor MRD in ALL by flow cytometry, and the only one that currently can be used to track MRD in B-lineage ALL. The use of this approach requires a deep understanding of the immunopheno-types expressed by normal hematopoietic cells, not only during steady-state condi-tions, but also during chemotherapy and active regeneration.

Targets for Polymerase Chain Reaction Studies

Two main categories of targets can be used to distinguish leukemic cells from normal cells with PCR. One is represented by gene fusions, such as BCR-ABL1, MLL-AFF1, TCF3-PBX1, and ETV6-RUNX1, which result in the expression of aberrant mRNA tran-scripts in leukemic cells.[24,25] Recurrent abnormalities suitable for amplification in clin-ical samples are present in approximately 40% of children and 50% of adults with ALL.[25,26] With the uncovering of genetic abnormalities afforded by the application of whole-genome screening technologies,[27,28] however, it is very likely that additional genetic targets will enrich the available gamut.

The second category of PCR targets for MRD studies in ALL is composed by the clonal rearrangement of immunoglobulin (IG) and T-cell receptor (TCR) genes whose junctional regions are unique to the leukemic clone, forming a molecular signature of sorts. The most commonly used way to target these rearrangements for MRD detection requires identification of the various IG or TCR gene rearrangements in each lymphoid malignancy at diagnosis.[29] Thus, the presence of rearranged genes typically is screened by using PCR primers matched to opposite sides of the junctions, to the V and J regions of various IG and TCR genes. If an apparently clonal rearrangement is found, one must ensure that it derives from ALL cells and not from contaminating normal cells by analyzing the PCR product for their clonal origin (eg, by heteroduplex analysis). The ALL-derived PCR products then are used for direct sequencing of the junctional regions of the IG/TCR gene rearrangements, which, in turn, are used to design junc-tional region-specific oligonucleotides, also called allele-specific oligonucleotides.[29] Clonal IG/TCR gene rearrangements also can be detected with high-resolution electro-phoresis systems, such as radioactive fingerprinting or fluorescent gene scanning, without the need for patient-specific oligonucleotides, but this approach has a consid-erably lower sensitivity, usually not better than 0.1%.[30,31]

Most (greater than 95%) of B-lineage ALL cases have IG gene rearrangements.[32,33] Cross-lineage TCR gene rearrangements also occur in up to 90% of B-lineage ALL cases.[34] TCR genes are rearranged in most cases of T-lineage ALL.[35–37] Cross-lineage IG gene rearrangements occur in approximately 20% of T-ALL cases.[32]

Quantitation of MRD by PCR using either fusion transcripts or IG/TCR gene rearrange-ments most is frequently performed by using real-time quantitative PCR (RQ-PCR).[38]

Strengths and Weaknesses of Various Minimal Residual Disease Assays

In virtually all patients with ALL, leukemia-associated immunophenotypes can be defined at diagnosis and then used to monitor MRD during treatment.

Immunophenotypes sufficiently dissimilar from those of normal cells to allow a sensitivity of detection of 0.01% are expressed by most cells in approximately 95% of cases.[22,39] In addition to their potential for accurate quantification of MRD, flow cytometric analysis also can be used to examine the status of normal hematopoietic cell maturation at the same time. This gives information about the degree of hemodilution in the sample studied and on the degree of lymphohematopoietic recovery.

The reliability of flow cytometric MRD assays depends on several factors. First, the immunophenotypes used to distinguish leukemic cells must not overlap with those of normal lymphoid cells. Certain immunophenotypes apparently absent among cells from a bone marrow sample from a healthy donor may become apparent if the bone marrow is actively proliferating after chemotherapy. The label leukemia-associated immunophenotype should be reserved to those marker combinations that truly never are expressed by normal hematopoietic cells, regardless of their proliferative and developmental status. A second factor that affects the reliability of flow cytometric MRD assays is the number of cells available for study. If one wants to detect one leukemic cell in 10,000, at least 100,000 mononuclear cells must be examined, because 10 leukemic events are the minimum required to interpret flow cytometry results.[22] Third, the markers used need to be expressed stably on leukemic cells, and the investigator must be aware of fluctuations that may occur during chemotherapy.[40] Finally, and perhaps most importantly, the laboratory performing the studies must have specific expertise in MRD assays. Simple availability of a flow cytometer and experience in leukemia immunophenotyping are not sufficient to perform MRD studies proficiently.

A strength of PCR amplification of fusion transcripts is the stable association between the molecular abnormality and the leukemic clone, regardless of cellular changes caused by therapy or clonal selection. Moreover, a positive MRD result with this technique may alert one to the presence of preleukemic or leukemia-initiating cells,[41] which might be missed by other methods. There are, however, some disadvantages in using fusion transcripts as a target for MRD studies. Perhaps the most worrisome is the imprecise estimate of the percentage of leukemic cells present. This is due to the fact that the amount of transcripts per leukemic cell may vary from patient to patient with the same genetic subtype of ALL, and could be affected by chemotherapy and the cell integrity when the sample is examined.[25] Because of these variables, it is practically impossible to establish a precise relation between quantity of PCR product and number of leukemic cells.

PCR amplification of antigen-receptor genes is a reliable and accurate method for monitoring MRD that can be used in most cases of childhood and adult ALL.[29,38,42] In contrast to fusion transcripts, rearranged IG and TCR genes are present in one copy per cell, which, with the use of RQ-PCR, allows a very precise quantitation of MRD to be achieved. IG and TCR genes in ALL might undergo continuing or secondary rearrangements,[43] resulting in oligoclonality (ie, the presence of subclones having distinct clonal IG/TCR gene rearrangements). IGH genes in B-lineage ALL are prone to subclone formation, with multiple gene rearrangements found in 30% to 40% of cases at diagnosis.[44] Minor clones that might be undetected at diagnosis may become predominant during the course of the disease,[45,46] an observation that has led to recommending targeting two or more different rearrangements.[29] Indeed, multiple targets are identifiable in most ALL cases, but multiple targets that allow detection of MRD with a high sensitivity (eg, 0.01%) are not identifiable in approximately 30% of cases.[47,48]

When applied in parallel to study MRD in the same samples, flow cytometry and PCR amplification of IG/TCR genes yield remarkably similar measurements, if MRD is present at a greater than or equal to 0.01% level (**Fig. 1**).[49–51]

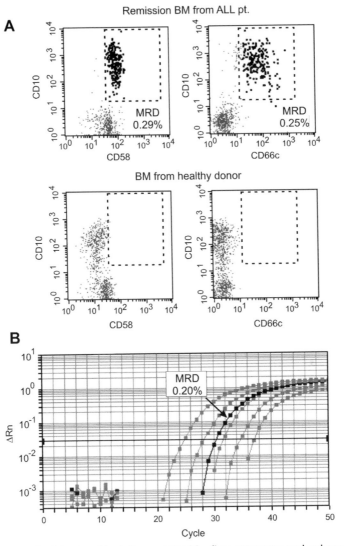

Fig. 1. Detection of minimal residual disease (MRD) by flow cytometry and polymerase chain reaction (PCR). A bone marrow sample collected at the end of remission induction therapy from a patient with B-lineage acute lymphoblastic leukemia (ALL) in morphologic remission was examined for MRD. (*A*) Flow cytometry studies of mononuclear cells using two different leukemia-associated markers (CD58 and CD66c) indicated the presence of 0.29% and 0.25% ALL cells, respectively (area within the dashed line in top panels). No cells (0.01%) within the equivalent areas of the dot plots were seen in the bone marrow of a healthy donor. (*B*) Molecular analysis of MRD was performed using real-time quantitative (RQ)-PCR amplification of a clonal immunoglobulin (IG) gene rearrangement determined at diagnosis. The *black line* corresponds to the amplification signal obtained in the patient sample; *gray lines* are the signal from serial dilutions of DNA extracted from the leukemic cell at diagnosis with that of peripheral blood from healthy donors. The estimated MRD level was 0.20%, similar to the estimates by flow cytometry.

Feasibility of Minimal Residual Disease Testing in Prospective Studies

MRD assays have been incorporated into clinical trials for children with ALL, and their feasibility for routine analysis of treatment response is established. Of the 2143 patients with B-lineage ALL enrolled on 9900 series treatment protocols of the Children's Oncology Group, day 29 samples were submitted from 2086 patients (97.3%) to be studied for MRD by flow cytometry.[52] In only 4% of cases, sample cellularity was too low, or the immunophenotype of the leukemic cells (determined at diagnosis) was not sufficiently distinct to allow a sensitivity of detection of 0.01%. MRD results were classified as indeterminate in 1.4% of cases. Overall, a test with the sensitivity of at least 0.01% was performed in 92% of patients.[52]

MRD was studied prospectively by PCR amplification of IG/TCR genes in pediatric patients enrolled in the Associazione Italiana Ematologia Oncologia Pediatrica-Berlin Frankfurt Munster (AIEOP-BFM) ALL 2000 trial.[48] Bone marrow samples were obtained at initial diagnosis and on days 33 and 78 of therapy. Of the 3341 diagnostic samples examined, 88 (3%) lacked suitable gene rearrangements targets for PCR analysis, and an additional 217 (7%) had a target but not sufficient to reach a sensitivity of 0.01%. In 671 patients (20%), there was only one sensitive target, whereas in the remaining 71% of patients, at least two sensitive targets were available for MRD analysis. At least one IG or TCR target could be identified in 98% of B-lineage ALL patients, with two or more targets detected in 93% of patients. In T-lineage ALL patients, these proportions were 93% and 88%, respectively. Overall, adequate data for MRD-based stratification were obtained in 2594 (78%) of the 3341 patients.

In the St Jude Total XV trial for children with newly diagnosed ALL, the author's laboratory monitored MRD by using flow cytometric detection of aberrant immunophenotypes or PCR amplification of antigen receptor genes. Flow cytometry was applied in patients with B-lineage ALL and T-ALL, whereas PCR studies were done only in patients with B-lineage ALL. Overall, 482 of 492 patients (98%) were monitored by flow cytometry, and 403 of 492 (82%) were monitored by PCR. As previously shown,[49-51] both methods yielded virtually identical results above the threshold level of 0.01% used to defined MRD positivity. In the few cases with discrepant results, the author's group used the highest MRD value. The two methods in combination could be applied to study 491 of 492 (99.8%) patients. The single patient with no available immunophenotypic or antigen receptor gene rearrangements had an MLL-AF9 fusion transcript and was monitored by RQ-PCR using that marker.

In adult ALL, 23% of B-lineage ALL cases lacked a IG targets for PCR analysis in one study.[53] In another study,[42] suitable IG or TCR clonal markers were lacking in 10% of cases.

CLINICAL SIGNIFICANCE OF MRD
Prognostic Significance of Minimal Residual Disease in Childhood Acute Lymphoblastic Leukemia

One of the most immediately obvious applications of MRD testing is its use in measuring early treatment response and identifying patients who achieve morphologic remission but still harbor considerable levels of disease. The prognostic value of such tests in childhood ALL was demonstrated most convincingly by three large prospective studies reported in the late 1990s by the European Organisation for Research and Treatment of Cancer (EORTC),[54] St Jude,[55] and BFM groups.[56] These and other reports[14,57] unequivocally demonstrated that MRD detected during the first 2 to 3 months of therapy is the strongest predictor of relapse. MRD also can help identify patients with a higher risk of relapse among those with specific ALL subtypes,[58–61] and among patients with first-relapse ALL who achieve a second remission,[62–64] and patients with isolated extramedullary relapse.[65] Detection of MRD before allogeneic hematopoietic stem cell transplantation (HSCT) is associated with an increase risk of relapse after HSCT.[31,66–70]

A commonly used cut-off level to define MRD positivity is 0.01% of bone marrow mononuclear cells. The selection of this level is due to the fact that this is the typical limit of detection for routine flow cytometric and molecular assays, and it has been shown to discriminate between patients with different risks of relapse. To this end, patients who had MRD of 0.01% or higher in bone marrow at any treatment interval monitored had a significantly higher risk of relapse in earlier St. Jude studies.[39,55,58] Likewise, MRD greater than or equal to 0.01% on day 29 was the strongest prognostic indicator in studies of the Children's Oncology Group.[52] Investigators of the EORTC, however, found that a cut-off level of 0.1% at the end of remission induction and at subsequent time points was very informative,[54] as did those of the Austrian BFM group,[71] and the Dana-Farber Cancer Institute ALL Consortium.[72]

During the early phases of treatment, levels of MRD are directly proportional to the risk of subsequent relapse. For example, MRD greater than or equal to 1% at the end of remission induction therapy was associated with an extremely high rate of relapse in St. Jude Studies.[58] Investigators of the I-BFM Study Group reported that patients whose bone marrow had MRD greater than or equal to 0.1% on both day 33 and day 78 of treatment had a relapse rate of 75%.[48,56]

An unexpected observation made while sequentially testing MRD in children with ALL was that, in a substantial proportion of patients, remission induction therapy induces a remarkable reduction in the leukemic cell burden, resulting in undetectable (less than 0.01%) MRD after only 2 to 3 weeks of therapy. In a recent analysis of 402 patients with B-lineage ALL, the author found that 183 (45.5%) had excellent response to treatment and were MRD less than 0.01% after 19 days of treatment.[73] Most patients who became MRD negative at an early stage of therapy had an excellent prognosis overall.[39,74] This led the author's group to develop a simplified flow cytometric MRD test that can detect residual leukemia on days 15 to 26 of treatment with a minimum panel of antibodies.[75] Although this test cannot be used beyond this treatment interval (owing to the high risk of false-positive results in recovering marrow samples) it is suited for identifying patients whose leukemic cells have the highest sensitivity to early treatment and are predicted to have good treatment responses overall.

It is known that genetic abnormalities in childhood ALL are associated with a different prevalence of MRD during remission induction therapy.[76,77] The author's laboratory found that among patients with B-lineage, ALL MRD on days 19 and 43 of treatment was much more prevalent in those with BCR-ABL1 ALL, and less prevalent overall in patients with ETV6-RUNX1, hyperdiploid (more than 50 chromosomes), and TCF3-PBX1 ALL.[73] Recent studies have identified novel subtypes of ALL with a significantly higher prevalence of MRD. Thus, patients with B-lineage ALL and mutations or deletions of Ikaros (IKZF1) were significantly more likely to have MRD detected during remission induction therapy than those without this abnormalitiy.[28] Among patients with T-lineage ALL, those classified as early thymic precursor (ETP)-ALL, had significantly higher levels of MRD during remission induction therapy than patients with typical T-ALL.[78] **Fig. 2** illustrates the prevalence of MRD among patients with various genetic subgroups of childhood ALL.

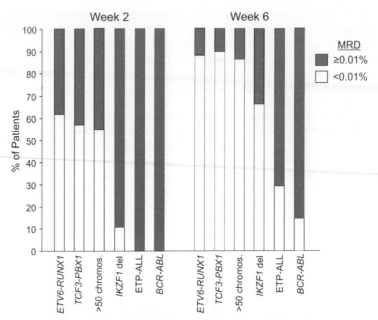

Fig. 2. Prevalence of minimal residual disease (MRD) in different subtypes of childhood acute lymphoblastic leukemia (ALL). The percentage of MRD-positive (greater than or equal to 0.01% of bone marrow mononuclear cells) and -negative as determined by flow cytometry 2 and 6 weeks from diagnosis is shown. The number of patients studied in each subgroups was 89 for ETV6-RUNX1, 21 for TCF3-PBX1, 115 for hyperdiploidy with more than 50 chromosomes, 100 for IKZF1 deletions/mutations, 14 for ETP-ALL, and 13 for BCR-ABL. More details are available elsewhere.[28,73,78]

Prognostic Significance of Minimal Residual Disease in Adult Acute Lymphoblastic Leukemia

Although the clinical significance of MRD has been studied less extensively in adult patients with ALL, there is considerable evidence supporting its potential usefulness. In an early study, Mortuza and colleagues[53] used PCR amplification of antigen receptor genes to study MRD in a group of 85 patients with Philadelphia chromosome-negative B-lineage ALL and found that its presence 3 to 5 months after induction therapy correlated with a poorer outcome. Subsequently, Bruggemann and colleagues[42] used PCR amplification of antigen receptor genes in 196 standard-risk patients to define three risk groups. A low-risk group included 10% of patients who had less than 0.01% MRD on day 11 and day 24; 3-year relapse rate was 0%. A high-risk group included 23% of patients defined by MRD greater than or equal to 0.01% until week 16; the relapse rate was 94%. Finally, an intermediate-risk group included all remaining patients; the relapse rate was 47%.

This team of investigators also reported results of a prospective analysis of postconsolidation samples in 105 patients enrolled in the German Multicenter Study Group for Adult ALL (GMALL) trial. Inclusion criteria were hematologic remission, completion of the first-year chemotherapy, and MRD-negativity before enrollment in the study. Conversion to MRD positivity was observed in 28 patients, 17 of whom relapsed (median time from MRD test to clinical relapse, 9.5 months); of the 77 patients who remained MRD-negative, only 5 had relapsed at the time of the report.[79] Holowiecki and colleagues[80] used flow cytometry to estimate MRD in 116 patients with

Philadelphia-negative ALL enrolled in the Polish Adult leukemia Group ALL 4-2002 MRD study and found that MRD greater than or equal to 0.1% after remission induction therapy was an independent predictor for relapse in both standard- and high-risk groups. Bassan and colleagues[81] studied MRD using fusion transcripts or IG/TCR gene rearrangements as targets. At the end of consolidation, 58 were MRD-negative (0.01%), and 54 were MRD-positive. Five-year overall disease-free survival estimates were 72% in the MRD-negative group versus 14% in MRD- positive group, regardless of clinical risk factors. MRD was the most significant risk factor for relapse.

Monitoring of MRD in adult patients with Philadelphia-positive ALL receiving HSCT or imatinib therapy has been shown to predict treatment outcome.[82–84] Similarly, in Philadelphia-negative ALL, MRD detected by flow cytometry in bone marrow samples of patients with ALL before initiation of conditioning for HSCT was a significant predictor of failure after HSCT.[85] Finally, in a study of 43 adult patients with ALL undergoing HSCT, the relapse rate at 36 months was 0% for the 12 patients who were MRD-negative before HSCT versus 46% for those who were MRD-positive.[86]

Uses of Minimal Residual Disease Testing for Risk Classification

There are numerous ways to include MRD studies in clinical trials, depending on treatment schedule, intensity, and previous experience. For example, the AIEOP-BFM group used MRD to classify patients into three risk groups: standard risk (MRD negative on days 33 and 78), intermediate risk (any MRD positivity on days 33 and 78 but less 0.1% on day 78), and high risk (MRD greater than or equal to 0.1% on day 78). Treatment intensity was regulated accordingly.[48] At St. Jude Children's Research Hospital, the current Total 16 study uses MRD levels on day 15 and day 42 for treatment assignment. Patients with MRD of greater than or equal to 1% on day 15 receive intensified remission induction therapy; further intensification is reserved for patients with greater than or equal to 5% leukemic cells. On the other hand, patients with MRD less than 0.01% on day 15 receive a slightly less intensive reinduction therapy and lower cumulative doses of anthracycline. Patients with standard-risk ALL who have MRD of greater than or equal to 0.01% on day 42 are reclassified as high-risk; patients with MRD greater than or equal to 1% are eligible for HSCT in first remission.

At St. Jude, MRD is also used to guide treatment for patients with first-relapse ALL who achieve a second remission. Those with persistent MRD are candidates for HSCT, whereas those who achieve MRD negativity (in the context of other favorable clinical features) are eligible for continuing chemotherapy. For patients who undergo HSCT, MRD is used to aid the timing of transplant. Thus, additional courses of chemotherapy may be administered in efforts to reduce MRD levels before HSCT. Monitoring MRD after HSCT may be helpful to make informed decisions about modulation of immunosuppressive therapy and administrations of donor lymphocyte infusions.

All the MRD methods described here are being used to monitor MRD by various groups, the selection depending primarily on existing expertise and strength of preclinical studies within the group. Flow cytometry results can be obtained within a few hours of sample collection. The development of a patient-specific PCR assay is time-consuming but, once the assay is developed, MRD estimates can also be obtained quite rapidly. Because of the time required to develop a patient-specific PCR assay (often more than 2 weeks), flow cytometry may be preferable for studies at very early time points during therapy, while PCR might be best for studies at the end of therapy or after HSCT because of its higher sensitivity. The author's current strategy is to use preferentially flow cytometry to monitor MRD during remission induction therapy, and develop a PCR assay for IG/TCR genes only if a suitable immunophenotype is not identified at diagnosis. After studying MRD with either one or the other method on days 15 and 42, MRD monitoring is stopped in patients with B-lineage ALL who are MRD-negative on day 42. Sequential MRD monitoring continues in patients with B-lineage ALL who are MRD-positive and in any patient with T-lineage ALL. Although it has been estimated that PCR is more expensive than flow cytometry,[87] in the author's experience, the two methods have comparable costs.

In patients with B-lineage ALL, MRD is usually present at higher levels in bone marrow than in peripheral blood.[88–90] This is not the case in T-lineage ALL, where MRD levels in peripheral blood are similar to those in bone marrow.[89,90] Based on these observations, it is the authors' current practice to use blood instead of marrow to monitor MRD after day 42 in patients with T-lineage ALL.

SUMMARY

It is unquestionable that MRD tests allow leukemia remission to be defined in a way that is much more accurate and rigorous than the one afforded by conventional morphologic techniques. In addition to their capacity to predict outcome on the basis of early response to therapy, MRD methods also can be used to recognize leukemia relapse before it is morphologically overt, to determine the leukemia burden before HSCT, and to measure the efficacy of a treatment regimen in relation to that of its predecessor. Current studies incorporating MRD to guide treatment decisions should clarify whether this approach produces significantly higher cure rates or lower toxicities. Beyond its direct clinical application, MRD measurements also can be used to reveal new molecular determinants of treatment response, as shown by correlative studies with the gene expression profiles of leukemic lymphoblasts,[91–93] and germline or leukemia-associated gene polymorphisms.[94,95]

MRD assays are complex and require expertise to be performed well. Therefore, simplification of the methodologies should be an objective for MRD researchers. Although MRD testing is relatively expensive compared with other routine laboratory assays performed at diagnosis in patients with ALL, it provides unique and powerful information that should not only improve treatment but, in the long run, also reduce overall clinical management costs.[87]

ACKNOWLEDGMENTS

I thank Elaine Coustan-Smith, Pat Stow, and Laura Key for providing **Fig. 1**, and all the staff, patients, and families at St. Jude Children's Research Hospital for their continuous support.

REFERENCES

1. Sandlund JT, Harrison PL, Rivera G, et al. Persistence of lymphoblasts in bone marrow on day 15 and days 22 to 25 of remission induction predicts a dismal treatment outcome in children with acute lymphoblastic leukemia. Blood 2002; 100(1):43–7.
2. Janossy G, Bollum FJ, Bradstock KF, et al. Cellular phenotypes of normal and leukemic hemopoietic cells determined by analysis with selected antibody combinations. Blood 1980;56(3):430–41.
3. Bradstock KF, Janossy G, Tidman N, et al. Immunological monitoring of residual disease in treated thymic acute lymphoblastic leukaemia. Leuk Res 1981;5: 301–9.

4. Hurwitz CA, Loken MR, Graham ML, et al. Asynchronous antigen expression in B lineage acute lymphoblastic leukemia. Blood 1988;72(1):299–307.

5. Terstappen LW, Loken MR. Myeloid cell differentiation in normal bone marrow and acute myeloid leukemia assessed by multidimensional flow cytometry. Anal Cell Pathol 1990;2(4):229–40.

6. Campana D, Coustan-Smith E, Janossy G. The immunologic detection of minimal residual disease in acute leukemia. Blood 1990;76(1):163–71.

7. Kawasaki ES, Clark SS, Coyne MY, et al. Diagnosis of chronic myeloid and acute lymphocytic leukemias by detection of leukemia-specific mRNA sequences amplified in vitro. Proc Natl Acad Sci U S A 1988;85(15):5698–702.

8. Hermans A, Gow J, Selleri L, et al. bcr-abl oncogene activation in Philadelphia chromosome-positive acute lymphoblastic leukemia. Leukemia 1988;2(10): 628–33.

9. d'Auriol L, MacIntyre E, Galibert F, et al. In vitro amplification of T-cell gamma gene rearrangements: a new tool for the assessment of minimal residual disease in acute lymphoblastic leukemias. Leukemia 1989;3(2):155–8.

10. Hansen-Hagge TE, Yokota S, Bartram CR. Detection of minimal residual disease in acute lymphoblastic leukemia by in vitro amplification of rearranged T-cell receptor delta chain sequences. Blood 1989;74(5):1762–7.

11. Yamada M, Hudson S, Tournay O, et al. Detection of minimal disease in hematopoietic malignancies of the B-cell lineage by using third complementary determining region (CDR-III)-specific probes. Proc Natl Acad Sci U S A 1989; 86(13):5123–7.

12. Brisco MJ, Condon J, Hughes E, et al. Outcome prediction in childhood acute lymphoblastic leukaemia by molecular quantification of residual disease at the end of induction. Lancet 1994;343(8891):196–200.

13. Szczepanski T, Orfao A, van der Velden VH, et al. Minimal residual disease in leukaemia patients. Lancet Oncol 2001;2:409–17.

14. Campana D. Determination of minimal residual disease in leukemia patients. Br J Haematol 2003;121:823–38.

15. Martens AC, Schultz FW, Hagenbeek A. Nonhomogeneous distribution of leukemia in the bone marrow during minimal residual disease. Blood 1987; 70(4):1073–8.

16. Mathe G, Schwarzenberg L, Mery AM, et al. Extensive histological and cytological survey of patients with acute leukaemia in complete remission. Br Med J 1966;5488:640–2.

17. Coustan-Smith E, Sandlund JT, Perkins SL, et al. Minimal disseminated disease in childhood T-cell lymphoblastic lymphoma: a report from the Children's Oncology Group. J Clin Oncol, 2009;27(21):3533–9.

18. Van Dijk MA, Voorhoeve PM, Murre C. Pbx1 is converted into a transcriptional activator upon acquiring the N-terminal region of E2A in pre-B-cell acute lymphoblastoid leukemia. Proc Natl Acad Sci U S A 1993;90(13):6061–5.

19. Behm FG, Smith FO, Raimondi SC, et al. Human homologue of the rat chondroitin sulfate proteoglycan, NG2, detected by monoclonal antibody 7.1, identifies childhood acute lymphoblastic leukemias with t(4;11)(q21;q23) or t(11;19)(q23;p13) and MLL gene rearrangements. Blood 1996;87(3):1134–9.

20. Smith FO, Rauch C, Williams DE, et al. The human homologue of rat NG2, a chondroitin sulfate proteoglycan, is not expressed on the cell surface of normal hematopoietic cells but is expressed by acute myeloid leukemia blasts from poor-prognosis patients with abnormalities of chromosome band 11q23. Blood 1996;87(3):1123–33.

21. Lucio P, Parreira A, van den Beemd MW, et al. Flow cytometric analysis of normal B-cell differentiation: a frame of reference for the detection of minimal residual disease in precursor-B- ALL. Leukemia 1999;13(3):419–27.

22. Campana D, Coustan-Smith E. Detection of minimal residual disease in acute leukemia by flow cytometry. Cytometry 1999;38:139–52.

23. Ciudad J, San Miguel JF, Lopez-Berges MC, et al. Prognostic value of immunophenotypic detection of minimal residual disease in acute lymphoblastic leukemia. J Clin Oncol 1998;16(12):3774–81.

24. van Dongen JJ, Macintyre EA, Gabert JA, et al. Standardized RT-PCR analysis of fusion gene transcripts from chromosome aberrations in acute leukemia for detection of minimal residual disease. Report of the BIOMED-1 concerted action: investigation of minimal residual disease in acute leukemia. Leukemia 1999;13(12):1901–28.

25. Gabert J, Beillard E, van der Velden V, et al. Standardization and quality control studies of real-time quantitative reverse transcriptase polymerase chain reaction of fusion gene transcripts for residual disease detection in leukemia—a Europe against cancer program. Leukemia 2003;17(12):2318–57.

26. Armstrong SA, Look AT. Molecular genetics of acute lymphoblastic leukemia. J Clin Oncol 2005;23(26):6306–15.

27. Mulligan CG, Goorha S, Radtke I, et al. Genome-wide analysis of genetic alterations in acute lymphoblastic leukaemia. Nature 2007;446(7137):758–64.

28. Mulligan CG, Su X, Zhang J, et al. Deletion of IKZF1 and prognosis in acute lymphoblastic leukemia. N Engl J Med 2009;360(5):470–80.

29. van der Velden V, Cazzaniga G, Schrauder A, et al. Analysis of minimal residual disease by IG/TCR gene rearrangements: guidelines for interpretation of real-time quantitative PCR data. Leukemia 2007;21(4):604–11.

30. Delabesse E, Burtin ML, Millien C, et al. Rapid, multifluorescent TCRG V-gamma and J-gamma typing: application to T-cell acute lymphoblastic leukemia and to the detection of minor clonal populations. Leukemia 2000;14(6):1143–52.

31. Knechtli CJC, Goulden NJ, Hancock JP, et al. Minimal residual disease status before allogeneic bone marrow transplantation is an important determinant of successful outcome for children and adolescents with acute lymphoblastic leukemia. Blood 1998;92(11):4072–9.

32. van Dongen JJ, Wolvers-Tettero IL. Analysis of immunoglobulin and T-cell receptor genes. Part II: possibilities and limitations in the diagnosis and management of lymphoproliferative diseases and related disorders. Clin Chim Acta 1991; 198(1-2):93–174.

33. Beishuizen A, Verhoeven MA, Mol EJ, et al. Detection of immunoglobulin heavy-chain gene rearrangements by Southern blot analysis: recommendations for optimal results. Leukemia 1993;7(12):2045–53.

34. Szczepanski T, Beishuizen A, Pongers-Willemse MJ, et al. Cross-lineage T-cell receptor gene rearrangements occur in more than ninety percent of childhood precursor-B acute lymphoblastic leukemias: alternative PCR targets for detection of minimal residual disease. Leukemia 1999;13(2):196–205.

35. Breit TM, Wolvers-Tettero IL, Beishuizen A, et al. Southern blot patterns, frequencies, and junctional diversity of T-cell receptor-delta gene rearrangements in acute lymphoblastic leukemia. Blood 1993;82(10):3063–74.

36. Szczepanski T, Langerak AW, Willemse MJ, et al. T-cell receptor gamma (TCRG) gene rearrangements in T-cell acute lymphoblastic leukemia reflect end-stage recombinations: implications for minimal residual disease monitoring. Leukemia 2000;14(7):1208–14.

37. Kneba M, Bolz I, Linke B, et al. Analysis of rearranged T-cell receptor beta-chain genes by polymerase chain reaction (PCR) DNA sequencing and automated high-resolution PCR fragment analysis. Blood 1995;86(10):3930–7.

38. van der Velden V, Hochhaus A, Cazzaniga G, et al. Detection of minimal residual disease in hematologic malignancies by real-time quantitative PCR: principles, approaches, and laboratory aspects. Leukemia 2003;17(6):1013–34.

39. Coustan-Smith E, Sancho J, Behm FG, et al. Prognostic importance of measuring early clearance of leukemic cells by flow cytometry in childhood acute lymphoblastic leukemia. Blood 2002;100(1):52–8.

40. Gaipa G, Basso G, Maglia O, et al. Drug-induced immunophenotypic modulation in childhood ALL: implications for minimal residual disease detection. Leukemia 2005;19(1):49–56.

41. Hong D, Gupta R, Ancliff P, et al. Initiating and cancer-propagating cells in TEL-AML1-associated childhood leukemia. Science 2008;319(5861):336–9.

42. Bruggemann M, Raff T, Flohr T, et al. Clinical significance of minimal residual disease quantification in adult patients with standard-risk acute lymphoblastic leukemia. Blood 2006;107(3):1116–23.

43. Szczepanski T, Pongers-Willemse MJ, Langerak AW, et al. Unusual immunoglobulin and T-cell receptor gene rearrangement patterns in acute lymphoblastic leukemias. Curr Top Microbiol Immunol 1999;246:205–13.

44. Beishuizen A, Hahlen K, Hagemeijer A, et al. Multiple rearranged immunoglobulin genes in childhood acute lymphoblastic leukemia of precursor B-cell origin. Leukemia 1991;5(8):657–67.

45. Szczepanski T, Willemse MJ, Brinkhof B, et al. Comparative analysis of IG and TCR gene rearrangements at diagnosis and at relapse of childhood precursor-B-ALL provides improved strategies for selection of stable PCR targets for monitoring of minimal residual disease. Blood 2002;99(7):2315–23.

46. van der Velden V, Bruggemann M, Hoogeveen PG, et al. TCRB gene rearrangements in childhood and adult precursor-B ALL: frequency, applicability as MRD-PCR target, and stability between diagnosis and relapse. Leukemia 2004;18(12):1971–80.

47. Pongers-Willemse MJ, Seriu T, Stolz F, et al. Primers and protocols for standardized detection of minimal residual disease in acute lymphoblastic leukemia using immunoglobulin and T-cell receptor gene rearrangements and TAL1 deletions as PCR targets. Leukemia 1999;13:110–8.

48. Flohr T, Schrauder A, Cazzaniga G, et al. Minimal residual disease-directed risk stratification using real-time quantitative PCR analysis of immunoglobulin and T-cell receptor gene rearrangements in the international multicenter trial AIEOP-BFM ALL 2000 for childhood acute lymphoblastic leukemia. Leukemia 2008;22:771–82.

49. Neale GA, Coustan-Smith E, Pan Q, et al. Tandem application of flow cytometry and polymerase chain reaction for comprehensive detection of minimal residual disease in childhood acute lymphoblastic leukemia. Leukemia 1999;13(8):1221–6.

50. Neale GA, Coustan-Smith E, Stow P, et al. Comparative analysis of flow cytometry and polymerase chain reaction for the detection of minimal residual disease in childhood acute lymphoblastic leukemia. Leukemia 2004;18:934–8.

51. Kerst G, Kreyenberg H, Roth C, et al. Concurrent detection of minimal residual disease (MRD) in childhood acute lymphoblastic leukaemia by flow cytometry and real-time PCR. Br J Haematol 2005;128(6):774–82.

52. Borowitz MJ, Devidas M, Hunger SP, et al. Clinical significance of minimal residual disease in childhood acute lymphoblastic leukemia and its relationship to other prognostic factors. A Children's Oncology Group Study. Blood 2008; 111(12):5477–85.

53. Mortuza FY, Papaioannou M, Moreira IM, et al. Minimal residual disease tests provide an independent predictor of clinical outcome in adult acute lymphoblastic leukemia. J Clin Oncol 2002;20(4):1094–104.

54. Cave H, van der Werff ten Bosch J, Suciu S, et al. Clinical significance of minimal residual disease in childhood acute lymphoblastic leukemia. European Organization for Research and Treatment of Cancer—Childhood Leukemia Cooperative Group. N Engl J Med 1998;339(9):591–8.

55. Coustan-Smith E, Behm FG, Sanchez J, et al. Immunological detection of minimal residual disease in children with acute lymphoblastic leukaemia. Lancet 1998; 351(9102):550–4.

56. van Dongen JJ, Seriu T, Panzer-Grumayer ER, et al. Prognostic value of minimal residual disease in acute lymphoblastic leukaemia in childhood. Lancet 1998; 352:1731–8.

57. Campana D. Minimal residual disease in acute lymphoblastic leukemia. Semin Hematol 2009;46(1):100–6.

58. Coustan-Smith E, Sancho J, Hancock ML, et al. Clinical importance of minimal residual disease in childhood acute lymphoblastic leukemia. Blood 2000;96:2691–6.

59. Biondi A, Valsecchi MG, Seriu T, et al. Molecular detection of minimal residual disease is a strong predictive factor of relapse in childhood B-lineage acute lymphoblastic leukemia with medium risk features. A case–control study of the International BFM Study Group. Leukemia 2000;14(11):1939–43.

60. Attarbaschi A, Mann G, Panzer-Grumayer R, et al. Minimal residual disease values discriminate between low and high relapse risk in children with B-cell precursor acute lymphoblastic leukemia and an intrachromosomal amplification of chromosome 21: the Austrian and German acute lymphoblastic leukemia Berlin-Frankfurt-Munster (ALL-BFM) trials. J Clin Oncol 2008;26(18):3046–50.

61. van der Velden V, Corral L, Valsecchi MG, et al. Prognostic significance of minimal residual disease in infants with acute lymphoblastic leukemia treated within the Interfant-99 protocol. Leukemia, 2009;23(6):1073–9.

62. Eckert C, Biondi A, Seeger K, et al. Prognostic value of minimal residual disease in relapsed childhood acute lymphoblastic leukaemia. Lancet 2001;358(9289): 1239–41.

63. Coustan-Smith E, Gajjar A, Hijiha N, et al. Clinical significance of minimal residual disease in childhood acute lymphoblastic leukemia after first relapse. Leukemia 2004;18:499–504.

64. Paganin M, Zecca M, Fabbri G, et al. Minimal residual disease is an important predictive factor of outcome in children with relapsed high-risk acute lymphoblastic leukemia. Leukemia 2008;22(12):2193–200.

65. Hagedorn N, Acquaviva C, Fronkova E, et al. Submicroscopic bone marrow involvement in isolated extramedullary relapses in childhood acute lymphoblastic leukemia: a more precise definition of isolated and its possible clinical implications, a collaborative study of the Resistant Disease Committee of the International BFM study group. Blood 2007;110(12):4022–9.

66. van der Velden V, Joosten SA, Willemse MJ, et al. Real-time quantitative PCR for detection of minimal residual disease before allogeneic stem cell transplantation predicts outcome in children with acute lymphoblastic leukemia. Leukemia 2001; 15(9):1485–7.

67. Bader P, Hancock J, Kreyenberg H, et al. Minimal residual disease (MRD) status prior to allogeneic stem cell transplantation is a powerful predictor for post-transplant outcome in children with ALL. Leukemia 2002;16(9):1668–72.
68. Uzunel M, Mattsson J, Jaksch M, et al. The significance of graft-versus-host disease and pretransplantation minimal residual disease status to outcome after allogeneic stem cell transplantation in patients with acute lymphoblastic leukemia. Blood 2001;98(6):1982–4.
69. Krejci O, van der Velden V, Bader P, et al. Level of minimal residual disease prior to haematopoietic stem cell transplantation predicts prognosis in paediatric patients with acute lymphoblastic leukaemia: a report of the Pre-BMT MRD Study Group. Bone Marrow Transplant 2003;32(8):849–51.
70. Goulden N, Bader P, van der Velden V, et al. Minimal residual disease prior to stem cell transplant for childhood acute lymphoblastic leukaemia. Br J Haematol 2003;122(1):24–9.
71. Dworzak MN, Froschl G, Printz D, et al. Prognostic significance and modalities of flow cytometric minimal residual disease detection in childhood acute lymphoblastic leukemia. Blood 2002;99(6):1952–8.
72. Zhou J, Goldwasser MA, Li A, et al. Quantitative analysis of minimal residual disease predicts relapse in children with B-lineage acute lymphoblastic leukemia in DFCI ALL Consortium Protocol 95-01. Blood 2007;110(5):1607–11.
73. Campana D. Molecular determinants of treatment response in acute lymphoblastic leukemia. Hematology Am Soc Hematol Educ Program 2008;366–73.
74. Panzer-Grumayer ER, Schneider M, Panzer S, et al. Rapid molecular response during early induction chemotherapy predicts a good outcome in childhood acute lymphoblastic leukemia. Blood 2000;95(3):790–4.
75. Coustan-Smith E, Ribeiro RC, Stow P, et al. A simplified flow cytometric assay identifies children with acute lymphoblastic leukemia who have a superior clinical outcome. Blood 2006;108(1):97–102.
76. Pui CH, Campana D, Evans WE. Childhood acute lymphoblastic leukemia—current status and future perspectives. Lancet Oncol 2001;2:597–607.
77. Borowitz MJ, Pullen DJ, Shuster JJ, et al. Minimal residual disease detection in childhood precursor B-cell acute lymphoblastic leukemia: relation to other risk factors. A Children's Oncology Group study. Leukemia 2003;17(8):1566–72.
78. Coustan-Smith E, Mullighan CG, Onciu M, et al. Early T-cell precursor leukaemia: a subtype of very high-risk acute lymphoblastic leukaemia. Lancet Oncol 2009;10(2):147–56.
79. Raff T, Gokbuget N, Luschen S, et al. Molecular relapse in adult standard-risk ALL patients detected by prospective MRD monitoring during and after maintenance treatment: data from the GMALL 06/99 and 07/03 trials. Blood 2007;109(3):910–5.
80. Holowiecki J, Krawczyk-Kulis M, Giebel S, et al. Status of minimal residual disease after induction predicts outcome in both standard and high-risk Ph-negative adult acute lymphoblastic leukaemia. The Polish Adult Leukemia Group ALL 4-2002 MRD Study. Br J Haematol 2008;142(2):227–37.
81. Bassan R, Spinelli O, Oldani E, et al. Improved risk classification for risk-specific therapy based on the molecular study of MRD in adult ALL. Blood 2009;113:4153–62.
82. Radich J, Gehly G, Lee A, et al. Detection of BCR-ABL transcripts in Philadelphia chromosome-positive acute lymphoblastic leukemia after marrow transplantation. Blood 1997;89(7):2602–9.

83. Wassmann B, Pfeifer H, Stadler M, et al. Early molecular response to post-transplantation imatinib determines outcome in MRD+ Philadelphia-positive acute lymphoblastic leukemia (Ph+ ALL). Blood 2005;106(2):458–63.

84. Pane F, Cimino G, Izzo B, et al. Significant reduction of the hybrid BCR/ABL transcripts after induction and consolidation therapy is a powerful predictor of treatment response in adult Philadelphia-positive acute lymphoblastic leukemia. Leukemia 2005;19(4):628–35.

85. Sanchez J, Serrano J, Gomez P, et al. Clinical value of immunological monitoring of minimal residual disease in acute lymphoblastic leukaemia after allogeneic transplantation. Br J Haematol 2002;116(3):686–94.

86. Spinelli O, Peruta B, Tosi M, et al. Clearance of minimal residual disease after allogeneic stem cell transplantation and the prediction of the clinical outcome of adult patients with high-risk acute lymphoblastic leukemia. Haematologica 2007;92(5):612–8.

87. Goulden N, Oakhill A, Steward C. Practical application of minimal residual disease assessment in childhood acute lymphoblastic leukaemia annotation. Br J Haematol 2001;112(2):275–81.

88. Brisco MJ, Sykes PJ, Hughes E, et al. Monitoring minimal residual disease in peripheral blood in B-lineage acute lymphoblastic leukaemia. Br J Haematol 1997;99(2):314–9.

89. Coustan-Smith E, Sancho J, Hancock ML, et al. Use of peripheral blood instead of bone marrow to monitor residual disease in children with acute lymphoblastic leukemia. Blood 2002;100:2399–402.

90. van der Velden V, Jacobs DC, Wijkhuijs AJ, et al. Minimal residual disease levels in bone marrow and peripheral blood are comparable in children with T cell acute lymphoblastic leukemia (ALL), but not in precursor-B-ALL. Leukemia 2002;16(8): 1432–6.

91. Cario G, Stanulla M, Fine BM, et al. Distinct gene expression profiles determine molecular treatment response in childhood acute lymphoblastic leukemia. Blood 2005;105(2):821–6.

92. Flotho C, Coustan-Smith E, Pei D, et al. Genes contributing to minimal residual disease in childhood acute lymphoblastic leukemia: prognostic significance of CASP8AP2. Blood 2006;108:1050–7.

93. Flotho C, Coustan-Smith E, Pei D, et al. A set of genes that regulate cell proliferation predicts treatment outcome in childhood acute lymphoblastic leukemia. Blood 2007;110(4):1271–7.

94. Rocha JC, Cheng C, Liu W, et al. Pharmacogenetics of outcome in children with acute lymphoblastic leukemia. Blood 2005;105(12):4752–8.

95. Yang JJ, Cheng C, Yang W, et al. Genome-wide interrogation of germline genetic variation associated with treatment response in childhood acute lymphoblastic leukemia. JAMA 2009;301(4):393–403.

Looking Toward the Future: Novel Strategies Based on Molecular Pathogenesis of Acute Lymphoblastic Leukemia

Syed A. Abutalib, MD[a], Meir Wetzler, MD, FACP[b], Wendy Stock, MD[c],*

KEYWORDS

- Prognostic factors • Risk-adapted therapies
- Novel therapeutics

There has been exponential growth in our understanding of the pathobiology of acute lymphoblastic leukemia (ALL) leading to the discovery of new prognostic markers and potential new treatment strategies. The inferior treatment outcome observed in adults with ALL in comparison with children with ALL means that new therapeutic approaches are required, preferably based on novel molecular insights. The use of highly effective pediatric ALL regimens for the treatment of adults with ALL may result in improved treatment outcomes, particularly for older adolescents and young adults (AYA) (see article by Ribera elsewhere in this issue). As greater insights into the molecular pathogenesis of the disease are revealed, significant advances in treatment risk stratification are anticipated based on new prognostic markers. Furthermore, the addition of molecularly targeted therapy to conventional chemotherapy regimens is already beginning to improve the treatment outcomes in ALL as demonstrated most dramatically for adults with Philadelphia chromosome positive (Ph[+]) ALL (see article by Ravandi elsewhere in this issue). Improved understanding about the use of quantitative minimal residual disease (MRD) assessments to assess prognosis and to evaluate treatment efficacy may also facilitate treatment stratification, including the decision to proceed with allogeneic stem cell transplant (SCT) in first remission (see

[a] Section of Hematology and Oncology, Cancer Treatment Centers of America, Zion, IL, USA
[b] Leukemia Section, Roswell Park Cancer Institute, Elm and Carlton Streets, Buffalo, NY 14263, USA
[c] University of Chicago Hospitals and Cancer Research Center, 5841 S Maryland, M/C 2115, Chicago, IL 60637, USA
* Corresponding author.
E-mail address: wstock@medicine.bsd.uchicago.edu (W. Stock).

Hematol Oncol Clin N Am 23 (2009) 1099–1119
doi:10.1016/j.hoc.2009.07.004
0889-8588/09/$ – see front matter © 2009 Elsevier Inc. All rights reserved.

the article by Campana elsewhere in this issue). In this concluding article, the important themes that have been discussed in earlier articles are reviewed. Looking toward the future, the authors highlight several of the new therapeutic agents and discuss some of the recently described molecular genetic aberrations that might serve as therapeutic targets for future drug development.

MOLECULAR INSIGHTS TO GUIDE TREATMENT
Unanswered Questions About Minimal Residual Disease: Can We Use it to Optimally Select Postremission Therapy for Patients with Acute Lymphoblastic Leukemia?

The evaluation of MRD provides independent prognostic information in children and adults with ALL. There is convincing evidence in pediatric and adult ALL that a high level of MRD at the end of induction therapy is associated with a higher relapse rate.[1-8] Furthermore, the continuous detection of high levels of MRD during consolidation and maintenance therapy, the re-emergence, or increase in MRD levels all seem to herald relapse. In contrast, declining or negative MRD results are associated with a favorable prognosis. The evaluation of MRD also has begun to provide important insights into the efficacy of current treatment of specific molecular/cytogenetic subsets of ALL. From the studies that have been completed in the last decade, there seem to be sufficient data to justify the incorporation of MRD status into decisions about postremission treatment assignment including whether to recommend hematopoietic stem cell transplantation (HSCT) in first remission.[1-10] Several large cooperative trails are now underway using this strategy in a prospective fashion. Two general strategies are being evaluated: (1) intensification of postremission treatment, that is, HSCT in first complete remission (CR1) for patients with high levels of MRD: escalation of therapy; and (2) decreased duration or intensity of treatment of patients with low or undetectable levels of MRD: de-escalation of therapy. From a practical standpoint, the latter approach seems to be more applicable to childhood ALL where excellent treatment outcomes have provided an opportunity to study less intensive therapies in certain subtypes of patients.

The Children's Oncology Group (COG) in North America is combining two prognostic markers to assign postremission therapy: (1) results of a remission induction day 14 bone marrow (BM) examination and (2) a day 29 MRD evaluation. MRD measurements will be performed using four-color flow postremission therapy, using a real-time quantitative polymerase chain reaction (RQ-PCR) technique following induction cytometric assay in two central reference laboratories. Patients defined as high risk based on these two test results will be assigned to an intensified postremission course of treatment. The Dana Farber ALL consortium also plans to use MRD detection to further stratify therapy; patients with a high level of MRD will be assigned additional postremission therapy with daunorubicin and/or cytarabine. In these North American studies, there will be no de-escalation of therapy based on MRD evaluation. In contrast, the ongoing European BFM-AEIOP uses the results of RQ-PCR, performed in reference laboratories, to assign MRD-high level patients to allogeneic HSCT in first remission, whereas MRD-low level patients will be de-escalated to receive a reduced course of postremission therapy.

In adult ALL, the ongoing prospective GMALL 07/2003 trial has provided some important insights into MRD evaluation in patients considered standard risk according to their definition of conventional risk factors, which precludes age as a risk factor.[8] In patients with low-risk (LR) MRD defined as MRD levels of $< 10^{-4}$ at all postremission time points, the maintenance therapy was omitted. Patients with high-risk (HR) MRD, defined as patients with MRD $>10^{-4}$ at any postremission time point, were allocated to allogeneic HSCT, whereas patients with intermediate-risk (IR) MRD, defined as "MRD evaluation was not possible," were either given intensified maintenance or less intensive therapy. Primarily, because of stringent quality standards, an unexpected majority was categorized into the IR MRD group. The relapsed risk in patients with LR MRD was between 20% and 30%. In the HR MRD group, less than half of the patients actually received allogeneic HSCT; however these patients had better disease-free survival (DFS) than those who did not receive allogeneic HSCT. Patients in the IR MRD group had a better prognosis if they received intensified maintenance therapy. These data indicate that improvement in the methodology is needed to properly assign patients to appropriate risk groups, several time points are needed to optimally stratify patients, and it might be difficult to justify complete omission of maintenance therapy in the LR MRD group. The final results of this prospective study are eagerly awaited.

As planned in the German trial, MRD measurements following remission induction therapy may serve as a useful strategy for selecting patients who may benefit from an allogeneic HSCT in first complete remission (CR1). As discussed by Forman and colleagues elsewhere in this issue, the recently published Medical Research Council (MRC)/Eastern Cooperative Oncology Group (ECOG) trial[11] demonstrated improved overall survival (OS) for patients who underwent an allogeneic HSCT in CR1 but did not result in survival advantage for high-risk ALL patients as a result of an increase in transplant-related mortality (TRM). In their study the high-risk group was defined as age >35 years, white blood cell count >30,000 cells/mm^3 for B cell lineage ALL or >100,000 cells/mm^3 for T cell lineage ALL. Thus, in addition to thinking about changes in the preparative regimen for future trials in adult ALL, MRD measurements in early remission may improve and refine the selection of patients who could benefit from an allogeneic HSCT in CR1.

The unresolved issues of technique standardization and quality control cannot be overemphasized and must be addressed if MRD measurements are to be incorporated into clinical trials and used for treatment stratification and evaluation of treatment efficacy, The Europe Against Cancer (EAC) and BIOMED initiatives have resulted in the development of standardized and validated methodology for quantitative PCR analysis to permit accurate comparison of MRD data.[9,10] Adoption of this approach in ongoing and future trials with standardization of methodologies will be essential to accurately evaluate data from different clinical trials and to answer important questions. Moreover, any MRD result must be interpreted in the context of the treatment administered and the clinical context in which it is being evaluated.

Recognition of Drug Resistance: Genome-wide Association Studies and Pharmacogenomics

The likelihood of cure of ALL is influenced by several disease and host-related factors. These include the patient's performance status, the type of treatment employed, adherence to treatment, and various disease-specific biologic factors.[12,13] Some of the biologic factors include molecular heterogeneity in subsets of ALL, polymorphisms in genes that metabolize drugs, and the influence of the BM microenvironment on leukemic cells that may result in interpatient variability in response to therapy. Acquired or inherent drug resistance also remains a major obstacle to successful treatment of ALL. Gene expression array studies are a relatively new tool for identifying potential pathways of resistance and identification of treatment strategies to overcome these obstacles. For example, Wei and colleagues[14] screened the database of drug-associated gene expression profiles for molecules whose profile overlapped with a gene expression signature of glucocorticoid sensitivity/resistance in ALL cell lines. The screen demonstrated that treatment of ALL cells with the *mTOR* inhibitor, rapamycin, resulted in a gene expression profile that matched the expression signature of glucocorticoid-sensitive ALL cell lines. This result led to the observation that treatment with rapamycin could restore glucocorticoid -induced apoptosis via modulation of antiapoptotic *MCL1*. These data indicate that genome-wide assessments of molecular changes in ALL could lead to promising new treatment strategies: for example, the addition of rapamycin to glucocorticoid-based therapy may represent a promising treatment strategy to overcome glucocorticoid resistance.

Other mechanisms of drug resistance have also been reported.[13] Expression of the multidrug resistance protein-1 (MDR-1) has been associated with a poorer prognosis in ALL.[15,16] Possible strategies to combine MDR-1 inhibitors with chemotherapy, therefore, may be an attractive therapeutic strategy in ALL; however, exploration of this strategy with various MDR-1 inhibitors has, overall, been unsuccessful in improving response rates or survival in several large randomized trials in adults with acute myelocytic leukemia (AML).[17,18]

Pharmacogenomic studies are also beginning to provide important insights into drug metabolism and differential drug sensitivity in ALL patients; to date, these studies have been largely been confined to the pediatric population.[19,20] Polymorphisms in the methylenetetrahydrofolate (*MTFHR*), thymidylate synthase (*TS*) and thiopurine methyltransferase (*TMPT*) genes affect sensitivity to active agents including methotrexate and 6-mercaptopurine[19–24] and may result in differences in toxicity and treatment outcomes in otherwise identical biologic subsets. Evans and colleagues[25] demonstrated that patients with rapid methotrexate clearance had inferior complete remission (CR) rates and shorter duration of remission, which is a reflection of interpatient variability in metabolism of methotrexate, possibly as a result of *MTFHR* polymorphisms that affect enzymatic activity. Homozygosity for a triple-tandem repeat polymorphism of the *TS* gene was associated with inferior prognosis.[21] The polymorphism of the *TMPT* gene may lead to increased sensitivity to 6-mercaptopurine (6-MP) and improved leukemia-free survival (LFS).[22] Patients with precursor B cell ALL harboring the *TEL-AML1* fusion gene and *MLL* gene rearrangements are more sensitive to asparaginase and cytarabine, respectively.[26,27] Unlike patients with hyperdiploid cytogenetics who are quite sensitive to antimetabolites,[28] patients with the *E2A-PBX1* fusion gene usually demonstrate resistance to antimetabolites.[29] However, this resistance is abrogated with more intensive chemotherapy regimens.[29–31] In the future, it might be possible to select a personalized, and more effective combination therapy based on these host- and disease-specific biologic variations. Little is known about the influence of age on drug metabolism. Insights into this area will be critical to understanding the inferior outcomes observed in older adults when compared with children and young adults with ALL.

IMPROVING ON EXISTING REGIMENS
Following the Lead of the Pediatricians: Can We Replicate Their Results in Young Adults with Acute Lymphoblastic Leukemia?

Increasing age is one of the most important poor prognostic factors of outcome in newly diagnosed patients with ALL.[32,33] The 5-year DFS is approximately 80% for children and 40% for adults with ALL. These divergent outcome results can be explained, in part, by the much higher incidence of poor risk cytogenetics (eg, the Philadelphia chromosome) and a lower incidence of favorable risk molecular genetics (eg, *TEL-AML1*) in older adults with ALL. In addition, older patients with ALL have a higher incidence of associated comorbid conditions with poorer baseline performance status, which frequently precludes the use of intensive chemotherapy regimens and enrollment into clinical trials.[33–35] Recent retrospective data suggest that younger patients between the ages of 16 and 21 years fare better when treated according to current intensive pediatric regimens rather than with conventional adult ALL treatment regimens.[36–41] Despite slight differences in treatment approaches across the different cooperative groups, all of the retrospective studies have demonstrated significantly better outcome for the patients when treated on pediatric studies where survival has been reported in the range of 60% to 65%.[36–41] In contrast, when the same age group is treated on adult cooperative group ALL treatment trials, survival has only been in the range of 30% to 40%.[42–44]

It seems that the major differences in treatment include more intensive use of the nonmyelosuppressive agents: glucocorticoids, L-asparaginase, and vincristine, earlier and more intensive central nervous system (CNS) directed therapy, and more prolonged maintenance therapy employed in the pediatric studies.[40,45] In addition to the obvious treatment differences between adult and pediatric trials, there has been much debate about potential differences in adherence to protocol therapy among pediatric or adult medical hematologists and the patients that they treat.[38,45]

Based on these insights, several groups have begun to treat younger adults using the pediatric treatment approach(see article by Ribera elsewhere in this issue). Several new prospective European and American studies that apply the pediatric approach to younger adults suggest very promising outcomes for those patients 18 to 50 years old.[46–48] In the United States, the three adult cooperative groups (Cancer and Leukemia Group B [CALGB], Southwest Oncology Group [SWOG], and ECOG) are performing a large (planned N = 300) phase 2 trial (C10403) for young adults with ALL (16–30 years old) that would replicate a successful COG study that has resulted in significant improvement in survival rates of more than 70% for high-risk children and adolescents with ALL. Results will be compared with those from a phase 3 COG study (AALL0232) in which pediatric hematologist will treat patients from 1 to 30 years of age with newly diagnosed B cell ALL. The older adults may not benefit from these pediatric style treatment approaches due, in part, to their inability to tolerate the intensive asparaginase, glucocorticoid, and vincristine dosing on which these regimens are based.[47]

EXPANSION OF THE THERAPEUTIC ARMAMENTARIUM: FOCUS ON OLDER ADULTS WITH ACUTE LYMPHOBLASTIC LEUKEMIA

The focus on new drug development may be particularly crucial for adults with ALL. Overall, only approximately one-third of all adult patients are disease-free at 5 years after diagnosis and for patients older than 60 years of age, the survival rate has been poor with only approximately 10% survival with frontline therapies.[42–44] The outcome of salvage chemotherapy also remains dismal.[49] Novel agents are desperately required to strengthen the backbone of current regimens or to form new therapeutic regimens based on disease biology. Promising results have already been demonstrated in relapsed disease using newer agents including clofarabine and nelarabine in precursor B cell and T cell ALL, respectively.[50–52] These agents are being incorporated into frontline therapy for pediatric ALL. Newer formulations of old chemotherapeutic agents including PEG-asparaginase are also being incorporated in clinical trials in an attempt to maximize efficacy and minimize treatment related toxicities (**Table 1**). These and other agents including tyrosine kinases inhibitors (TKIs) that target *BCR/ABL* monoclonal antibodies, including rituxan and alemtuzumab, which are the subject of active investigation and are discussed in more detail in the article by Thomas et al, elsewhere in this issue. Several of the newest subset-specific

Table 1
Novel chemotherapeutic agents in acute lymphoblastic leukemia

Category	Agents	Comments
New formulations of old drugs	Pegylated asparaginase[53]	Long half-life (6 days) Decreased immunogenicity
	Sphingosomal vincristine[54]	Decreased neuropathy Higher tissue concentration
	Liposomal annamycin[55]	Decreased cardiotoxicity
	Liposomal cytarabine[56]	Long half-life Caution is advised with use for CNS prophylaxis[56]
Antifolates	Trimetrexate[57]	Lipophilic analogues of methotrexate
	Aminopterin[58]	Excellent oral bioavailability
Antimicrotubule agents	ABT-751[59]	Oral bioavailability
Nucleoside analogues	Nelarabine[52]	T cell ALL
	Clofarabine[50]	B and T cell ALL
	Forodesine (BCX-1777)[60]	Oral phosphorylase (PNP) inhibitor

treatment strategies that are being explored are reviewed in the following paragraphs. Other agents that have been tested recently for patients with ALL are summarized in **Table 2**.

Newer Monoclonal Antibodies for Acute Lymphoblastic Leukemia

As demonstrated so convincingly in other lymphoid malignancies, the addition of targeted antibody therapy to combination chemotherapy offers the potential to increase the efficacy of conventional frontline therapy with minimal added toxicity (see **Table 2**). Several other monoclonal antibodies targeting epitopes commonly expressed on lymphoblasts are actively being explored. The rationale and early clinical results of the addition of rituximab to frontline therapy are described in the article by Thomas elsewhere in this issue; early clinical efforts describing the feasibility and efficacy of other targeted monoclonal antibodies for treatment of ALL are discussed later.

Alemtuzumab

Alemtuzumab (Campath-1H) is a humanized version of a rat monoclonal antibody directed against the CD52 antigen which is found on all mononuclear leukocytes.

Table 2
Novel antibodies in acute lymphoblastic leukemia trials

Antibody	Comment
Rituximab (anti-CD20)[61]	Potentiate chemotherapy in B cell malignancies
Alemtuzumab (anti-CD52)[62]	Subcutaneous injections
Epratuzumab (anti-CD22)[63,64]	May have a synergistic effect with anti-CD20 antibody
Anti-CD19[65,66]	Conjugated to immunotoxins
Anti-CD7[67]	Positive in vitro data in combination with ricin
Gemtuzamab ozagamicin (anti-CD33)[68,69]	Conjugated with calicheamicin
Antibodies to FLT3 ie, IMC-EB10 and IMC-NC7[70]	Positive in vitro and in vivo data in NOD/SCID mice

The CD52 antigen is expressed on normal and malignant lymphocytes. Approved for the treatment of B cell chronic lymphocytic leukemia, this antibody has also shown single-agent activity in a small number of patients with refractory ALL.[71,72] A phase 1/2 study has been completed by the Cancer and Leukemia Group B (CALGB 10,102) and demonstrated the safety of administering 30 mg of alemtuzumab subcutaneously three times a week for 4 weeks between courses of intensive consolidation chemotherapy with the aim of eradicating MRD with this novel agent.[73] Approximately 70% of adult ALL cases have been shown to express CD52 thus, if reductions in MRD levels can be demonstrated, alemtuzumab might be considered for further testing for both precursor B and T cell ALL on >10% of the blasts.[62]

Ofatumumab
Ofatumumab is a unique monoclonal antibody that targets a distinct small loop epitope on the CD20 molecule, different from rituximab. Preclinical data have shown that it is active against B cell lymphoma/chronic lymphocytic leukemia cells with low CD20-antigen density and high expression of complement inhibitory molecules. It was recently approved for patients with refractory follicular lymphoma who have failed treatment with rituximab,[74] and it may be of consideration in the future for ALL patients who express CD20.

Epratuzumab
Epratuzumab, a humanized monoclonal antibody against CD22 located in the cytoplasm of precursor B cells and on the surface of mature B cells, may also have activity in previously untreated patients. Epratuzumab has activity in children with relapsed ALL.[63,64] Unlike the anti-CD20 antibody, which has antiproliferative effects, epratuzumab seems to function more by an immunomodulatory mechanism.[75] Combination of rituximab and epratuzumab has shown promising results in non-Hodgkin lymphoma[76] and seems to be an attractive investigational approach in ALL.

CD19-directed antibodies
CD19 is a B-lineage specific transmembrane signaling protein expressed at high surface density on most ALL cells and therefore might be a prime target in this disease. Prior approaches with anti-CD19 antibodies have shown minimal benefits but 3 recently developed approaches are worth mentioning. The first is a bispecific antibody composed of a single chain of the anti-CD19 antibody and a single chain for the trigger molecule CD16 (present on natural killer cells and macrophages) connected by a peptide linker.[77] A similar approach consists of a humanized anti-CD19 antibody with an engineered Fc domain generated to increase the binding to Fc receptors on immune cells and thus increase Fc-mediated effector functions.[78] Finally, a microtubule destabilizing agent (monomethyl auristatin) was conjugated to the humanized anti-CD19 antibody via a protease-sensitive valine-citruline dipeptide linker.[79] A phase 1 trial that will begin to test the feasibility and toxicity of using a novel anti-CD19 antibody is planned for initiation in late 2009–2010.

Targeting Aberrant Signaling Pathways

BCR/ABL: beyond imatinib
Recent data demonstrate a clear therapeutic benefit of incorporating imatinib into frontline therapy for patients with Ph+ ALL, as discussed extensively in the article by Ravandi elsewhere in this issue. However, relapses are still common in Ph+ ALL as a result of the emergence of resistant clones. Understanding the mechanisms underlying imatinib resistance will provide key insights needed for more effective future treatment strategies in Ph+ ALL. The most common cause of resistance in

ALL seems to be mutations in the kinase domain of *BCR-ABL* that prevent binding of imatinib.[80] In Ph[+] ALL, the most frequently occurring imatinib-resistant mutations seem to be P-loop mutations and the T315I point mutation at the contact site.[81,82] These mutations represent a significant clinical issue, as both P-loop and T315I mutations are highly resistant to imatinib and have been associated with particularly poor prognosis.[83–85] Furthermore, the T315I mutation confers resistance to second-generation *BCR-ABL* inhibitors, including nilotinib and dasatinib. Persistent clones often emerge after an initial response to therapy ultimately leading to morphologic relapse. Primary imatinib refractory Ph[+] ALL has also been described[86] leading to the rational of incorporating second- and third-generation *BCR-ABL* inhibitors in the frontline therapy. Ongoing efforts to develop the next generation of targeted *ABL* inhibitors will be required to overcome drug resistance caused by the T315I, and other kinase domain mutations (**Table 3**).

Other mechanisms of imatinib resistance have also been described, such as overexpression or amplification of *BCR-ABL* and alterations in drug efflux or influx via alterations in Pgp or OCT-1, respectively.[86,87] In addition, *BCR-ABL*-independent pathways have been implicated to cause imatinib resistance including perturbation in the *SRC-LYN* kinase pathway and/or expression of oncogenic Ikaros isoforms.[88,89] It has been shown that combined inhibition of *BCR-ABL* and *SF kinases* improved the long-term survival in mice, whereas imatinib alone had a weaker inhibitory effect.[88] Therefore, a combined strategy of inhibiting *BCR-ABL* and other critical kinases may prove to be a promising treatment strategy for Ph[+] ALL patients.

Strategies to overcome imatinib resistance

Given these data, early phase trials have demonstrated significant activity of the second-generation *ABL* tyrosine kinase inhibitors, nilotinib and dasatinib, in Ph[+] ALL patients who were intolerant to, or relapsed after, imatinib-based therapy.[90–92] Therapy with dasatinib results in complete cytogenetic remissions (CcyR), but the responses were generally not durable with median progression-free survival of only 3.3 months. Nevertheless, these results and the ability of dasatinib to penetrate the CNS have led to trials of this agent as initial therapy for patients with Ph[+] ALL with excellent response rates approaching 100% with minimal toxicity.[93] The US Cooperative Groups will be incorporating dasatinib into combination chemotherapy as frontline therapy for patients with Ph[+] ALL in their next series of trials.

In addition to these agents, the dual *SRC/BCR-ABL* inhibitors SKI-606 and INNO-406 are currently being evaluated in clinical trials and have shown promise in imatinib-resistant patients with chronic myelocytic leukemia (CML) and Ph[+] ALL.[94–96] These agents are more potent against native *BCR-ABL* compared with imatinib and are active in a most imatinib-resistant *BCR-ABL* mutations except the T315I mutation.[95] The aurora kinase inhibitor Merck-0457 is the first TKI that has demonstrated activity against T315I mutation.[97–100] Early results from a phase 1/2 study show that Merck-0457 achieved a complete hematologic remission (CHR) in 1 patient with Ph[+] ALL harboring the T315I mutation.[98]

BCR-ABL and IKZF1 deletion

Approximately 85% of patients with *BCR-ABL* positive ALL have *IKZF1* deletion (*IKAROS*) suggesting its critical role in the pathogenesis of Ph[+] ALL.[101] Recently, Mullighan and colleagues have demonstrated that deletions and inactivating mutations of *IKZF1* also occur in a subset of cases of standard-risk Ph− precursor B cell ALL (approximately 29%) and confer a poor prognosis. These leukemias have a gene expression profile almost identical to Ph+ ALL[102,103] which suggests that *IKZF1* loss plays a crucial role in the pathogenesis of precursor B cell ALL. From a therapeutic standpoint, these fascinating observations present the immediate challenge of whether a clinical test to screen newly diagnosed patients with precursor B cell ALL for *IKZF1* mutations can be developed and whether more intensive therapy, including proceeding to an allogeneic HSCT in CR1 should be recommended for these patients. In addition, given the similarity of the gene expression signatures of this subset of *BCR-ABL* negative cases with *IKZF1* mutations and *BCR-ABL* positive ALL, there is a suggestion that these cases may have unidentified activating mutations in other tyrosine kinases that could be the target for drug development.

FLT3 signaling pathway inhibition

The receptor tyrosine kinase FLT3 is an important regulatory molecule in early hematopoiesis and seems to be, in part, responsible for cell proliferation, differentiation, and survival.[104,105] In normal hematopoietic cells, activation of the *FLT3* receptor by its ligand (FL) results in receptor dimerization and autophosphorylation with downstream phosphorylation of various signaling proteins, including the Janus kinase (*JAK*) 2 activated kinase (*JAK2*), signal transducer and activator of transcription (*STAT*) 5, and mitogen-activated protein kinase (*MAPK*) and *P13K/AKT* pathways.[105]

The *FLT3* protein is almost universally overexpressed in precursor B cell ALL, particularly in patients with *MLL* gene rearrangements and those with high hyperdiploidy (>50 chromosomes).[106] The *FLT3* gene mutations are observed in approximately 18% and 28% of patients with *MLL* gene rearrangement and hyperdiploid patients, respectively. In adults harboring t(4;11), overexpression of wild-type *FLT3* gene has also been observed.[107] The *FLT3* inhibitor CEP701 demonstrated antileukemic activity in ALL cell lines with inhibition proportional to the level of *FLT3* expression. Experience from AML and in vitro studies indicate that *FLT3* inhibitors are beneficial when used concomitantly with conventional chemotherapy.[108] Specific inhibition by PKC412 decreased ligand-induced phosphorylation and reduced the survival of leukemic cells when compared with untreated cells. Recently, Levis and colleagues demonstrated that *FLT3* inhibitors, when combined with conventional cytotoxic agents, were synergistic if added concomitantly but antagonistic if added before conventional therapy. Overall, these data indicate that inhibition of the *FLT3* protein might have a therapeutic role in combination with chemotherapy for certain subtypes of ALL and warrants further investigation.

Mammalian target of rapamycin (mTOR) inhibitors

The mammalian target of rapamycin (*mTOR*), an atypical serine/threonine kinase, plays a central role in the regulation of cell proliferation, growth, differentiation, migration and survival. Increasing evidence suggests that deregulation of the *mTOR* pathway is associated with hematological malignancies. Rapamycin targets *PI3K/AKT* pathways governed by *mTOR*, which are involved in the survival and chemoresistance of malignant lymphoblasts. The *mTOR* inhibitors such as rapamycin have been shown to induce apoptosis, overcome glucocorticoid resistance and enhance doxorubicin-induced cell death, provided *NF-κB* is not overexpressed, in ALL cell lines.[109] In vitro experiments have shown antiproliferative and pro-apoptotic effects of *mTOR* inhibitors in B-ALL cell lines.[110] All inhibitors have so far shown a safe toxicity profile in early clinical trials, with skin rashes and mucositis being the most common complications. Sporadic activity with no evidence of a dose-effect relationship has been reported. Chan and colleagues[111] demonstrated that concurrent inhibition of both *NOTCH1* and *mTOR* pathways have synergistic effects in T-ALL cell lines. On the contrary, when *mTOR* inhibitors are combined with cell cycle–specific cytotoxic drugs, the efficacy of chemotherapy may be compromised by inducing cell cycle arrest. Therefore, concomitant administration of *mTOR* inhibitors with cytotoxic agents will require carefully designed schedules based on preclinical modeling of dose and schedule. The *mTOR* inhibitor rapamycin is currently being explored in the post allogeneic HSCT setting for relapsed/refractory ALL patients (NCT00795886). The primary hypothesis in this setting is to evaluate addition of rapamycin to graft versus host disease (GVHD) prophylaxis and potentially increase LFS through the novel benefit of using a drug that has the potential to control GVHD and suppress leukemic blasts.

JAK2 mutations in ALL patients with Down syndrome

Children with Down syndrome have a greatly increased risk of ALL. A specific genotype-phenotype association was recently discovered between the somatic mutation with JAK2 pseudokinase domain *(R683)* and ALL development.[112,113] These mutations immortalized primary mouse hematopoietic stem cells and caused constitutive JAK activation and cytokine-independent growth of BaF3 cells.[112] Therefore, JAK2 inhibitors could be useful for the treatment of this type of leukemia.

Other Novel Targets

Heat shock protein 90

Heat shock protein 90 (Hsp90) is a molecular chaperone that affects the stability and function of multiple oncogenic proteins including *BCR-ABL*. Geldanamycin (GA) specifically inhibits Hsp90 by competitively binding to an ATP-binding pocket in the amino terminus of Hsp90. Disruption of Hsp90 function by GA or its less toxic analogue, 17-allylaminogeldanamycin (17-AAG), in *BCR-ABL* expressing leukemia cells has been shown to induce *BCR-ABL* protein degradation and suppress cell proliferation even in T315I mutant cells.[114] Another Hsp90 inhibitor, IPI-504 degraded BCR-ABL protein, decreased numbers of leukemia stem cells, and prolonged survival of leukemic mice bearing the T315I mutation.[115] Concurrent administration of suberanoylanilide hydroxamic acid (SAHA), a histone deacetylase (HDAC) inhibitor with 17-AAG synergistically induces apoptosis in *BCR-ABL* positive cells.[116] These findings may represent a novel therapeutic strategy for Ph+ ALL (see **Table 3**).

Proteasome inhibition

The ubiquitin-proteasome pathway is the most important intracellular pathway for protein degradation. Important proteins affected by this pathway are, for example, cyclins and the transcription factor nuclear factor-κB. The process is needed for cells to proceed through the cell cycle and its inhibition results in apoptosis. Bortezomib is a potent and selective proteasome inhibitor already approved in the treatment of multiple myeloma (MM). A phase 1 clinical trial of bortezomib in refractory or relapse acute leukemia was recently conducted.[117] However, it was associated with neurologic toxicity, one of the most common toxicities associated with this drug. Because ALL patients are treated with vincristine, application of bortezomib into the ALL armamentarium is unlikely. However, the recently developed proteasome inhibitors carfilzomib[118] or its derivative PR-047[119] are believed to be devoid of the neurologic toxicity and, therefore, proteasome inhibition could be tested again in ALL in the near future.

Targeting NOTCH1 in precursor T cell ALL

NOTCH receptors participate in a conserved signaling pathway that controls the development of diverse tissues and cell types, including lymphoid cells. Signaling is normally initiated through one or more ligand-mediated proteolytic cleavage enzymes.

One of the critical enzymes, γ-secretase, is responsible for releasing the intracellular portion of NOTCH1 receptor (ICN1) on its activation. This permits release of nuclear translocation of the *NOTCH1* which then binds and activates transcription factors of the *Su(H)/CBF1* family and results in normal lymphoid development.[120–122] Aberrant activation of the *NOTCH1* pathway has been implicated in the pathogenesis of both childhood and adult precursor T cell ALL.[120,122,123] Activating mutations in *NOTCH1* signaling have been identified in more than 50% of human T cell ALL.[122] A phase 1 clinical trial of a γ-secretase inhibitor (GSI) in relapsed precursor T cell ALL was initiated.[124] The agent demonstrated some pharmacodynamic activity in the leukemia cells, but the trial was stopped early because of significant gastrointestinal toxicities and an inability to perform dose escalation. It has recently been shown that inhibition of NOTCH1 signaling in glucocorticoid-resistant precursor T cell ALL restored glucocorticoid receptor autoupregulation and apoptotic cell death. Furthermore, in murine models, the gastrointestinal toxicity induced by GSIs could be overcome by the addition of glucocorticoids.[125] Thus, there is an excellent rationale for testing the combination of a GSI with glucocorticoids in the treatment of glucocorticoid-resistant T-ALL.[126]

Epigenetic modulation

Drugs that modulate the epigenome of ALL cells may be another interesting approach to expand the therapeutic armamentarium. Epigenetic silencing of the key regulatory genes in lymphoid development, through aberrant methylation of CpG islands of the promoter region and/or aberrant deacetylation of histones has been described.[127,128] Both mechanisms are hypothesized to lead to a survival advantage. Approximately 80% of the ALL cases demonstrate aberrant methylation both at presentation and relapse.[129–135] In the past several years, subsets of patients with specific hypermethylated genes have been identified,[129–132,135] particularly the cell cycle regulatory genes, *p16* and *p15*. Abnormal silencing of *p16*, *p15* and other genes[133] has been linked to worse outcome in ALL.[129–132,135] In this study methylation status of 15 genes (*CDH1*, *p73*, *p16*, *p15*, *p57*, *NES-1*, *DKK-3*, *CDH13*, *p14*, *TMS-1*, *APAF-1*, *DAPK*, *PARKIN*, *LATS-1*, and *PTEN*) was analyzed in 251 patients with ALL. In 77% of the patients at least 1 gene was hypermethylated and ≥ 3 genes were hypermethylated in approximately 35% of the patients. The DFS was 75.5% in the nonmethylated group compared with only 9.4% in the hypermethylated group (≥ 3 methylated genes), respectively. The OS was also adversely affected in the hypermethylated group with an OS of only 7.8% compared with an OS of 66.1% in the nonmethylated group. Multivariate analysis demonstrated that the methylation profile was an independent prognostic factor in predicting DFS ($P<.0001$) and OS ($P = .003$). Another study by Shen and colleagues[134] showed that methylation of at least two genes involved in the cell cycle regulatory pathways are needed to result in unfavorable OS ($P = .02$) in patients with Ph$^-$ ALL. Based on these insights, a phase 1/2 study at the MD Anderson Cancer Center is currently testing the addition of the hypomethylating agent decitabine to standard chemotherapy in patients with relapsed ALL.

Improved knowledge about epigenetic phenomena in ALL, including careful identification of involved tumor-related genes and activation of oncogenes, is imperative to effectively restore normal hematopoiesis and to improve treatment outcomes. Finally, recent data also suggest that epigenetic evaluation may become another novel strategy for evaluation of MRD.[136]

WHERE DO WE STAND NOW?

ALL in adults remains a challenging disease that will require innovative strategies for cure (**Table 4**). Whereas adoption of pediatric-inspired regimens focusing on intensive

Table 3
Molecular targeted agents for treatment of acute lymphoblastic leukemia

Selected Molecular Targets	Inhibitor	Comment(s)
Tyrosine Kinases[86,96]	Dasatinib (BMS-354/825) Nilotinib MK0457 (VX-680) Aurora kinase inhibitor Bosutinib (SKI-606)	-Multi-targeted ABL/Src inhibitor -20- to 50-fold greater potency than imatinib -Effective in T315I-mutated Ph+ ALL -Oral Src inhibitor with anti-Abl activities
Fms-like tyrosine kinase-3 (FLT-3)[101]	CEP-701 Midostaurin Tandutinib	-Positive in-vitro data
Histone deacetylase[107]	Vorinostat High dose Valproic acid Depsipeptide	-Positive in-vitro data -Positive anecdotal data in childhood ALL
DNA methyltransferase[117,123]	Decitabine Azacytidine	-Possibly in combination with HDACi*
mTOR[104]	Rapamycin Temsirolimus Everolimus	-Positive in-vitro data
NOTCH-1[112]	γ-secretase inhibitor (GSI)	Ongoing Trials in T-ALL
Heat shock protein-90[107]	17-AAG**	-Positive in-vitro data in combination with other molecular pathways inhibitors
NFκB[126]	Bortezomib Carfilzomib PR-047	-Rational to combine with mTOR inhibitors and Anthracyclines -Carfilzomib and PR-047 may be less neurotoxic.

* HDACi: Histone deacetylase inhibitors
** 17-AAG:17-allylamino-17-demethoxygeldanamycin

use of glucocorticoids, vincristine, and L-asparaginase may significantly improve the outcome of younger adults with ALL, alternative strategies may be required for improved survival of older adults. Options for the immediate future include testing alternative (perhaps reduced intensity conditioning) allogeneic HSCT for high-risk adults in CR1. Prospective MRD measurements may refine our ability to select patients at high risk for relapse for whom allogeneic transplant may currently represent the only potential curative approach. Increasingly, improvements in outcome may come from insights into disease pathogenesis and testing of specifically targeted agents in biologically selected subsets of patients. A wonderful example of this progress is already occurring for the large percentage of adults with ALL who are Ph+; the first and second-generation ABL TKIs are already refining and improving treatment strategies and survival. In the clinic currently, nelarabine, an approved agent for relapsed precursor T cell ALL, has also been incorporated into pediatric frontline regimens with promising results (and little additional toxicity) and should also be tested in this manner in adults with precursor T cell ALL. Targeting specific subsets of ALL with appropriate monoclonal antibodies such as rituximab and alemtuzumab are also being examined as adjuncts to frontline therapy, and results from these trials are forthcoming. Newer antibodies, such as epratuzumab, already tested in relapsed disease,

Table 4	
Possible Strategies to Improve Treatment Outcomes in Acute Lymphoblastic Leukemia Treatment	
Treatment Phase	**Possible Strategies**
General	• Understanding of disease subtype/molecular basis of the disease • Insights into pharmacogenomics • Understanding the pharmacokinetics and pharmacodynamics of each agent employed in the treatment regimens • Implications of MRD status in each phase of treatment • Stringent remission criteria • Understanding and overcoming drug resistance • Regimen selection based on molecular genetic features • Optimization of therapy with addition of selected targeted agents such as BCR/ABL inhibitors and monoclonal antibodies • Development of age adapted regimens esp. for elderly population: validation of pediatric inspired approach in younger adults with ALL • Optimization of intracranial prophylaxis • Further improvement in the supportive care measures: minimize treatment toxicity
Induction	• Enhancement of induction regimens with non-myelotoxic and targeted agents without incurring greater TRM
Consolidation	• Clarification of HSCT indications with advent of molecular targets esp. Ph + ALL • MRD-based treatment stratification • Incorporation of new agents into post-remission therapy based on disease biology
Maintenance	• Duration and type of maintenance therapy; can this also be biologically defined? • Role of BCR/ABL inhibition post-HSCT and duration of TKI therapy in Ph+ patients who are not transplanted e.g. Role of demethylating agents and Histone deacetylase inhibitors

are also excellent candidates for incorporation into frontline treatment strategies, An exciting new era of individualized treatment based on disease pathogenesis is on the horizon; potential targets include aberrant signaling pathways (*FLT3, mTOR, JAK2*), transcription factors (*NOTCH1*), and epigenetic deregulation. Critical to the success of any molecular subset-based approach will be improved molecular diagnostic tools, and participation in cooperative group and/or multicenter studies designed to test targeted agents in carefully selected disease subsets of this relatively rare disease.

REFERENCES

1. Bruggemann M, et al. Clinical significance of minimal residual disease quantification in adult patients with standard-risk acute lymphoblastic leukemia. Blood 2006;107:1116–23.
2. Cave H, van der Werff ten Bosch J, Suciu S, et al. Clinical significance of minimal residual disease in childhood acute lymphoblastic leukemia. European Organization for Research and Treatment of Cancer–Childhood Leukemia Cooperative Group. N Engl J Med 1998;339:591–8.
3. Coustan-Smith E, et al. Prognostic importance of measuring early clearance of leukemic cells by flow cytometry in childhood acute lymphoblastic leukemia. Blood 2002;100:52–8.

4. Dworzak MN, et al. Prognostic significance and modalities of flow cytometric minimal residual disease detection in childhood acute lymphoblastic leukemia. Blood 2002;99:1952-8.

5. Marshall GM, et al. Importance of minimal residual disease testing during the second year of therapy for children with acute lymphoblastic leukemia. J Clin Oncol 2003;21:704-9.

6. Mortuza FY, et al. Minimal residual disease tests provide an independent predictor of clinical outcome in adult acute lymphoblastic leukemia. J Clin Oncol 2002;20:1094-104.

7. Nyvold C, et al. Precise quantification of minimal residual disease at day 29 allows identification of children with acute lymphoblastic leukemia and an excellent outcome. Blood 2002;99:1253-8.

8. Raff T, et al. Molecular relapse in adult standard-risk ALL patients detected by prospective MRD monitoring during and after maintenance treatment: data from the GMALL 06/99 and 07/03 trials. Blood 2007;109:910-5.

9. van der Velden VH, et al. Analysis of minimal residual disease by Ig/TCR gene rearrangements: guidelines for interpretation of real-time quantitative PCR data. Leukemia 2007;21:604-11.

10. van Dongen JJ, et al. Design and standardization of PCR primers and protocols for detection of clonal immunoglobulin and T-cell receptor gene recombinations in suspect lymphoproliferations: report of the BIOMED-2 Concerted Action BMH4-CT98-3936. Leukemia 2003;17:2257-317.

11. Goldstone AH, et al. In adults with standard-risk acute lymphoblastic leukemia, the greatest benefit is achieved from a matched sibling allogeneic transplantation in first complete remission, and an autologous transplantation is less effective than conventional consolidation/maintenance chemotherapy in all patients: final results of the International ALL Trial (MRC UKALL XII/ECOG E2993). Blood 2008;111:1827-33.

12. Campana D. Molecular determinants of treatment response in acute lymphoblastic leukemia. Hematology Am Soc Hematol Educ Program 2008;2008:366-73.

13. Pui CH, Robison LL, Look AT. Acute lymphoblastic leukaemia. Lancet 2008;371:1030-43.

14. Wei G, et al. Gene expression-based chemical genomics identifies rapamycin as a modulator of MCL1 and glucocorticoid resistance. Cancer Cell 2006;10:331-42.

15. Steinbach D, et al. The multidrug resistance-associated protein 3 (MRP3) is associated with a poor outcome in childhood ALL and may account for the worse prognosis in male patients and T-cell immunophenotype. Blood 2003;102:4493-8.

16. Tafuri A, et al. MDR1 protein expression is an independent predictor of complete remission in newly diagnosed adult acute lymphoblastic leukemia. Blood 2002;100:974-81.

17. Baer MR, et al. Phase 3 study of the multidrug resistance modulator PSC-833 in previously untreated patients 60 years of age and older with acute myeloid leukemia: Cancer and Leukemia Group B Study 9720. Blood 2002;100:1224-32.

18. Solary E, et al. Quinine as a multidrug resistance inhibitor: a phase 3 multicentric randomized study in adult de novo acute myelogenous leukemia. Blood 2003;102:1202-10.

19. Evans WE, Relling MV. Moving towards individualized medicine with pharmacogenomics. Nature 2004;429:464-8.

20. Pui CH, Relling MV, Evans WE. Role of pharmacogenomics and pharmacody-namics in the treatment of acute lymphoblastic leukaemia. Best Pract Res Clin Haematol 2002;15:741–56.
21. Krajinovic M, Costea I, Chiasson S. Polymorphism of the thymidylate synthase gene and outcome of acute lymphoblastic leukaemia. Lancet 2002;359:1033–4.
22. Relling MV, et al. Mercaptopurine therapy intolerance and heterozygosity at the thiopurine S-methyltransferase gene locus. J Natl Cancer Inst 1999;91:2001–8.
23. Taub JW, et al. Polymorphisms in methylenetetrahydrofolate reductase and methotrexate sensitivity in childhood acute lymphoblastic leukemia. Leukemia 2002;16:764–5.
24. Ulrich CM, et al. Pharmacogenetics of methotrexate: toxicity among marrow transplantation patients varies with the methylenetetrahydrofolate reductase C677T polymorphism. Blood 2001;98:231–4.
25. Evans WE, et al. Clinical pharmacodynamics of high-dose methotrexate in acute lymphocytic leukemia. Identification of a relation between concentration and effect. N Engl J Med 1986;314:471–7.
26. Ramakers-van Woerden NL, et al. TEL/AML1 gene fusion is related to in vitro drug sensitivity for L-asparaginase in childhood acute lymphoblastic leukemia. Blood 2000;96:1094–9.
27. Stam RW, et al. Differential mRNA expression of Ara-C-metabolizing enzymes explains Ara-C sensitivity in MLL gene-rearranged infant acute lymphoblastic leukemia. Blood 2003;101:1270–6.
28. Kaspers GJ, et al. Favorable prognosis of hyperdiploid common acute lympho-blastic leukemia may be explained by sensitivity to antimetabolites and other drugs: results of an in vitro study. Blood 1995;85:751–6.
29. Kager L, et al. Folate pathway gene expression differs in subtypes of acute lymphoblastic leukemia and influences methotrexate pharmacodynamics. J Clin Invest 2005;115:110–7.
30. Lampert F, et al. Karyotypes in acute childhood leukemias may lose prognostic significance with more intensive and specific chemotherapy. Cancer Genet Cytogenet 1991;54:277–9.
31. Raimondi SC, et al. Cytogenetics of pre-B-cell acute lymphoblastic leukemia with emphasis on prognostic implications of the t(1;19). J Clin Oncol 1990;8:1380–8.
32. Moorman AV, et al. Karyotype is an independent prognostic factor in adult acute lymphoblastic leukemia (ALL): analysis of cytogenetic data from patients treated on the Medical Research Council (MRC) UKALLXII/Eastern Cooperative Oncology Group (ECOG) 2993 trial. Blood 2007;109:3189–97.
33. Secker-Walker LM, et al. Cytogenetics adds independent prognostic information in adults with acute lymphoblastic leukaemia on MRC trial UKALL XA. MRC Adult Leukaemia Working Party. Br J Haematol 1997;96:601–10.
34. Appelbaum FR. Impact of age on the biology of acute leukemia. In: Perry MC, editor. American Society of Clinical Oncology Educational Book Alexandria (VA): Society of Clinical Oncology; 2005. p. 528–32.
35. Wetzler M, et al. Prospective karyotype analysis in adult acute lymphoblastic leukemia: the cancer and leukemia Group B experience. Blood 1999;93:3983–93.
36. Boissel N, et al. Should adolescents with acute lymphoblastic leukemia be treated as old children or young adults? Comparison of the French FRALLE-93 and LALA-94 trials. J Clin Oncol 2003;21:774–80.

37. Haiat S, Vekhoff A, Marzac C, et al. Improved outcome of adult acute lympho-blastic leukemia treated with a pediatric protocol: results of a pilot study. [ASH Annual Meeting Abstracts]. Blood 2007;110:2822a.

38. Nachman J, Sather HN, Buckley JD, et al. Young adults 16–21 years of age at diagnosis entered on Childrens Cancer Group acute lymphoblastic leukemia and acute myeloblastic leukemia protocols, results of treatment. Cancer 1993; 71(10 suppl):3377–85.

39. Ramanujachar R, et al. Adolescents with acute lymphoblastic leukaemia: outcome on UK national paediatric (ALL97) and adult (UKALLXII/E2993) trials. Pediatr Blood Cancer 2007;48:254–61.

40. Schiffer CA. Differences in outcome in adolescents with acute lymphoblastic leukemia: a consequence of better regimens? Better doctors? Both? J Clin Oncol 2003;21:760–1.

41. Stock W, et al. What determines the outcomes for adolescents and young adults with acute lymphoblastic leukemia treated on cooperative group protocols? A comparison of Children's Cancer Group and Cancer and Leukemia Group B studies. Blood 2008;112:1646–54.

42. Larson RA, et al. A randomized controlled trial of filgrastim during remission induction and consolidation chemotherapy for adults with acute lymphoblastic leukemia: CALGB study 9111. Blood 1998;92:1556–64.

43. Takeuchi J, et al. Induction therapy by frequent administration of doxorubicin with four other drugs, followed by intensive consolidation and maintenance therapy for adult acute lymphoblastic leukemia: the JALSG-ALL93 study. Leukemia 2002;16:1259–66.

44. Thiebaut A, et al. Adult acute lymphocytic leukemia study testing chemotherapy and autologous and allogeneic transplantation. A follow-up report of the French protocol LALA 87. x. Hematol Oncol Clin North Am 2000;14:1353–66.

45. Sallan SE. Myths and lessons from the adult/pediatric interface in acute lymphoblastic leukemia. Hematology Am Soc Hematol Educ Program 2006;128–32.

46. DeAngelo DJ, Dahlberg S, Silverman LB, et al. A multicenter phase II study using a dose intensified pediatric regimen in adults with untreated acute lymphoblastic leukemia [ASH Annual Meeting Abstracts]. Blood 2007;110: 587.

47. Huguet F, et al. Pediatric-inspired therapy in adults with Philadelphia chromo-some-negative acute lymphoblastic leukemia: the GRAALL-2003 study. J Clin Oncol 2009;27:911–8.

48. Ribera JM, et al. Comparison of the results of the treatment of adolescents and young adults with standard-risk acute lymphoblastic leukemia with the Programa Espanol de Tratamiento en Hematologia pediatric-based protocol ALL-96. J Clin Oncol 2008;26:1843–9.

49. Advani A, et al. A prognostic scoring system for adult patients less than 60 years of age with acute lymphoblastic leukemia in first relapse. Leuk Lymphoma 2009; 50:1126–31.

50. Berg SL, et al. Phase II study of nelarabine (compound 506U78) in children and young adults with refractory T-cell malignancies: a report from the Children's Oncology Group. J Clin Oncol 2005;23:3376–82.

51. Jeha S, et al. Phase II study of clofarabine in pediatric patients with refractory or relapsed acute lymphoblastic leukemia. J Clin Oncol 2006;24:1917–23.

52. Kantarjian H, et al. Phase 2 clinical and pharmacologic study of clofarabine in patients with refractory or relapsed acute leukemia. Blood 2003;102:2379–86.

53. Douer D, et al. Pharmacodynamics and safety of intravenous pegaspargase during remission induction in adults aged 55 years or younger with newly diagnosed acute lymphoblastic leukemia. Blood 2007;109:2744–50.
54. Krishna R, Webb MS, St Onge G, et al. Liposomal and nonliposomal drug pharmacokinetics after administration of liposome-encapsulated vincristine and their contribution to drug tissue distribution properties. J Pharmacol Exp Ther 2001; 298:1206–12.
55. Andreeff M, Giles F, Korblau S, et al. Phase I study of annamycin, a novel anthracycline, in patients with relapsed/refractory acute myeloid leukemia and lymphoid leukemias. Proc Am Soc Clin Oncol 2001;20:303a.
56. Jabbour E, et al. Neurologic complications associated with intrathecal liposomal cytarabine given prophylactically in combination with high-dose methotrexate and cytarabine to patients with acute lymphocytic leukemia. Blood 2007;109: 3214–8.
57. Sarris AH, et al. Trimetrexate in relapsed T-cell lymphoma with skin involvement. J Clin Oncol 2002;20:2876–80.
58. Kang MH, Harutyunyan N, Hall CP, et al. Methotrexate and aminopterin exhibit similar in vitro and in vivo preclinical activity against acute lymphoblastic leukaemia and lymphoma. Br J Haematol 2009;145:389–93.
59. Yee KW, et al. Phase 1 study of ABT-751, a novel microtubule inhibitor, in patients with refractory hematologic malignancies. Clin Cancer Res 2005;11:6615–24.
60. Furman RR, Gore L, Ravandi F, et al. Forodesine IV (Bcx-1777) is clinically active in relapsed/refractory T-cell leukemia: results of a Phase II Study (Interim Report). [ASH Annual Meeting Abstracts]. Blood 2006;108:1851.
61. Thomas DA, et al. Chemoimmunotherapy with hyper-CVAD plus rituximab for the treatment of adult Burkitt and Burkitt-type lymphoma or acute lymphoblastic leukemia. Cancer 2006;106:1569–80.
62. Lozanski G, et al. Quantitative measurement of CD52 expression and alemtuzumab bindings in adult acute lymphoblastic leukemia (ALL): correlation with immunophenotype and cytogenetics in patients (Pts) enrolled on a phase I/II trial from the Cancer and Leukemia Group G (CALGB 10102). [ASH Annual Meeting Abstracts]. Blood 2007;110:2386.
63. Borowitz MJ, Carrol WL, Adamson PC, et al. Effective targeting of leukemic cells in children with B-precursor acute lymphoblastic leukemia treated with anti-CD22 (Epratuzumab). a Children's Oncology Group (COG) Study. Blood 2006; 108:2585a.
64. Raetz EA, et al. Chemoimmunotherapy reinduction with epratuzumab in children with acute lymphoblastic leukemia in marrow relapse: a Children's Oncology Group Pilot Study. J Clin Oncol 2008;26:3756–62.
65. Goulet AC, et al. Conjugation of blocked ricin to an anti-CD19 monoclonal antibody increases antibody-induced cell calcium mobilization and CD19 internalization. Blood 1997;90:2364–75.
66. Stone MJ, et al. A phase I study of bolus versus continuous infusion of the anti-CD19 immunotoxin, IgG-HD37-dgA, in patients with B-cell lymphoma. Blood 1996;88:1188–97.
67. Peipp M, et al. A recombinant CD7-specific single-chain immunotoxin is a potent inducer of apoptosis in acute leukemic T cells. Cancer Res 2002; 62:2848–55.
68. Golay J, et al. Gemtuzumab ozogamicin (Mylotarg) has therapeutic activity against CD33 acute lymphoblastic leukaemias in vitro and in vivo. Br J Haematol 2005;128:310–7.

69. Zwaan CM, et al. Gemtuzumab ozogamicin in pediatric CD33-positive acute lymphoblastic leukemia: first clinical experiences and relation with cellular sensitivity to single agent calicheamicin. Leukemia 2003;17:468–70.

70. Piloto O, et al. IMC-EB10, an anti-FLT3 monoclonal antibody, prolongs survival and reduces nonobese diabetic/severe combined immunodeficient engraftment of some acute lymphoblastic leukemia cell lines and primary leukemic samples. Cancer Res 2006;66:4843–51.

71. Laporte JP, Isnard F, Garderet L, et al. Remission of adult acute lymphocytic leukaemia with alemtuzumab. Leukemia 2004;18:1557–8.

72. Tibes R, et al. Activity of alemtuzumab in patients with CD52-positive acute leukemia. Cancer 2006;106:2645–51.

73. Stock W, et al. Incorporation of Alemtuzumab into front-line therapy of adult acute lympholbastic leukemia (ALL) is feasible: a phase I/II study from the Cancer and Leukemia Group B (CALGB 10102). Blood 2005;106:145a.

74. Hagenbeek A, et al. First clinical use of ofatumumab, a novel fully human anti-CD20 monoclonal antibody in relapsed or refractory follicular lymphoma: results of a phase 1/2 trial. Blood 2008;111:5486–95.

75. Carnahan J, et al. Epratuzumab, a CD22-targeting recombinant humanized antibody with a different mode of action from rituximab. Mol Immunol 2007;44:1331–41.

76. Leonard JP, et al. Durable complete responses from therapy with combined epratuzumab and rituximab: final results from an international multicenter, phase 2 study in recurrent, indolent, non-Hodgkin lymphoma. Cancer 2008;113:2714–23.

77. Kellner C, et al. A novel CD19-directed recombinant bispecific antibody derivative with enhanced immune effector functions for human leukemic cells. J Immunother 2008;31:871–84.

78. Horton HM, et al. Potent in vitro and in vivo activity of an Fc-engineered anti-CD19 monoclonal antibody against lymphoma and leukemia. Cancer Res 2008;68:8049–57.

79. Gerber HP, et al. Potent antitumor activity of the anti-CD19 auristatin antibody drug conjugate hBU12-vcMMAE against rituximab-sensitive and -resistant lymphomas. Blood 2009;113:4352–61.

80. Hofmann WK, Komor M, Hoelzer D, et al. Mechanisms of resistance to STI571 (imatinib) in Philadelphia-chromosome positive acute lymphoblastic leukemia. Leuk Lymphoma 2004;45:655–60.

81. Branford S, et al. Detection of BCR-ABL mutations in patients with CML treated with imatinib is virtually always accompanied by clinical resistance, and mutations in the ATP phosphate-binding loop (P-loop) are associated with a poor prognosis. Blood 2003;102:276–83.

82. Soverini S, et al. Contribution of ABL kinase domain mutations to imatinib resistance in different subsets of Philadelphia-positive patients: by the GIMEMA Working Party on Chronic Myeloid Leukemia. Clin Cancer Res 2006;12:7374–9.

83. Druker BJ, et al. Activity of a specific inhibitor of the BCR-ABL tyrosine kinase in the blast crisis of chronic myeloid leukemia and acute lymphoblastic leukemia with the Philadelphia chromosome. N Engl J Med 2001;344:1038–42.

84. Mahon FX, et al. Selection and characterization of BCR-ABL positive cell lines with differential sensitivity to the tyrosine kinase inhibitor STI571: diverse mechanisms of resistance. Blood 2000;96:1070–9.

85. Soverini S, et al. ABL mutations in late chronic phase chronic myeloid leukemia patients with up-front cytogenetic resistance to imatinib are associated with a greater likelihood of progression to blast crisis and shorter survival: a Study

by the GIMEMA Working Party on Chronic Myeloid Leukemia. J Clin Oncol 2005; 23:4100–9.

86. Illmer T, et al. P-glycoprotein-mediated drug efflux is a resistance mechanism of chronic myelogenous leukemia cells to treatment with imatinib mesylate. Leukemia 2004;18:401–8.

87. Hochhaus A, La Rosee P. Imatinib therapy in chronic myelogenous leukemia: strategies to avoid and overcome resistance. Leukemia 2004;18:1321–31.

88. Hu Y, et al. Targeting multiple kinase pathways in leukemic progenitors and stem cells is essential for improved treatment of Ph+ leukemia in mice. Proc Natl Acad Sci U S A 2006;103:16870–5.

89. Iacobucci I, et al. Expression of spliced oncogenic Ikaros isoforms in Philadelphia-positive acute lymphoblastic leukemia patients treated with tyrosine kinase inhibitors: implications for a new mechanism of resistance. Blood 2008;112: 3847–55.

90. Kantarjian HM, Talpaz M, Giles F, et al. New insights into the pathophysiology of chronic myeloid leukemia and imatinib resistance. Ann Intern Med 2006;145:913–23.

91. Ottmann O, et al. Dasatinib induces rapid hematologic and cytogenetic responses in adult patients with Philadelphia chromosome positive acute lymphoblastic leukemia with resistance or intolerance to imatinib: interim results of a phase 2 study. Blood 2007;110:2309–15.

92. Talpaz M, et al. Dasatinib in imatinib-resistant Philadelphia chromosome-positive leukemias. N Engl J Med 2006;354:2531–41.

93. Foa R, Vitale A, Meloni G, et al. Dasatinib as front-line monotherapy for the induction treatment of adult and elderly PH+ acute lymphoblastic leukemia (ALL) patients: interim analysis of the GIMEMA prospective study LAL 12205. [ASH Annual Meeting Abstracts]. Blood 2007;110:7a.

94. Golas JM, et al. SKI-606, a 4-anilino-3-quinolinecarbonitrile dual inhibitor of Src and Abl kinases, is a potent antiproliferative agent against chronic myelogenous leukemia cells in culture and causes regression of K562 xenografts in nude mice. Cancer Res 2003;63:375–81.

95. Kimura S, et al. NS-187, a potent and selective dual Bcr-Abl/Lyn tyrosine kinase inhibitor, is a novel agent for imatinib-resistant leukemia. Blood 2005;106: 3948–54.

96. Naito H, et al. In vivo antiproliferative effect of NS-187, a dual Bcr-Abl/Lyn tyrosine kinase inhibitor, on leukemic cells harbouring Abl kinase domain mutations. Leuk Res 2006;30:1443–6.

97. Carter BZ, et al. Regulation of survivin expression through Bcr-Abl/MAPK cascade: targeting survivin overcomes imatinib resistance and increases imatinib sensitivity in imatinib-responsive CML cells. Blood 2006;107:1555–63.

98. Giles FJ, et al. MK-0457, a novel kinase inhibitor, is active in patients with chronic myeloid leukemia or acute lymphocytic leukemia with the T315I BCR-ABL mutation. Blood 2007;109:500–2.

99. Harrington EA, et al. VX-680, a potent and selective small-molecule inhibitor of the Aurora kinases, suppresses tumor growth in vivo. Nat Med 2004;10:262–7.

100. Young MA, et al. Structure of the kinase domain of an imatinib-resistant Abl mutant in complex with the Aurora kinase inhibitor VX-680. Cancer Res 2006; 66:1007–14.

101. Mullighan CG, et al. BCR-ABL1 lymphoblastic leukaemia is characterized by the deletion of Ikaros. Nature 2008;453:110–4.

102. Mullighan CG, et al. Genome-wide analysis of genetic alterations in acute lymphoblastic leukaemia. Nature 2007;446:758–64.

103. Mullighan CG, et al. Deletion of IKZF1 and prognosis in acute lymphoblastic leukemia. N Engl J Med 2009;360:470–80.
104. Gilliland DG, Griffin JD. The roles of FLT3 in hematopoiesis and leukemia. Blood 2002;100:1532–42.
105. Levis M, Small D. FLT3: ITDoes matter in leukemia. Leukemia 2003;17:1738–52.
106. Brown P, et al. FLT3 inhibition selectively kills childhood acute lymphoblastic leukemia cells with high levels of FLT3 expression. Blood 2005;105:812–20.
107. Torelli GF, et al. FLT3 inhibition in t(4;11)+ adult acute lymphoid leukaemia. Br J Haematol 2005;130:43–50.
108. Levis M, Pham R, Smith BD, et al. In vitro studies of a FLT3 inhibitor combined with chemotherapy: sequence of administration is important to achieve synergistic cytotoxic effects. Blood 2004;104:1145–50.
109. Avellino R, et al. Rapamycin stimulates apoptosis of childhood acute lymphoblastic leukemia cells. Blood 2005;106:1400–6.
110. Teachey DT, et al. The mTOR inhibitor CCI-779 induces apoptosis and inhibits growth in preclinical models of primary adult human ALL. Blood 2006;107: 1149–55.
111. Chan SM, Weng AP, Tibshirani R, et al. Notch signals positively regulate activity of the mTOR pathway in T-cell acute lymphoblastic leukemia. Blood 2007;110: 278–86.
112. Bercovich D, et al. Mutations of JAK2 in acute lymphoblastic leukaemias associated with Down's syndrome. Lancet 2008;372:1484–92.
113. Kearney L, et al. Specific JAK2 mutation (JAK2R683) and multiple gene deletions in Down syndrome acute lymphoblastic leukemia. Blood 2009;113:646–8.
114. Gorre ME, Ellwood-Yen K, Chiosis G, et al. BCR-ABL point mutants isolated from patients with imatinib mesylate-resistant chronic myeloid leukemia remain sensitive to inhibitors of the BCR-ABL chaperone heat shock protein 90. Blood 2002; 100:3041–4.
115. Peng C, et al. Inhibition of heat shock protein 90 prolongs survival of mice with BCR-ABL-T315I-induced leukemia and suppresses leukemic stem cells. Blood 2007;110:678–85.
116. Rahmani M, et al. Cotreatment with suberanoylanilide hydroxamic acid and 17-allylamino 17-demethoxygeldanamycin synergistically induces apoptosis in Bcr-Abl+ cells sensitive and resistant to STI571 (imatinib mesylate) in association with down-regulation of Bcr-Abl, abrogation of signal transducer and activator of transcription 5 activity, and Bax conformational change. Mol Pharmacol 2005;67:1166–76.
117. Cortes J, et al. Phase I study of bortezomib in refractory or relapsed acute leukemias. Clin Cancer Res 2004;10:3371–6.
118. Kuhn DJ, et al. Potent activity of carfilzomib, a novel, irreversible inhibitor of the ubiquitin-proteasome pathway, against preclinical models of multiple myeloma. Blood 2007;110:3281–90.
119. Zhou HJ, et al. Design and synthesis of an orally bioavailable and selective peptide epoxyketone proteasome inhibitor (PR-047). J Med Chem 2009;52:3028–38.
120. Ellisen LW, et al. TAN-1, the human homolog of the *Drosophila notch* gene, is broken by chromosomal translocations in T lymphoblastic neoplasms. Cell 1991;66:649–61.
121. O'Neil J, et al. Activating Notch1 mutations in mouse models of T-ALL. Blood 2006;107:781–5.
122. Weng AP, et al. Activating mutations of NOTCH1 in human T cell acute lymphoblastic leukemia. Science 2004;306:269–71.

123. Lee SY, et al. Mutations of the Notch1 gene in T-cell acute lymphoblastic leukemia: analysis in adults and children. Leukemia 2005;19:1841–3.
124. DeAngelo DJ, et al. A phase I clinical trial of the notch inhibitor MK-0752 in patients with T-cell acute lymphoblastic leukemia/lymphoma. J Clin Oncol 2006;24:357a.
125. Palomero T, et al. Mutational loss of PTEN induces resistance to NOTCH1 inhibition in T-cell leukemia. Nat Med 2007;13:1203–10.
126. Real PJ, et al. Gamma-secretase inhibitors reverse glucocorticoid resistance in T cell acute lymphoblastic leukemia. Nat Med 2009;15:50–8.
127. Bird A. DNA methylation patterns and epigenetic memory. Genes Dev 2002;16:6–21.
128. Jones PA, Baylin SB. The fundamental role of epigenetic events in cancer. Nat Rev Genet 2002;3:415–28.
129. Faderl S, et al. The prognostic significance of p16INK4a/p14ARF and p15INK4b deletions in adult acute lymphoblastic leukemia. Clin Cancer Res 1999;5:1855–61.
130. Fizzotti M, et al. Detection of homozygous deletions of the cyclin-dependent kinase 4 inhibitor (p16) gene in acute lymphoblastic leukemia and association with adverse prognostic features. Blood 1995;85:2685–90.
131. Heyman M, et al. Prognostic importance of p15INK4B and p16INK4 gene inactivation in childhood acute lymphocytic leukemia. J Clin Oncol 1996;14:1512–20.
132. Maloney KW, McGavran L, Odom LF, et al. Acquisition of p16(INK4A) and p15(INK4B) gene abnormalities between initial diagnosis and relapse in children with acute lymphoblastic leukemia. Blood 1999;93:2380–5.
133. Roman-Gomez J, et al. Promoter hypermethylation of cancer-related genes: a strong independent prognostic factor in acute lymphoblastic leukemia. Blood 2004;104:2492–8.
134. Shen L, et al. Aberrant DNA methylation of p57KIP2 identifies a cell-cycle regulatory pathway with prognostic impact in adult acute lymphocytic leukemia. Blood 2003;101:4131–6.
135. Wong IH, Ng MH, Huang DP, et al. Aberrant p15 promoter methylation in adult and childhood acute leukemias of nearly all morphologic subtypes: potential prognostic implications. Blood 2000;95:1942–9.
136. Nowak D, Stewart D, Koeffler HP. Differentiation therapy of leukemia: 3 decades of development. Blood 2009;113:3655–65.

Nelarabine for the Treatment of Patients with Relapsed or Refractory T-cell Acute Lymphoblastic Leukemia or Lymphoblastic Lymphoma

Daniel J. DeAngelo, MD, PhD

KEYWORDS

- Nelarabine • Compound 506078 • Arranon
- T-cell acute lymphoblastic leukemia
- T-cell lymphoblastic lymphoma

RELAPSED T-CELL ACUTE LYMPHOBLASTIC LEUKEMIA AND LYMPHOMA

T-cell acute lymphoblastic leukemia/lymphoblastic lymphoma (T-ALL/LBL) is an aggressive disease affecting a small number of adult and pediatric patients that progresses rapidly in the absence of effective therapy. There are an estimated 4300 patients diagnosed with ALL annually in the United States, approximately one third of whom are over 20 years of age[1] and approximately 20% to 25% of whom have T-cell disease.[2,3] Approximately 54,000 patients are diagnosed with non-Hodgkin's lymphoma annually in the United States,[1] 1.7% of whom have T-LBL.[4] Although historically classified separately, T-ALL and T-LBL are now considered different manifestations of the same disease entity and are treated according to the same regimens.

Optimal first-line therapy consists of intensive multiagent systemic chemotherapy (induction, consolidation, and maintenance) together with central nervous system

Department of Medical Oncology, Dana-Farber Cancer Institute, Harvard Medical School, 44 Binney Street, Boston, MA 02115, USA
E-mail address: ddeangelo@partners.org

Hematol Oncol Clin N Am 23 (2009) 1121–1135
doi:10.1016/j.hoc.2009.07.008   hemonc.theclinics.com
0889-8588/09/$ – see front matter © 2009 Elsevier Inc. All rights reserved.

(CNS)-directed treatment, usually consisting of intrathecal (IT) chemotherapy and cranial irradiation. Patients with T-ALL/LBL receiving first-line therapy with a five-drug induction regimen and intensive consolidation had a complete remission (CR) rate of 97% with 69% survival at 3 years.[5] Subsequent studies have estimated that the relapse rate is 30% to 40% in adults and 10% to 20% in children. Unlike pre-B cell ALL, relapses in patients with pre–T-ALL/LBL usually occur within the first 2 years.[6]

Patients who are refractory or relapse shortly after first-line therapy have an especially poor prognosis. These patients tend to have biologically aggressive disease and, as a result, they often have residual bone marrow compromise and comorbidity from their initial therapy and underlying disease. No standard second-line therapy has emerged for refractory or relapsed adult patients, and second remission rates are low with standard and high-dose chemotherapy and with high-dose therapy with autologous stem cell transplant (SCT). Second remission rates in the relapsed/refractory adult T-ALL population are less than 35% with high- or intermediate-dose cytarabine-based combination chemotherapy with anthracyclines and 10% to 15% with amsacrine, teniposide, and etoposide,[7] and remissions are short-lived.[8–11] After salvage chemotherapy, allogeneic hematopoietic SCT remains the only treatment offering long-term survival, and those patients undergoing SCT while in remission have the best chance for prolonged survival.

There are remarkably few studies in adult and pediatric T-ALL/LBL patients in second or greater relapse due to a small and difficult patient population. Outcomes are expected to be no better and probably inferior to results for patients in first relapse.[11] Based on the collective results of multiple studies, the most effective strategy in relapsed/refractory patients seems to be allogeneic SCT after induction of a second or greater CR, but the benefit of such therapy has not been demonstrated in a randomized study. Furthermore, because of age limitations, disease-related comorbidity, and the need for histocompatible donors, only a fraction of subjects are candidates for allogeneic SCT.

NELARABINE

Nelarabine (compound 506U78; Arranon) is a prodrug, which is demethylated by adenosine deaminase to the deoxyguanosine analog, 9-β-D-arabinofuranosylguanine (ara-G).[12] T lymphoblasts are exquisitely sensitive to the cytotoxic effects of deoxyguanosine (**Fig. 1**).[12–18] The accumulation of deoxyguanosine triphosphate and subsequent inhibition of ribonucleotide reductase, inhibition of DNA synthesis, and resultant cell death account for nelarabine's T-cell activity.[14–18]

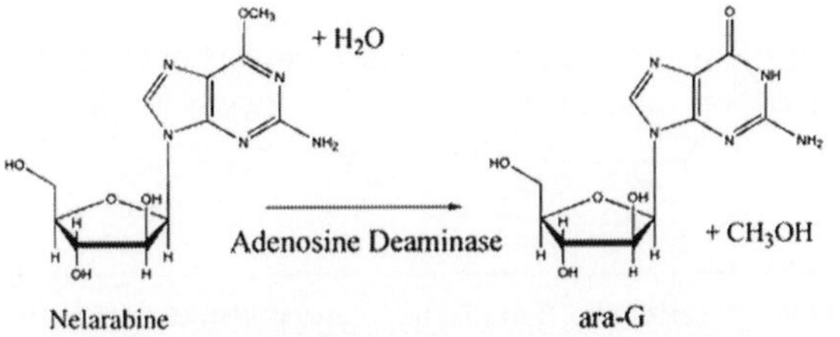

Fig. 1. The chemical structures of nelarabine and ara-G on conversion via adenosine deaminase. (*From* Kisor DF, Plunkett W, Kurtzberg J, et al. Pharmacokinetics of nelarabine and 9-beta-D-arabinofuranosyl guanine in pediatric and adult patients during a phase I study of nelarabine for the treatment of refractory hematologic malignancies. J Clin Oncol 2000;18:995–1003; with permission.)

The clinical use of deoxyguanosine is limited because it is rapidly degraded by purine nucleoside phosphorylase, which is present in high quantities within red blood cells. In 1983, Cohen and colleagues[13] reported that the prodrug, ara-G, was resistant to degradation by purine nucleoside phosphorylase and toxic to T lymphoblasts at micromolar concentrations. Laboratory studies demonstrated that conversion of ara-G to its 5'-triphosphate, ara-GTP, is required for lymphocytotoxicity mediated by the inhibition of DNA synthesis.[16–18] Ara-G is phosphorylated via deoxycytidine kinase and mitochondrial deoxyguanosine kinase.[15–19]

The increased activity of ara-G against T cells as compared with B cells was initially thought to be due to decreased catabolism of ara-GTP in T cells relative to B cells. Recent studies suggest, however, that the rate of ara-GTP catabolism is similar in T and B cells but that initial ara-G concentrations are higher in T cells for a given dose. Thus, T cells have a greater intracellular exposure to ara-GTP.[17]

Unfortunately, ara-G is difficult to synthesize and is poorly water-soluble.[20] For these reasons, there have been no clinical studies using ara-G. Use of advanced enzyme technology has allowed synthesis of nelarabine, a compound 10 times more water-soluble than ara-G.[21] Nelarabine is rapidly demethylated in blood by adenosine deaminase to ara-G. Thus, many of the obstacles to the use of ara-G have been circumvented by the development of nelarabine.

PHASE I TRIALS WITH NELARABINE

A phase I study explored the administration of nelarabine as a 1-hour intravenous infusion daily for 5 consecutive days.[22] Ninety-three adult and pediatric patients with refractory hematologic malignancies were enrolled on this multi-institutional trial. The half-life of nelarabine was determined to be approximately 20 minutes due to rapid conversion of the drug to ara-G. The half-life of ara-G is approximately 3 hours, but the intracellular half-life of the active ara-GTP is more than 24 hours.[23,24]

The pharmacokinetics of nelarabine in adult and pediatric subjects is characterized by a rapid decline in plasma concentrations with a half-life of approximately 13 minutes in pediatric subjects and 18 minutes in adult subjects (**Table 1**).[25] Virtually all nelarabine is converted to ara–G. The average maximum concentration (C_{max}) and area under the curve (AUC) for nelarabine are essentially proportional to the administered dose. The mean C_{max} and AUC for ara-GTP was 3- to 4-fold higher in responders than nonresponders, whereas the C_{max} and AUC for nelarabine were comparable in responders and nonresponders. Similarly, the C_{max} and AUC for ara-GTP, but not nelarbine, were higher in patients who experienced neurologic toxicity. The steady-state volume of distribution of ara–G is similar in adult and pediatric subjects. The weight-normalized clearance of ara–G is approximately one third less in adult

Table 1
Comparative pharmacokinetics of ara-G

Species	Injection Time (min)	Dose (mg/m^2)	AUC$_{0-\infty}$ (μmol/L/h)	C_{max} (μmol/L)	Half-Life (min)	Clearance (L/h/m^2)
Mice	Bolus	369	38	19	50	34
Rabbits	10–20	192	63.4	57.3	52	11
Rats	Bolus	375	24	39	15	55
Dogs	Bolus	500	31.3	93.4	14	57
Monkeys	Bolus	1800	1203	288	120–240	5
Humans	120	1500	579	111	120–240	9

subjects, however, as compared with pediatric subjects. No dose adjustments are required for elderly patients and there seems to be no effect on pharmacokinetics based on gender or race. Furthermore, nelarabine is a substrate for neither the cytochrome P450 nor the efflux transporter, P-glycoprotein.[25]

A response rate of 35% in adults and children with relapsed and refractory hematologic malignancies was observed in the initial phase I trial.[22] The maximally tolerated doses for children and adults determined from the phase I clinical trials were reduced early in phase II studies due to neurotoxicity. Regardless of dosing schedule, the most frequently reported adverse events (AEs) at any grade were malaise and fatigue, fever, hypnagogic effects (somnolence), nausea, vomiting, musculoskeletal pain, and hematologic abnormalities (neutropenia/thrombocytopenia).

As predicted by preclinical in vitro studies, the highest response rates were observed in patients with T-ALL (CR 23%, partial remission [PR] 31%), patients with T-cell chronic lymphoblastic leukemia (T-CLL) (PR 29%), and patients with T-cell lymphoma (PR 13%). Responses were seen at all dose levels tested. The maximum tolerated dose was 40 mg/kg/day in adults and 60 mg/kg/day in children when given for 5 days. Neurotoxicity, consisting of somnolence, encephalopathy, seizures, mental status changes, obtundation, and ascending paralysis, was dose limiting.[22] Subsequent phase I studies evaluated further dose escalation using this schedule and reported a maximum tolerated dose of 2.2 g/m^2/day.

PHASE II STUDIES WITH NELARABINE IN ADULT PATIENTS WITH RELAPSED/REFRACTORY T-CELL ACUTE LYMPHOBLASTIC LEUKEMIA/LYMPHOBLASTIC LYMPHOMA

A phase II, open-label, multicenter, clinical trial was initiated to evaluate the efficacy and safety of single-agent nelarabine in adult subjects with refractory or relapsed T-ALL/LBL.[26] Although a dose of 2.2 g/m^2/day was initially chosen, the study was amended after three patients received therapy to a dose of 1.5 g/m^2/day on days one, three, and five to decrease the potential risk of neurologic toxicities. Three subjects received the 2.2 g/m^2 dose, and data from these subjects were included in all analyses. Thirty-six of the 39 subjects received 1.5 g/m^2 on days one, three, and five. All 39 subjects completed at least one course; 14 received only one course; 17 received two courses; five received three courses; two received five courses, and one patient received six courses. The range of cumulative doses of nelarabine for all subjects was 4.3 to 26.9 g/m^2.

Patients were assessed for disease response on day 22, and if residual leukemia or lymphoma was present, a second course of nelarabine was administered at the same dose and schedule. Patients achieving a CR were eligible to receive two additional courses of nelarabine as consolidation therapy at the same dose and schedule as described previously. A calculated creatinine clearance of 50 mL/minute or greater using the Cockcroft equation was documented before drug administration for each cycle. Patients who achieved a response and were candidates for an allogeneic SCT were removed from the protocol.

Because T-cell antigens are often aberrantly expressed, all patients were required to express at least two of the following cell surface antigens: CD1a, CD2, CD3 (surface or cytoplasmic), CD4, CD5, CD7, and CD8. In an effort to exclude cases of biphenotypic and bilineal leukemia, the immature cells were also required to be negative for myeloperoxidase or Sudan black B histochemical stains. Furthermore, if the only T-cell markers present were CD4 and CD7, the leukemia cells must also have lacked the myeloid markers CD33 or CD13. Patients with greater than 25% lymphoblasts in the bone marrow at initial diagnosis or at study entry were considered to have ALL rather than LBL.

Twenty-six patients (67%) had T-ALL at study entry and 13 (33%) had T-LBL (**Table 2**). Eleven patients (28%) had received one prior multiagent induction regimen and 28 (72%) had received two or more prior regimens. Moreover, of the 28 patients with two or more prior inductions, 17 (61%) had not achieved a CR with the most recent induction attempt. Nineteen patients (49%) had disease that was refractory to their most recent therapy. Twenty-six patients (67%) had extramedullary disease, which was lymphadenopathy or splenomegaly.

Ten patients (26%) achieved a CR with full hematologic recovery; two additional patients achieved CR without complete hematologic recovery (CRi). There were no differences in response rates between T-ALL and T-LBL. Eight of 26 patients (31%)

Table 2	
Summary of response in adult patients with relapsed/refractory T-ALL/LBL	
Overall response	
CR + CRi + PR, n (%)	16 (41%)
[95% CI]	[26%–58%]
Complete remission (with or without hematologic recovery)	
CR + CRi, n (%)	12 (31%)
[95% CI]	[17%–48%]
Median duration of CR + CRi	20.5 wk
Minimum to maximum	3.8–273.3 wk
Complete remission	
CR, n%	10 (26%)
[95% CI]	[13%–42%]
Median duration of CR	27 wk
Minimum to maximum	4.1–273.3 wk
Complete remission without hematologic recovery	
CRi, n (%)	2 (5%)
Responses in patients with T-ALL ($N = 26$)	
CR + CRi, n (%)	8 (31%)
[95% CI]	[14%–52%]
Responses in patients with T-LBL ($N = 13$)	
CR, n (%)	4 (31%)
[95% CI]	[9%–61%]
Disease-free survival	
Median DFS (wk)	20 wk
[95% CI]	[11%–56%]
DFS at 1 year	25%
[95% CI]	[6%–50%]
Overall survival	
Median OS (wk)	20 wk
[95% CI]	[13%–36%]
Survival at 1 y	28%
[95% CI]	[15%–43%]

Abbreviations: DFS, disease-free survival; OS, overall survival.

with T-ALL and 4 of 13 patients (31%) with T-LBL had a CR/CRi. The median survival for all treated patients was 20 weeks, with a 95% CI of 13 to 36 weeks. The Kaplan-Meier estimate for survival is shown in (**Fig. 2**). The 1-year survival rate for all treated patients was 28% (95% CI, 15%–43%) (see **Table 2** and **Fig. 2**).[26]

Of the 28 patients who had previously received at least two prior induction regimens, 10 (36%) experienced a CR, Cri, or PR (**Table 3**). In comparison, 6 of 11 (55%) patients who had received only one prior induction regimen demonstrated a CR, Cri, or PR to nelarabine. Nineteen patients had previously failed to respond to their most recent prior induction attempt. Of those 19 patients, four (21%) experienced a CR after nelarabine, and all of these CRs were confirmed 1 month later. All four of these patients had received two or more prior induction regimens.

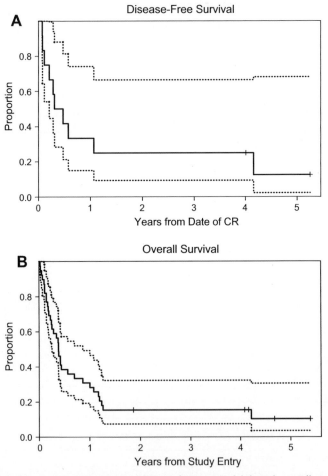

Fig. 2. Kaplan-Meier curve representing disease-free survival (A) and overall survival (B) of adult patients with relapsed/refractory T-ALL/LBL, with the dotted curves representing the 95% CI limits. (*From* DeAngelo DJ, Yu D, Johnson JL, et al. Nelarabine induces complete remissions in adults with relapsed or refractory T-cell acute lymphoblastic leukemia or lymphoblastic lymphoma: cancer and Leukemia Group B study 19801. Blood 2007;109:5136–42; with permission.)

Table 3
Summary of response rates by number of prior multiagent regimens in adult patients

n (%)	1 Prior Induction (N = 11)	≥2 Prior Inductions (N = 28)	Total (N = 39)
Overall response			
CR + Cri + PR	6 (55%)	10 (36%)	16 (41%)
[95% CI]	[23%–82%]	[19%–56%]	[26%–58%]
Complete response with or without hematologic recovery			
CR + CRi	4 (36%)	8 (29%)	12 (31%)
[95% CI]	[11%–69%]	[13%–49%]	[17%–48%]
Survival			
Median OS (wk)	19.8 wk	20.3 wk	19.8 wk
[95% CI]	[12.0–219.4]	[10.4–36.4]	[13.0–36.4]
Survival at 1 year	36%	25%	28%
[95% CI]	[11%–63%]	[11%–42%]	[15%–43%]

Abbreviation: OS, overall survival.

Toxicity data using nelarabine in adult patients revealed that the most frequent grade 3 or higher nonhematologic events were fatigue (18%) and muscle weakness (11%) (**Table 4**). Although gastrointestinal symptoms (nausea, diarrhea, stomatitis, or vomiting) were reported in 51% of subjects, only one of these events was severe (diarrhea grade 3). Peripheral sensory neuropathy was reported in 37% of patients, but all of the events were grade 1 or 2. Peripheral motor neuropathy was reported in 21% of patients, but most of the events were grade 1 or 2 with only one grade 3 AE. In addition, there was only one grade 4 AE of the nervous system, which was a reversible depressed level of consciousness.

An expanded adult safety database was reported on 103 patients treated at the same dose as in the Cancer and Leukemia Group B (CALGB) study.[25] As expected, grade 3 or 4 hematologic toxicity was observed in approximately 70% of the patients. Grade 3 or 4 gastrointestinal disorders, including nausea, diaarhea, vomiting, and stomatitis, occurred in less than 1% of treated patients. Overall, 72% patients had neurologic events; 10% were grade 3 and 3% grade 4 (**Table 5**).

NELARABINE BEFORE STEM CELL TRANSPLANT

Successful engraftment after SCT was not an endpoint in the adult phase II study design,[26] but data were collected and reported retrospectively. Seven subjects who were treated with nelarabine subsequently received a SCT. Only five patients who achieved a CR or a CRi and two subjects who did not respond to nelarabine underwent a SCT. Engraftment data for five of these seven patients were collected and full hematopoietic engraftment was documented on days 7, 11, and 18 post transplant in three of the seven patients who underwent a SCT.

The use of nelarabine has been tested in a German ALL study group in heavily pretreated relapsed T-ALL and T-LBL patients followed by SCT. Nelarabine was administered as a single agent at a dose of 1.5 g/m² on days 1, 3, and 5. The median age was 31 years (range 19–81). Forty-seven (89%) patients had T-ALL and six had T-LBL. All patients were heavily pretreated, and seven (13%) relapsed after SCT.[27]

Twenty-five of 53 patients (47%) achieved a CR, and an additional seven patients (13%) achieved PR. A higher CR rate was observed in patients with pre–T-ALL

Table 4
Summary of adverse events (all treated adult subjects with available toxicity data, *n* = 38)

	Grade 3, *N* (%)	Grade 4, *N* (%)	Grade 5, *N* (%)
Blood/bone marrow			
Netropenia	5 (13%)	11 (29%)	0
Thrombocytopenia	7 (18%)	6 (16%)	0
Anemia	6 (16%)	2 (5%)	0
Cardiovascular			
Hypertension	1 (3%)	0	0
Hepatic			
AST (AST)	1 (3%)	1 (3%)	0
ALT (ALT)	1 (3%)	1 (3%)	0
Bilirubin	2 (5%)	0	0
Infection/febrile neutropenia			
Infection (ANC >500)	1 (3%)	1 (3%)	0
Febrile neutropenia	3 (8%)	0	0
Neurologic			
Aphasia	1 (3%)	0	0
Hallucinations	1 (3%)	0	0
Depressed consciousness	0	1 (3%)	0
Depression	1 (3%)	0	0
Confusion	1 (3%)	0	0
Neuropathy, peripheral	1 (3%)	0	0
Seizure	1 (3%)	0	0
Constitutional/other			
Diarrhea	1 (3%)	0	0
Fatigue	6 (16%)	1 (3%)	0
Muscle weakness	4 (11%)	0	0
Myalgia	1 (3%)	0	0

Abbreviations: ALT, alanine aminotransferase; ANC, absolute neutrophil count per microliter; AST, aspartate aminotransferase.

phenotype. Nineteen of 25 patients (76%) who achieved CR went on to receive a SCT. Four had a sibling transplant, 14 underwent a matched unrelated donor SCT, and one patient had an autologous SCT. Time to SCT was 41 days on average (range, 20–83 days). Seven of the 25 patients are in continuous CR with a median follow-up of 13 months. Only two patients suffered neurologic toxicity consisting of reversible agitation and somnolence. The use of nelarabine as a bridge toward SCT in patients with relapsed T-ALL and T-LBL is being pursued.[28]

THE USE OF NELARABINE IN PEDIATRIC PATIENTS

A total of 121 pediatric patients were enrolled on a phase II study of nelarabine.[29] There were four different patient strata analyzed. Stratum 1 consisted of patients in first relapse with greater than 25% bone marrow involvement. Stratum 2 included patients in second relapse with greater than 25% bone marrow involvement. The third stratam included patients with CNS relapse, and the fourth stratum included patients with extramedullary, non-CNS relapse. Unfortunately, significant neurotoxicity was

Table 5
Neurologic adverse events ($\geq 2\%$) in adult patients

System Organ Class (Preferred Term)	Patients (%), $N = 103$				
	Grade 1	Grade 2	Grade 3	Grade 4	All Grades
Somnolence	20	3	0	0	23
Dizziness	14	8	0	0	21
Peripheral neurologic disorders, any event	8	12	2	0	21
Neuropathy	0	4	0	0	4
Peripheral neuropathy	2	2	1	0	5
Peripheral motor neuropathy	3	3	1	0	7
Peripheral sensory neuropathy	7	6	0	0	13
Hypoesthesia	5	10	2	0	17
Headache	11	3	1	0	15
Paresthesia	11	4	0	0	15
Ataxia	1	6	2	0	9
Depressed level of consciousness	4	1	0	1	6
Tremor	2	3	0	0	5
Amnesia	2	1	0	0	3
Dysgeusia	2	1	0	0	3
Balance disorder	1	1	0	0	2
Sensory loss	0	2	0	0	2

One patient had a fatal neurologic event, cerebral hemorrhage/coma/leukoencephalopathy.

seen at the initial dose of 1.2 g/m^2 daily for 5 days; therefore, two dose reductions were mandated. The final doses were 650 mg/m^2 per day for stratum 1 and stratum 2 and 400 mg/m^2 per day for strata 3 and 4.

The CR and PR rate at the final dose level was 55% in stratum 1, 25% in stratum 2, 33% in stratum 3, and 14% in stratum 4 (**Table 6**). From all strata, 31 episodes of grade 3 or higher neurologic toxicity were identified, corresponding to 18% of all patients treated. Within the pediatric population, patients with first and second or greater relapse were analyzed separately with a 55% versus 27% response rate between the two subgroups (see **Table 6**). The difference in response rates was statistically significant and likely related to the amount of prior therapy that was received. Mechanisms of acquired resistance of nelarabine are thought to involve decreased expression of deoxyguanosine kinase and possibly deoxycytidine kinase.[30,31] It is possible that in heavily pretreated patients the predominant leukemic clone that has been selected contains one of these nelarabine resistance traits.

Nelarabine was also tested in pediatric patients with CNS relapse based on cerebrospinal fluid (CSF) cytology. These patients were excluded from the adult strata.[26] Antimetabolites and nucleoside analogs, including methotrexate and cytarabine, are typically administered at high systemic doses to treat CNS leukemia. Patients in this stratum were allowed to receive additional chemotherapy; therefore, single-agent activity cannot be accurately defined. The eight patients who cleared the CSF cytology, however, suggest that nelarabine may play a role in the treatment or possibly the prevention of CNS leukemia. The fourth stratum analyzed included patients with minimal bone marrow involvement defined as less than 25% blast cells. These patients typically presented with a lymphomatous presentation and would be classified in most

Table 6
Response to nelarabine in pediatric patients by stratum at all dose levels

Stratum/ Dose (mg/m²)	Total Patients	Assessable Patients	CR	PR	Response Rate, CR + PR (%)	95% CI (%)
1. T-ALL, first relapse						
900	6	6	2	0	33	(0–71)
650	34	33	16	2	55	(38–72)
2. T-ALL, second relapse						
≥900	10	10	3	0	30	(2–47)
650	36	30	7	1	27	(11–43)
3. CNS relapse						
900	2	1	0	0	0	N/A
650	6	6	1	0	17	(0–47)
400	24	21	5	2	33	(13–53)
4. Lymphoma						
650	8	7	1	2	43	(6–80)
400	27	22	0	3	14	(0–28)
Overall	153	136	35	10	33	(25–41)

The final dose levels used to determine response rate are indicated in bold.
Abbreviation: N/A, not applicable.

cases as having T-LBL. There was minimal hematologic toxicity within this stratum with only 4 of 29 patients developing grade 4 thrombocytopenia or neutropenia. The importance of this observation suggests that nelarabine may be combined with other cytotoxic agents without inducing significant or excessive myelosuppression.

Similar neurologic toxicity was seen in children and adult patients with primary toxicities, including tremors, weakness, and ataxia. As expected within the phase I study, dose-limiting neurotoxicities did consist of weakness and ataxia and confusion and coma. These were principally seen in patients treated at higher doses, however. For example, neurologic toxicity was seen in 3 of 4 adults and 1 of 11 children treated at the 60-mg/kg dose level, which corresponds to approximately 1.8 g/m². In 2 of 31 adults treated at the 40-mg/kg dose level (approximately 1.2 g/m²), neurologic toxicity was also identified. There was only one child treated at a dose of 75 mg/kg (approximately 2.25 g/m²), and this individual experienced severe somnolence that resolved after 10 days and was followed by generalized seizure on day 11 and ascending paralysis and coma. The patient later died of progressive leukemia.

An expanded adult safety database was reported on 84 pediatric patients treated at the approved dose and schedule (**Table 7**).[25] As expected, grade 3 or 4 hematologic toxicity was observed in approximately 90% of the patients. The most frequent neurologic toxicity was headache. Other neurologic side effects included somnolence, hypoesthesia, and neuropathy. Sensory and motor peripheral neuropathies were noted in this database. Seizures, paresthesias, tremor, and ataxia were also noted, but these were extremely uncommon.

Although it is difficult to definitively know the relationship of neurotoxicity to nelarabine, the most commonly seen neurologic AEs were somnolence and peripheral neuropathy that occurred typically within the first course of nelarabine therapy. It is possible that the peripheral neuropathy was related to prior chemotherapy drug exposure and cumulative drug dosing. It was typically gradual in onset and reversible.

Table 7
Neurologic adverse events in pediatric patients

Nervous System Disorders (Preferred Term)	Patients (%), N = 84				
	Grade 1	Grade 2	Grade 3	Grade 4+	All Grades
Headache	8	2	4	2	17
Peripheral neurologic disorders, any event	1	4	7	0	12
Peripheral neuropathy	0	4	2	0	6
Peripheral motor neuropathy	1	0	2	0	4
Peripheral sensory neuropathy	0	0	6	0	6
Somnolence	1	4	1	1	7
Hypoesthesia	1	1	4	0	6
Seizures, any event	0	0	0	6	6
Convulsions	0	0	0	4	4
Grand mal convulsions	0	0	0	1	1
Status epilepticus	0	0	0	1	1
Motor dysfunction	1	1	1	0	4
Nervous system disorder	1	2	0	0	4
Paresthesia	0	2	1	0	4
Tremor	1	2	0	0	4
Ataxia	1	0	1	0	2

Note: grade 4+ = grade 4 and grade 5. One patient had a fatal neurologic event, status epilepticus.

Given the small number of patients on the study, it is difficult to draw definitive conclusions about the toxicities and the reversibility of some of the more severe complications. The mechanism of nelarabine-induced toxicity is unclear. Similar side effects are seen with other antimetabolites, such as methotrexate and high-dose cytarabine. IT chemotherapy is also known to induce neurologic cytotoxicities, including leukoencephalopathy and paralysis. The development of ascending peripheral neuropathy in a Guillain-Barré syndrome pattern is an unusual side effect. It has been reported in patients after receiving high-dose cytarabine in a bone marrow transplant preparative regimen, but several cases of the Guillain-Barré–like syndrome were seen using nelarabine at high doses in adult and pediatric patients. Therefore, although this is not unique to nelarabine, it may be associated with purine nucleoside toxicity in general. Furthermore, purine nucleoside phosphorylase deficiency can be associated with spasticity and other neurologic abnormalities, which may reflect on abnormal purine metabolism. It is known that brain and nerve tissue expresses high levels of deoxyguanosine kinase activity, which may lead to high concentrations of cytotoxic ara-GTP within these tissues. The mechanisms involving this pathway are, however, speculative and need to be pursued further to elucidate the risk factors and therefore the management of nelarabine-related neurologic toxicity.

NEW TREATMENT STRATEGIES

Combination therapy in young patients with newly diagnosed T-ALL is currently being tested within the Children's Oncology Group. Patients receive multiagent chemotherapy with the addition of nelarabine to assess toxicity and safety. As the trial began enrollment in January 2007[33], other proposals include stratification within the newly diagnosed adult patients with T-ALL to receive nelarabine during a component of consolidation chemotherapy.

THE USE OF NELARABINE IN INDOLENT NON-HODGKIN'S LYMPHOMA

A large phase I trial was conducted at the MD Anderson Cancer Center in 35 patients with B-cell chronic lymphocytic leukemia and T-cell prolymphocytic leukemia (T-PLL).[32] Two different schedules were used with or without the addition of fludarabine. Twenty percent of patients with CLL, 15% with T-PLL, and 63% of patients treated with a combination of nelarabine plus fludarabine achieved a response. In keeping with the treatment in patients with ALL, peripheral neuropathy was the most frequent nonhematologic toxicity. The plasma pharmacokinetic profiles of nelarabine and ara-G in indolent leukemias were comparable with those observed in ALL and lymphoma.

The CALGB conducted a phase II study of nelarabine in cutaneous T-cell lymphoma and peripheral T-cell lymphomas using the same dosing cycle that was used for T-ALL and T-LBL.[34] A total of 19 patients were enrolled in the study, 11 with cutaneous T-cell lymphoma and 8 with systemic T-cell lymphoma. Thirty-three percent of patients experienced grade 3 or 4 neurologic toxicity, and only two PRs, lasting 3 and 5.5 months, respectively, were noted. Given the lack of efficacy and excessive toxicity, specifically neurotoxicity, nelarabine is not recommended as monotherapy for patients with cutaneous T-cell lymphoma or systemic T-cell lymphoma, at least in this dosing schedule.

SUMMARY

Nelarabine is now approved in pediatric and adult T-ALL and T-LBL patients with relapsed refractory disease after two or more prior treatment regimens. Although T-ALL and T-LBL are chemotherapy-sensitive diseases, response rates in patients with relapsed/refractory disease are low and durations are short, especially in patients with second or greater relapse. This group of patients typically proceeds toward SCT. This approach may produce prolonged remissions in a fraction of the patients who achieve CR. In addition, SCT is often performed before complete blood count recovery or disease assessment; therefore, the actual CR rate may be difficult to ascertain given the propensity to rapidly send patients to SCT. The overall response rate (CR and CRi) in pediatric patients was 23% and in adult patients was 31%. Although SCT was performed in many patients, nontransplanted patients who achieved a clinical remission had significant durability with one case of DFS as long as 195 weeks.

The median survival for adult relapsed T-ALL/LBL patients treated with nelarabine with two or more prior inductions was 20 weeks, and 25% of this group of patients was still alive at 1 year. Historical survival data for patients in this population are not known, but the results observed here are similar to those reported for children and adults treated with multiagent regimens after failure of one prior regimen.[8–11] For example, Thomas and colleagues[11] reported 24% 1-year survival in 57 relapsed/refractory T-ALL patients treated with various multiagent regimens. Four of the 19 subjects (21%) who had failed to respond after their most recent induction attempt exhibited a CR or CRi after treatment with nelarabine, suggesting that the mechanism of action of nelarabine differs from that of the other standard agents that these patients had previously received.

Neurotoxicity from nelarabine has been an ongoing concern since the early phase I studies. The majority of the neurologic events reported in the trial in adult patients were reversible grade 1 or 2. There were seven severe (grade 3 or 4) neurologic AEs, however, in four patients among 38 treated patients whose toxicity data were available. In two of these cases, the events had other likely causes and were thought to be unrelated to nelarabine. Thus, although neurologic AEs have been reported, the number of severe neurologic AEs likely related to nelarabine was low.

The neurologic AEs that occurred on this study may have been at least in part related to prior chemotherapy with other neurotoxic agents, such as vincristine, methotrexate, cytarabine, or IT therapy. Because patients with active CNS disease were excluded, patients did not receive concurrent IT chemotherapy on this study. Possibly, the relatively low rate of neurologic events observed on this study was due to the lack of concurrent IT treatment.

The treatment goal for patients with relapsed or refractory ALL/LBL is to prepare patients for allogeneic SCT. Therefore, the response must be of sufficient duration to allow for a transplant evaluation. The durations of responses (CR + CRi) observed in the adult and pediatric studies were in excess of 4 weeks. When time to response is added to the duration of response, an adequate period of disease control was obtained. Recently, Gökbuget[27] reported results from a similar phase II study with nelarabine by the German Multicenter Study Group for Adult ALL wherein 47% of patients with relapsed T-ALL or T-LBL achieved a CR. Impressively, 76% of the patients achieving a CR were able to proceed to a SCT.

In summary, nelarabine demonstrated clinically significant antineoplastic activity with acceptable neurotoxicity in adult and pediatric patients with relapsed/refractory T-ALL/LBL. These data led to the approval of nelarabine for this indication in the United States by the Food and Drug Administration. Nelarabine has the potential to provide an alternative chemotherapeutic approach and should be evaluated in frontline regimens in sequence with other standard chemotherapy agents in an attempt to increase the cure rates of patients with T-ALL/LBL.

REFERENCES

1. Jemal A, Tiwari RC, Murray T, et al. Cancer statistics, 2004. CA Cancer J Clin 2004;54:8–29.
2. Ludwig WD, Raghavachar A, Thiel E. Immunophenotypic classification of acute lymphoblastic leukaemia. Baillieres Clin Haematol 1994;7:235–62.
3. Ludwig WD, Reiter A, Loffler H, et al. Immunophenotypic features of childhood and adult acute lymphoblastic leukemia (ALL): experience of the German Multicentre Trials ALL-BFM and GMALL. Leuk Lymphoma 1994;13(Suppl 1):71–6.
4. Hoelzer D, Gokbuget N. Acute lymphoblastic leukemia in adults. In: Lister TA, Greaves M, Henderson E, editors. Leukemia. 7th edition. Philadelphia: Elsevier Science; 2002. p. 621–55.
5. Larson RA, Dodge RK, Burns CP, et al. A five-drug remission induction regimen with intensive consolidation for adults with acute lymphoblastic leukemia: cancer and leukemia group B study 8811. Blood 1995;85:2025–37.
6. Laport GF, Larson RA. Treatment of adult acute lymphoblastic leukemia. Semin Oncol 1997;24:70–82.
7. Hoelzer D, Gokbuget N, Digel W, et al. Outcome of adult patients with T-lymphoblastic lymphoma treated according to protocols for acute lymphoblastic leukemia. Blood 2002;99:4379–85.
8. Giona F, Testi AM, Rondelli R, et al. ALL R-87 protocol in the treatment of children with acute lymphoblastic leukaemia in early bone marrow relapse. Br J Haematol 1997;99:671–7.

9. Giona F, Annino L, Rondelli R, et al. Treatment of adults with acute lymphoblastic leukaemia in first bone marrow relapse: results of the ALL R-87 protocol. Br J Haematol 1997;97:896–903.

10. Testi AM, Del Giudice I, Arcese W, et al. A single high dose of idarubicin combined with high-dose ARA-C for treatment of first relapse in childhood 'high-risk' acute lymphoblastic leukaemia: a study of the AIEOP group. Br J Haematol 2002;118:741–7.

11. Thomas DA, Kantarjian H, Smith TL, et al. Primary refractory and relapsed adult acute lymphoblastic leukemia: characteristics, treatment results, and prognosis with salvage therapy. Cancer 1999;86:1216–30.

12. Lambe CU, Averett DR, Paff MT, et al. 2-Amino-6-methoxypurine arabinoside: an agent for T-cell malignancies. Cancer Res 1995;55:3352–6.

13. Cohen A, Lee JW, Gelfand EW. Selective toxicity of deoxyguanosine and arabinosyl guanine for T-leukemic cells. Blood 1983;61:660–6.

14. Gelfand EW, Lee JW, Cohen A. Sensitivity of T-leukemic cells to deoxyguanosine and arabinosyl guanine. Adv Exp Med Biol 1984;165(Pt B):309–14.

15. Shewach DS, Mitchell BS. Differential metabolism of 9-beta-D-arabinofuranosylguanine in human leukemic cells. Cancer Res 1989;49:6498–502.

16. Shewach DS, Daddona PE, Ashcraft E, et al. Metabolism and selective cytotoxicity of 9-beta-D-arabinofuranosylguanine in human lymphoblasts. Cancer Res 1985;45:1008–14.

17. Verhoef V, Fridland A. Metabolic basis of arabinonucleoside selectivity for human leukemic T- and B-lymphoblasts. Cancer Res 1985;45:3646–50.

18. Ullman B, Martin DW Jr. Specific cytotoxicity of arabinosylguanine toward cultured T lymphoblasts. J Clin Invest 1984;74:951–5.

19. Hebert ME, Greenberg ML, Chaffee S, et al. Pharmacologic purging of malignant T cells from human bone marrow using 9-beta-D-arabinofuranosylguanine. Transplantation 1991;52:634–40.

20. Reist EJ, Goodman L. Synthesis of 9-beta-D-arabinofuranosylguanine. Biochemistry 1964;3:15–8.

21. Krenitsky TA, Koszalka GW, Tuttle JV. Purine nucleoside synthesis, an efficient method employing nucleoside phosphorylases. Biochemistry 1981;20:3615–21.

22. Kurtzberg J, Ernst TJ, Keating MJ, et al. Phase I study of 506U78 administered on a consecutive 5-day schedule in children and adults with refractory hematologic malignancies. J Clin Oncol 2005;23:3396–403.

23. Kisor DF, Plunkett W, Kurtzberg J, et al. Pharmacokinetics of nelarabine and 9-beta-D-arabinofuranosyl guanine in pediatric and adult patients during a phase I study of nelarabine for the treatment of refractory hematologic malignancies. J Clin Oncol 2000;18:995–1003.

24. Gandhi V, Plunkett W, Rodriguez CO Jr, et al. Compound GW506U78 in refractory hematologic malignancies: relationship between cellular pharmacokinetics and clinical response. J Clin Oncol 1998;16:3607–15.

25. Cohen MH, Johnson JR, Massie T, et al. Approval summary: nelarabine for the treatment of T-cell lymphoblastic leukemia/lymphoma. Clin Cancer Res 2006; 12:5329–35.

26. DeAngelo DJ, Yu D, Johnson JL, et al. Nelarabine induces complete remissions in adults with relapsed or refractory T-lineage acute lymphoblastic leukemia or lymphoblastic lymphoma: cancer and Leukemia Group B study 19801. Blood 2007;109:5136–42.

27. Gökbuget N, Arnold R, Atta J, et al. Compound GW506U78 has high single-drug activity and good feasibility in heavily pretreated relapsed T-lymphoblastic

leukemias (T-ALL) and T-lymphoblastic lymphoma (T-LBL) and offers the option for cure with stem cell transplantation (SCT) [abstract]. Blood 2005;106:47a.

28. NCT 00,684,619. Available at: http://www.clinicaltrials.gov.
29. Berg SL, Blaney SM, Devidas M, et al. Phase II study of nelarabine (compound 506U78) in children and young adults with refractory T-cell malignancies: a report from the Children's Oncology Group. J Clin Oncol 2005;23:3376–82.
30. Lotfi K, Mansson E, Peterson C, et al. Low level of mitochondrial deoxyguanosine kinase is the dominant factor in acquired resistance to 9-beta-D-arabinofurano-sylguanine cytotoxicity. Biochem Biophys Res Commun 2002;293:1489–96.
31. Kakihara T, Fukuda T, Tanaka A, et al. Expression of deoxycytidine kinase (dCK) gene in leukemic cells in childhood: decreased expression of dCK gene in relapsed leukemia. Leuk Lymphoma 1998;31:405–9.
32. Gandhi V, Tam C, O'Brien S, et al. Phase I trial of nelarabine in indolent leukemias. J Clin Oncol 2008;26:1098–105.
33. NCT 00,408,005. Available at: http://www.clinicaltrials.gov.
34. Czuczman MS, Porcu P, Johnson J, et al. Results of a phase II study of 506U78 in cutaneous T-cell lymphoma and peripheral T-cell lymphoma: CALGB 59901. Leuk Lymphoma 2007;48:97–103.

Recent Progress in the Treatment of Acute Lymphoblastic Leukemia: Clofarabine

Sima Jeha, MD[a,b],*

KEYWORDS

- Acute lymphoblastic leukemia therapy • Novel agents
- Nucleoside analogs • Relapsed acute lymphoblastic leukemia
- High-risk acute lymphoblastic leukemia

Acute lymphoblastic leukemia (ALL) is a heterogeneous disease with an age-adjusted incidence rate of 1.5 per 100,000 per year. Approximately two thirds of cases are diagnosed in patients younger than 20 years old, making ALL the most common pediatric malignancy.[1] Significant progress has been achieved in the treatment of ALL mainly by better use of the same chemotherapeutic agents that have been around for over 30 years. Although 80% of children with ALL are cured with contemporary regimens incorporating risk group–adjusted therapy and central nervous system prophylaxis,[2] relapsed leukemia remains the fourth most common pediatric malignancy and the leading cause of death from a disease in children. The challenge is even bigger in adults with ALL, who have less than 50% chance of surviving their disease.[3–5] Salvage regimens, mostly based on different combinations of the same agents used in front-line therapy, have a dismal outcome in patients who have refractory disease, early medullary relapse, or multiple relapses.[6–8] Several promising new therapeutic strategies are being developed. While most target a specific biologic or genetic ALL subtype, improving the therapeutic index of existing agents is also being explored. The new-generation deoxyadenosine analog clofarabine has demonstrated significant activity in various ALL subtypes and was granted approval for use in children with ALL

This work was supported in part by a Cancer Center Support Grant (CA21765) from the National Cancer Institute and by the American Lebanese Syrian Associated Charities (ALSAC).
[a] Department of Oncology, St. Jude Children's Research Hospital, 262 Danny Thomas Place, Memphis, Memphis, TN 38105, USA
[b] Leukemia/Lymphoma Developmental Therapeutics, Department of Oncology, St. Jude Children's Research Hospital, Memphis, TN, USA
* Department of Oncology, St. Jude Children's Research Hospital, 262 Danny Thomas Place, Memphis, Memphis, TN 38105, USA.
E-mail address: sima.jeha@stjude.org

in second or higher relapse. Ongoing trials are integrating clofarabine into salvage regimens, as well as into front-line high-risk ALL regimens.

CLOFARABINE

The nucleoside analogs family contains the guanosine analogs thioguanine and mercaptopurine, which were among the first agents to show activity against ALL and which continue to play a central role in contemporary regimens. The cytosine analog cytarabine, introduced shortly after thioguanine and mercaptopurine, has been an integral part of leukemia protocols for decades. Neurotoxicity has restricted the use of the deoxyadenosine analogs cladribine and fludarabine to indolent lymphoproliferative disorders and at doses lower than those with activity against acute leukemias.[9–11] Clofarabine was rationally synthesized to improve the activity and overcome the toxicity associated with fludarabine and cladribine.

Molecular Structure and Mechanism of Action

Structurally similar to cladribine and fludarabine, clofarabine (2-chloro-2′-fluoro-deoxy-9-β-D-arabinofuranosyladenine [CAFdA]) retains the halogen atom at the 2 position of the purine ring, rendering the molecule resistant to cellular degradation by adenosine deaminase.[12] Unlike other purine analogs, clofarabine incorporates an additional fluorine at the 2′carbon in the arabinofuranosyl ring, which stabilizes the glycosidic bond by conferring resistance to bacterial purine nucleoside phosphorylase and to acid hydrolysis. These changes improve clofarabine bioavailability and prevent the release of the halogenated adenine, an inactive compound associated with neurotoxicity. Further differentiating clofarabine from its congeners is its greater affinity for deoxycytidine kinase, the rate-limiting activating enzyme required for intracellular phosphorylation of the nucleoside analogs to the active triphosphate form.[13–15] While fludarabine primarily inhibits DNA polymerases and cladribine mostly inhibits ribonucleotide reductase, clofarabine inhibits DNA synthesis through both mechanisms. In preclinical models, clofarabine has demonstrated the ability to inhibit DNA repair by incorporation into the DNA chain during the repair process. In addition to its effects on cell division, clofarabine results in cell death in noncycling cells by disrupting mitochondrial function and releasing cytochrome C and other apoptosis-inducing factors.[13,14,16]

Pharmacokinetics, Pharmacodynamics, and Metabolism

The peak level of clofarabine in plasma occurs at the end of the infusion. Despite heterogeneity among patients, there is a linear increase in plasma clofarabine concentration with increasing doses. Cellular pharmacokinetics also vary among patients and are dose-proportional at lower doses. At doses of 30 mg/m^2 and 40 mg/m^2, there seems to be saturation in the accumulation of intracellular clofarabine triphosphate. Blasts from patients with ALL or acute myeloid leukemia (AML) treated with clofarabine retain more than one half of the initial concentration of clofarabine triphosphate for 24 hours, in contrast to the mean half-life of 8 to 10 hours for fludarabine and cladribine in similar patient populations.[17] Clofarabine is 47% bound to plasma proteins, predominantly to albumin. Elimination is primarily via renal excretion with 49% to 60% of the dose excreted unchanged in the urine. The pathways of nonrenal excretion are unknown. Clofarabine is not likely metabolized by the CYP450 enzyme system. The terminal half-life was estimated to be 5.2 hours. Once intracellular, clofarabine is phosphorylated by deoxycytidine kinase to its monophosphate form. The activity of deoxycytidine kinase, the rate-limiting enzyme for many of the adenosine analogs, is not rate limiting with clofarabine, and the drug accumulation in leukemic blasts appears to be dependent upon phosphorylation of clofarabine monophosphate.[17,18] The degree and duration of DNA synthesis inhibition during therapy with clofarabine is dose-related.[17] DNA synthesis is 75% to 95% inhibited at the end of infusion with clofarabine at doses ranging from 22.5 mg/m^2 to 55 mg/m^2. At 24 hours, partial recovery of DNA synthesis is observed before the next administration of clofarabine in the blasts of patients treated with 22.5 mg/m^2 and 30 mg/m^2. In contrast, the inhibition of DNA synthesis is maintained 24 hours in samples from patients treated at 40 mg/m^2 and 55 mg/m^2.

ACTIVITY OF SINGLE-AGENT CLOFARABINE IN ACUTE LYMPHOBLASTIC LEUKEMIA

In an initial phase I trial conducted at the M.D. Anderson Cancer Center, 32 adult patients with leukemia were treated with clofarabine at five dose-levels ranging between 4 mg/m^2 to 55 mg/m^2 administered intravenously over 1 hour daily for five consecutive days.[19] Overall response rate was 15% for the 13 patients with ALL enrolled on the study: 1 complete remission (CR) was reported at the 40-mg/m^2 dose level, and 1 CR without platelet recovery to 100×10^9/L (CRp) was achieved in a patient with t(9;22) ALL in fourth relapse treated on the 11.25-mg/m^2 dose level. A parallel single-center phase I pediatric study enrolled 25 children with leukemia at dose levels ranging between 11.25 mg/m^2 and 70 mg/m^2 administered intravenously over 1 hour for 5 consecutive days. CR was reported in 4 (24%) of 17 children with ALL: 1 at the 30-mg/m^2 dose level, 2 at the 40-mg/m^2 dose level, and 1 at the 50-mg/m^2 dose level.[20] Dose limiting toxicity was transient elevation in liver transaminases, and the maximum tolerated dose was 40 mg/m^2/d for 5 days in adults and 52 mg/m^2/d for 5 days in children.

Of 12 adults with ALL treated with single-agent clofarabine at 40 mg/m^2/d $\times$ 5 days on a phase II study,[21] 1 achieved CR and 1 achieved CRp for an overall response rate of 17%. A pediatric multicenter single-agent phase II clofarabine trial enrolled 61 children with ALL at 52 mg/m^2/d $\times$ 5 days.[22] The patients had received a median of three prior regimens (range 2–6) including prior stem cell transplantation in 30%. Two thirds of the patients had not responded to the last salvage regimen received before clofarabine. Of these heavily pretreated children, 7 (12%) achieved CR and 5 (8%) CRp for an overall response rate of 20%. An additional 10% had a partial response. Responses were observed in various ALL subtypes, allowing several patients to proceed to transplant. No increase in posttransplant complications was noted, and the median CR duration was 7 months in patients receiving transplant. Responders who did not proceed to transplant maintained their response for a median of over 2 months, with 2 patients remaining in CR on single-agent clofarabine for over 9 months.[23]

In these early single-agent clofarabine trials, responses were observed in precursor B- and T-cell ALL, and in a variety of genetic subtypes in children and adults (**Table 1**). Resistance to other nucleoside analogs, including cytarabine, fludarabine, and nelarabine, did not preclude response to clofarabine. Treatment was associated with nausea, vomiting, and myelosuppression. Drug fever, skin rash, and palmoplantar erythrodysethesia occurred in 5% to 10% of patients.[19–22] Levels of liver transaminases usually peak around day 5 to 7 and normalize by day 15 of the clofarabine course. Some children experienced infusion-related irritability, which resolved when the clofarabine was infused over 2 hours instead of one. In some patients, the first course of treatment caused tumor lysis syndrome, cytokine release, or systemic inflammatory response–like syndromes that resulted in capillary leak. None of the patients developed neurotoxicity.[22] Myelosuppression and infections were comparable to those seen with other salvage regimens. No extramedullary cumulative toxicity was

Table 1
Characteristics of patients with acute lymphoblastic leukemia achieving complete recovery or complete recovery without platelet recovery in phase I and II studies of single-agent clofarabine

Age (y)	ALL Subtype	Prior Induction Regimens	Most Recent Therapy Before Clofarabine	Clofarabine Dosage (mg/m²/d × 5 d)	Response	Response Duration (wk)	References
25	t(9;22)	4	NA	11.25	CRp	4	19
13	t(9;22)	4[a]	Ida/FLAG[b]	30[a]	CR	70	20
31	t(9;22), -7	1	DEX/VCR/ADRIA[b]	40	CR	16	21
12	T-ALL	4	VP/Ifos/Carbo[b]	52	CR	4	22
17	T-ALL	3	Nelarabine[b]	52[a]	CR	11	20
20	T-ALL	3	Mito/ara-C	52	CRp	5	22
2	t(1;19)	3[a]	ara-C/CTX/TBI/BMT	52[a]	CRp	29	22
17	t(1;19)	2[a]	VP/ara-C/CTX/TBI/BMT	52[a]	CR	10	22
12	Diploid	2	Ifos/VP/DEX[b]	40[a]	CR	57	20
14	Diploid	3	MTX/ara-C/VP	52	CR	59	23
16	Diploid	4[c]	VCR[b]	52	CR	47	23
19	Diploid	4	FLAG[b]	52	CR	1+	22
9	Hypodiploid	4[c]	Ida/ara-C/BMT	52	CRp	12	22
11	Hypodiploid	2	DEX/VCR/ADRIA/ASP	52[a]	CR	37+	22
64	Hyperdiploid	3	NA	40	CR	12	19
10	Random	2	MP/MTX[b]	40[a]	CR	76+	20
23	Complex	3	Prednisone/VCR/ASP[b]	40	CRp	4	21
7	Pseudo	2[a]	ICE/MTX/ara-C	52	CRp	8+	22
12	Pseudo	6	VCR/Ida/ASP/DEX[b]	52[a]	CRp	23+	22
18	Pre-B	3	Ida/ara-C[b]	52	CR	6	22

Abbreviations: ADRIA, adriamycin; ASP, asparaginase; BMT, bone marrow transplant; Carbo, carboplatinum; CTX, Cyclophosphamide; DEX, dexamethasone; FLAG, fludarabine, cytarabine, G-CSF, Granulocyte colony-stimulating factor; ICE, ifosfamide, ara-C, etoposide; Ida, idarubicin; Ifos, ifosfamide; Mito, mitoxantrone; MP, mercaptopurine; MTX, methotrexate; NA, not available; TBI, total body irradiation; VCR, vincristine; VP, etoposide.
[a] Received transplant in addition to chemotherapy listed.
[b] Refractory to chemotherapy listed.
[c] Received two transplants in addition to chemotherapy listed.

observed with repeated cycles, but dose adjustments were needed in some patients secondary to prolonged myelosupression with repeated administration.[22]

The phase II pediatric study was the basis for accelerated approval of clofarabine in the United States and Europe for treatment of pediatric ALL in second or higher relapse. Significant activity was also reported in AML, myelodysplastic syndrome, and chronic myeloid leukemia in blastic phase.[19,21]

CLOFARABINE COMBINATIONS IN ACUTE LYMPHOBLASTIC LEUKEMIA TREATMENT

The responses reported in heavily pretreated children and adults with leukemia, as well as the favorable toxicity profile, encouraged investigators to incorporate clofarabine in rational combinations.

Clofarabine in Combination with DNA-Damaging Agents

Because clofarabine inhibits both DNA synthesis and repair,[24] several trials are exploring the benefits of combining clofarabine with DNA-damaging agents. In vitro, biochemical synergy has been demonstrated between the triphosphate form of clofarabine, which inhibits DNA polymerases and ribonucleotide reductase, and the alkylating agent cyclophosphamide.[24] Cells pretreated with clofarabine impeded repair of cyclophosphamide-induced DNA damage, which in turn resulted in a more than additive apoptotic cell death. A phase I study of clofarabine followed by cyclophosphamide in adults with refractory acute leukemias showed increased DNA damage with clofarabine and cyclophosphamide combined compared with cyclophosphamide alone.[25]

A pediatric phase I trial (CLO218) explored the safe dose of clofarabine when given in combination with etoposide and cyclophosphamide over five consecutive days.[26] Clofarabine was administered over 2 hours at an initial dosage of 20 mg/m^2/d, followed by a 2-hour infusion of etoposide at an initial dosage of 75 mg/m^2/d, and a 30-minute infusion of cyclophosphamide at an initial dosage of 340 mg/m^2/d, daily for 5 days. After etoposide and cyclophosphamide were escalated to their target dosages of 100 mg/m^2/d and 440 mg/m^2/d respectively, the dosage of clofarabine was increased in subsequent cohorts to its target dosage of 40 mg/m^2/d (**Table 2**). Twenty-five patients (20 ALL, 5 AML) were enrolled in five cohorts. The dosages evaluated in the target cohort (cohort 5) were found to be tolerable. A maximum tolerated dosage was not reached, and the recommended phase II dosages of clofarabine, etoposide, and cyclophosphamide were determined to be 40 mg/m^2/d, 100 mg/m^2/d, and 440 mg/m^2/d, respectively, each given for 5 consecutive days. Of the 20 patients with ALL enrolled into the study, 9 achieved CR and 2 a CRp for an overall response rate 55% (**Table 2**). Responses were observed among patients in all dosage cohorts.

Table 2
Patients with acute lymphoblastic leukemia enrolled on CLO218 study

Clofarabine (mg/m^2/d × 5)	Etoposide (mg/m^2/d × 5)	Cyclophosphamide (mg/m^2/d × 5)	Number of Patients Treated	CR	CRp
20	75	340	3	1	1
20	100	440	3	2	0
20	100	440	1	1	0
30	100	440	8	3	1
40	100	440	5	2	0

The phase II study is ongoing, and the activity of this regimen is encouraging investigators to offer it in front-line pediatric ALL regimens for high-risk patients.[26]

A combination regimen with an anthracycline would combine the ability of clofarabine to inhibit DNA strand elongation with anthracycline's ability to induce DNA intercalation and strand break. Faderl and colleagues[27] are studying the combination of clofarabine with idarubicin alone and with cytarabine in patients with relapsed/refractory leukemias.

Clofarabine-Cytarabine Combinations

In an ongoing Children Oncology Group trial, clofarabine is administered in combination with cytarabine in children with relapsed ALL and AML based on the ability of clofarabine to potentiate cytarabine triphosphate accumulation into leukemic blasts.[28] The activity and tolerability of a regimen combining 40 mg/m^2/d clofarabine with 1 g/m^2/d cytarabine for five consecutive days has been reported in adults with relapsed AML and myelodysplastic syndromes and in elderly patients with untreated AML who are at high risk of anthracycline toxicity.[29] In addition to extending this regimen to patients with ALL, the Children Oncology Group study will also explore the feasibility of escalating the clofarabine dosage to the pediatric maximum tolerated dosage of 52 mg/m^2/d for 5 days (keeping cytarabine at the same dose) in a two-stage dose-escalation design.

FUTURE DIRECTIONS

Based on the promising results reported above, clofarabine is being incorporated into relapsed ALL regimens as well as into front-line regimens for high-risk ALL. It remains to be determined whether these approaches will improve the historically poor outcome in these patients. Investigators are also exploring the use of clofarabine as a conditioning agent in hematopoietic stem cell transplantation,[30] and studying different dose schedules of intravenous or oral clofarabine in patients with myelodysplastic syndrome, non-Hodgkin lymphomas, chronic lymphocytic leukemia, refractory Langerhans cell histiocytosis, and solid tumors. The activity of clofarabine seems to extend beyond relapsed ALL for which it has been approved. However, its efficacy in other malignancies, as well as the optimal dose schedule to be used, remain to be determined.[31,32]

REFERENCES

1. Redaelli A, Laskin BL, Stephens JM, et al. A systematic literature review of the clinical and epidemiological burden of acute lymphoblastic leukaemia (ALL). Eur J Cancer Care (Engl) 2005;14(1):53–62.
2. Pui CH, Evans WE. Treatment of acute lymphoblastic leukemia. N Engl J Med 2006;354(2):166–78.
3. Hoelzer D, Gokbuget N. New approaches to acute lymphoblastic leukemia in adults: Where do we go? Semin Oncol 2000;27(5):540–59.
4. Kantarjian H, Thomas D, O'Brien S, et al. Long-term follow-up results of hyperfractionated cyclophosphamide, vincristine, doxorubicin, and dexamethasone (Hyper-CVAD), a dose-intensive regimen, in adult acute lymphocytic leukemia. Cancer 2004;101(12):2788–801.
5. Linker C, Damon L, Ries C, et al. Intensified and shortened cyclical chemotherapy for adult acute lymphoblastic leukemia. J Clin Oncol 2002;20(10):2464–71.

6. Fielding AK, Richards SM, Chopra R, et al. Outcome of 609 adults after relapse of acute lymphoblastic leukemia (ALL); an MRC UKALL12/ECOG 2993 study. Blood 2007;109(3):944–50.
7. Gaynon PS. Childhood acute lymphoblastic leukaemia and relapse. Br J Haematol 2005;131(5):579–87.
8. Bailey LC, Lange BJ, Rheingold SR, et al. Bone-marrow relapse in pediatric acute lymphoblastic leukaemia. Lancet Oncol 2008;9(9):873–83.
9. Kornblau SM, Gandhi V, Andreeff HM, et al. Clinical and laboratory studies of 2-chlorodeoxyadenosine +/− cytosine arabinoside for relapsed or refractory acute myelogenous leukemia in adults. Leukemia 1996;10(10):1563–9.
10. Vahdat L, Wong ET, Wile MJ, et al. Therapeutic and neurotoxic effects of 2-chlorodeoxyadenosine in adults with acute myeloid leukemia. Blood 1994;84(10):3429–34.
11. Warrell RP Jr, Berman E. Phase I and II study of fludarabine phosphate in leukemia: therapeutic efficacy with delayed central nervous system toxicity. J Clin Oncol 1986;4(1):74–9.
12. Montgomery JA, Shortnacy-Fowler AT, Clayton SD, et al. Synthesis and biologic activity of 2'-fluoro-2-halo derivatives of 9-beta-D-arabinofuranosyladenine. J Med Chem 1992;35(2):397–401.
13. Xie KC, Plunkett W. Deoxynucleotide pool depletion and sustained inhibition of ribonucleotide reductase and DNA synthesis after treatment of human lymphoblastoid cells with 2-chloro-9-(2-deoxy-2-fluoro-beta-D-arabinofuranosyl) adenine. Cancer Res 1996;56(13):3030–7.
14. Lotfi K, Mansson E, Spasokoukotskaja T, et al. Biochemical pharmacology and resistance to 2-chloro-2'-arabino-fluoro-2'-deoxyadenosine, a novel analogue of cladribine in human leukemic cells. Clin Cancer Res 1999;5(9):2438–44.
15. Parker WB, Shaddix SC, Rose LM, et al. Comparison of the mechanism of cytotoxicity of 2-chloro-9-(2-deoxy-2-fluoro-beta-D-arabinofuranosyl)adenine, 2-chloro-9-(2-deoxy-2-fluoro-beta-D-ribofuranosyl)adenine, and 2-chloro-9-(2-deoxy-2,2-difluoro-beta-D-ribofuranosyl)adenine in CEM cells. Mol Pharmacol 1999;55(3):515–20.
16. Parker WB, Shaddix SC, Chang CH, et al. Effects of 2-chloro-9-(2-deoxy-2-fluoro-beta-D-arabinofuranosyl)adenine on K562 cellular metabolism and the inhibition of human ribonucleotide reductase and DNA polymerases by its 5'-triphosphate. Cancer Res 1991;51(9):2386–94.
17. Gandhi V, Kantarjian H, Faderl S, et al. Pharmacokinetics and pharmacodynamics of plasma clofarabine and cellular clofarabine triphosphate in patients with acute leukemias. Clin Cancer Res 2003;9(17):6335–42.
18. Bonate PL, Craig A, Gaynon P, et al. Population pharmacokinetics of clofarabine, a second-generation nucleoside analog, in pediatric patients with acute leukemia. J Clin Pharmacol 2004;44(11):1309–22.
19. Kantarjian HM, Gandhi V, Kozuch P, et al. Phase I clinical and pharmacology study of clofarabine in patients with solid and hematologic cancers. J Clin Oncol 2003;21(6):1167–73.
20. Jeha S, Gandhi V, Chan KW, et al. Clofarabine, a novel nucleoside analog, is active in pediatric patients with advanced leukemia. Blood 2004;103(3):784–9.
21. Kantarjian H, Gandhi V, Cortes J, et al. Phase 2 clinical and pharmacologic study of clofarabine in patients with refractory or relapsed acute leukemia. Blood 2003;102(7):2379–86.
22. Jeha S, Gaynon PS, Razzouk BI, et al. Phase II study of clofarabine in pediatric patients with refractory or relapsed acute lymphoblastic leukemia. J Clin Oncol 2006;24(12):1917–23.

23. Steinherz PG, Meyers PA, Steinherz LJ, et al. Clofarabine induced durable complete remission in heavily pretreated adolescents with relapsed and refractory leukemia. J Pediatr Hematol Oncol 2007;29(9):656–8.

24. Yamauchi T, Nowak BJ, Keating MJ, et al. DNA repair initiated in chronic lymphocytic leukemia lymphocytes by 4-hydroperoxycyclophosphamide is inhibited by fludarabine and clofarabine. Clin Cancer Res 2001;7(11):3580–9.

25. Karp JE, Ricklis RM, Balakrishnan K, et al. A phase 1 clinical-laboratory study of clofarabine followed by cyclophosphamide for adults with refractory acute leukemias. Blood 2007;110(6):1762–9.

26. Hijiya N, Gaynon PS, Fernandez M, et al. Durable remissions observed in a phase I/II study of clofarabine in combination with etoposide and cyclophosphamide in pediatric patients with refractory or relapsed acute leukemia. Blood 2008;112(11):2925.

27. Faderl S, Ferrajoli A, Wierda W, et al. Clofarabine combinations as acute myeloid leukemia salvage therapy. Cancer 2008;113(8):1995–8.

28. Cooper T, Ayres M, Nowak B, et al. Biochemical modulation of cytarabine triphosphate by clofarabine. Cancer Chemother Pharmacol 2005;55(4):361–8.

29. Faderl S, Verstovsek S, Cortes J, et al. Clofarabine and cytarabine combination as induction therapy for acute myeloid leukemia (AML) in patients 50 years of age or older. Blood 2006;108(1):45–51.

30. Bacher U, Klyuchnikov E, Wiedemann B, et al. Safety of conditioning agents for allogeneic haematopoietic transplantation. Expert Opin Drug Saf 2009;8(3): 305–15.

31. Rodriguez-Galindo C, Jeng M, Khuu P, et al. Clofarabine in refractory Langerhans cell histiocytosis. Pediatr Blood Cancer 2008;51(5):703–6.

32. Blum KA, Hamadani M, Phillips GS, et al. Prolonged myelosuppression with clofarabine in the treatment of patients with relapsed or refractory, aggressive non-Hodgkin lymphoma. Leuk Lymphoma 2009;50(3):349–56.

Index

Note: Page numbers of article titles are in **boldface** type.

A

Aberrations, genetic, success rates for detection in ALL, 994
Acute lymphoblastic leukemia (ALL). *See* Leukemia, acute lymphoblastic.
Adolescents, ALL in young adults and, **1033–1042**
    clinical and biological characteristics in, 1033–1034
    pediatric-based *vs.* adult-based treatments, 1034–1038
    role of hematopoietic stem cell transplantation in, 1038–1039
    when should adolescents be treated, 1039–1040
Adults, allogeneic hematopoietic cell transplantation for ALL in, **1011–1032**
    young, ALL in adolescents and, **1033–1042**
Age, at diagnosis, in prognosis of pediatric ALL, 974–975
Alemtuzumab, 1104–1105
ALL. *See* Leukemia, acute lymphoblastic.
Allogeneic stem cell transplantation, for ALL in adults, **1011–1032**
    for Ph+ ALL before and after imatinib era, 1049–1052
    with rituximab-based chemoimmunotherapy for ALL, 961
Anti-CD20 monoclonal antibodies, 964–965
Array-based comparative genomic hybridization, in ALL, 999
Autologous hematopoietic stem cell transplantation, for adult ALL, 1024–1025

B

BCR-ABL gene, and IKZF1 deletion, 1106
    in Ph+ ALL, 1043
    targeting aberrant signaling pathways, 1105–1106
Bone toxicities, long-term outcomes in survivors of childhood ALL, 1071–1072
Burkitt-type leukemia/lymphoma, rituximab-based chemoimmunotherapy for, 954–958, 960
    adult, 954–958
    pediatric, 960

C

Cancer survivors. *See* Survivors, cancer.
Candidate genes, resequencing of, in ALL, 1001–1003
Cardiotoxicity, in survivors of childhood ALL, 1072–1073
CD19-directed antibodies, 1105
CD20 expression, in precursor B-cell ALL, 950–953
    prognostic significance of, 950–951
    upregulation of, 951–953
Central nervous system (CNS), disease of, in Ph+ ALL, 1055–1056
    therapy directed at, in pediatric ALL, 980–981

Hematol Oncol Clin N Am 23 (2009) 1145–1154
doi:10.1016/S0889-8588(09)00158-0
0889-8588/09/$ – see front matter © 2009 Elsevier Inc. All rights reserved.

hemonc.theclinics.com

Central nervous system disease, in ALL, rituximab intrathecally for, 962
Chemoimmunotherapy, rituximab-based, 954–959
        for adult Burkitt-type leukemia/lymphoma, 954–958
        for adult Ph-negative precursor B-cell ALL, 958–959
        with allogeneic stem cell transplant for ALL, 961
Childhood cancers, long-term outcomes in survivors of childhood ALL, **1065–1082**
Chromosome aberrations, success rates for detection in ALL, 994
Clofarabine, for ALL, **1137–1144**
        activity of single-agent, 1139–1141
        in combinations, 1141–1142
            with cytarabine, 1142
            with DNA-damaging agents, 1141–1142
        molecular structure and mechanism of action, 1138
        pharmacology of, 1138–1139
Comparative genomic hybridization, array-based. in ALL, 999
Consolidation, in treatment of pediatric ALL, 978–979
Continuation regimen, in treatment of pediatric ALL, 979–980
Cyclophosphamide, in combination with clofarabine for ALL, 1141
Cytarabine, in combination with clofarabine for ALL, 1142
Cytogenetics, in prognosis of pediatric ALL, 975–976
    of acute lymphoblastic leukemia, 992–998
        fluorescence in situ hybridization, 993
        multicolor fluorescence in situ hybridization, 993–994
        prognostic relevance of, 994–998
        standard cytogenetic analysis, 992–993
        success rates of, 994

    D

Down syndrome, JAK2 mutations in ALL patients with, 1108
Drug resistance. *See* Resistance, drug.

    E

Early response, to therapy, in prognosis of pediatric ALL, 976–977
Epigenetic changes, associated with ALL, 1003
Epigenetic modulation, 1109
Epratuzumab, 1105
Etoposide, in combination with clofarabine for ALL, 1141
Expression microarray analysis, in ALL, 998–999

    F

Fertility, in survivors of childhood ALL, 1073
Flow cytometry, monitoring minimal residual disease in adult and pediatric ALL with,
        1084–1085
FLT3 signaling pathway inhibition, 1107
Fluorescence in situ hybridization (FISH), in ALL, 993
        multicolor, 993–994

G

Genetics, cytogenetics. *See* Cytogenetics.
   molecular. *See* Molecular genetic.
Genome-wide association studies, recognition of drug resistance in ALL, 1101–1102
Graft-*versus*-leukemia effect, role in hematopoietic stem cell transplantation for ALL, 1019–1020

H

Heat shock protein 90, 1108
Hematopoietic stem cell transplantation. *See* Stem cell transplantation.

I

Idarubucin, in combination with clofarabine for ALL, 1142
Imatinib, for Ph+ ALL, 1045–1049
   in elderly patients, 1048–1049
   in younger patients, 1045–1048
   resistance to, 1052–1053
   role of allogeneic stem cell transplantation after era of, 1050–1052
Immunophenotype, in prognosis of pediatric ALL, 975
   of ALL, 949–950
Intensification and reinduction regimen, in treatment of pediatric ALL, 978–979
Intrathecal administration, of rituximab, for CNS disease in ALL, 962

J

JAK2 mutations, in ALL patients with Down syndrome, 1108

L

Late effects, long-term outcomes in survivors of childhood ALL, **1065–1082**
   bone toxicities, 1071–1072
   neurocognitive, 1066–1068
   neuroendocrine, 1068–1069
   neurologic, 1068
   obesity and metabolic, 1069–1071
   other serious late effects of therapy, 1072–1073
   providing life-long risk-based care for, 1073–1074
Leukemia, acute lymphoblastic, 949–1144
   allogeneic hematopoietic cell transplantation in adults, **1011–1032**
      autologous, 1024–1025
      cell sources for, 1025
      for Ph+ ALL, 1014–1018
      for relapsed or primary refractory ALL, 1018
      future considerations, 1026–1027
      in first complete remission, 1013–1014
      management of relapse after, 1023–1024
      prognostic factors, 1012
      reduced intensity conditioning, 1020–1021

Leukemia (*continued*)
  regimen development for, 1021–1023
  role of graft *versus* leukemia effect in, 1019–1020
  role of minimal residual disease, 1012–1013
  treatment strategy for, 1026
  umbilical cord transplantation, 1025–1026
  unrelated, 1019
clofarabine for, **1137–1144**
  activity of single-agent, 1139–1141
  in combinations, 1141–1142
  molecular structure and mechanism of action, 1138
  pharmacology of, 1138–1139
cytogenetics and molecular genetics, **991–1010**
  cytogenetics, 992–998
    fluorescence in situ hybridization, 993
    multicolor fluorescence in situ hybridization, 993–994
    prognostic relevance of, 994–998
    standard cytogenetic analysis, 992–993
    success rates of, 994
  molecular genetics, 998–1003
    array-based comparative genomic hybridization, 999
    epigenetic changes associated with, 1003
    expression microarray analysis, 998–999
    perspectives for future, 1003
    resequencing of candidate genes, 1001–1003
    single nucleotide polymorphism array analysis, 999–1001
    timing of mutations associated with, 1003
in adolescents and young adults, **1033–1042**
  clinical and biological characteristics in, 1033–1034
  pediatric-based *vs.* adult-based treatments, 1034–1038
  role of hematopoietic stem cell transplantation in, 1038–1039
  when should adolescents be treated, 1039–1040
long-term outcomes in survivors of childhood, **1065–1082**
  bone toxicities, 1071–1072
  neurocognitive, 1066–1068
  neuroendocrine, 1068–1069
  neurologic, 1068
  obesity and metabolic, 1069–1071
  other serious late effects of therapy, 1072–1073
  providing life-long risk-based care for, 1073–1074
minimal residual disease monitoring, **1083–1098**
  assays for, 1084–1088
  clinical significance of, 1088–1092
nelarabine for relapsed or refractory T-lineage, **1121–1135**
  before stem cell transplant, 1127–1128
  in indolent non-Hodgkin's lymphoma, 1132
  in pediatric patients, 1128–1132
  new treatment strategies, 1132
  phase I trials, 1123–1124
  phase II trials, 1124–1127
novel strategies based on molecular pathogenesis, **1099–1119**

current status, 1109–1111
expansion of therapeutic armamentarium in older adults, 1103–1109
improving on existing regimens, 1102–1103
molecular insights to guide treatment, 1100–1102
pediatric, risk-adapted treatment, **973–990**
prognostic factors, age and leukocyte count at diagnosis, 974
cytogenetics, 975–976
early response to therapy, 976–977
immunophenotype, 975
treatment, 977–982
CNS-directed therapy, 880–981
continuation (maintenance), 979–880
intensification (consolidation) and reinduction, 978–979
remission induction, 977–978
stem cell transplantation, 981–982
targeted therapy, 982
Philadelphia (Ph) chromosome-positive, **1043–1063**
Philadelphia chromosome-positive (Ph+), biology, 1043
treatment of adults and children with, 1044–1056
rituximab for, **949–971**
effects on detection of minimal residual disease, 962–963
for adult Burkitt-type leukemia/lymphoma, 954–958
for adult Ph-negative precursor B-cell ALL, 958–960
for CNS disease in ALL, 962
for pediatric Burkitt-type leukemia/lymphoma and precursor B-cell ALL, 960
future directions, 965
immunophenotypic classification of ALL, 949–950
mechanisms of resistance to, 963–964
novel anti-CD20 monoclonal antibodies, 964–965
principles of monoclonal antibody therapy with, 953–954
prognostic significance of CD20 expression in precursor B-cell ALL, 950–951
toxicity of, 963
upregulation if CD20 expression in precursor B-cell ALL, 951–953
with allogeneic stem cell transplant, 961
Leukocyte count, at diagnosis, in prognosis of pediatric ALL, 974–975
Lymphoblastic lymphoma, nelarabine for relapsed or refractory, **1121–1135**
Lymphoblastic leukemia, acute (ALL). See Leukemia, acute lymphoblastic.
Lymphoma, Burkitt-type leukemia/lymphoma, rituximab-based chemoimmunotherapy
for, 954–958, 960
adult, 954–958
pediatric, 960
lymphoblastic, nelarabine for relapsed or refractory, **1121–1135**

M

Maintenance regimen, in treatment of pediatric ALL, 979–980
Mammalian target of rapamycin (mTOR) inhibitors, 1107–1108
Metabolic outcomes, long-term, and obesity in survivors of childhood ALL, 1069–1071
Minimal residual disease, effects of rituximab on detection of, in precursor B-cell ALL,
962–963
monitoring in adult and pediatric ALL, **1083–1098**

Minimal (*continued*)
    assays for, 1084–1088
        feasibility of testing in prospective studies, 1088
        strengths and weaknesses of, 1085–1087
        targets for flow cytometric studies, 1084–1085
        targets for polymerase chain reaction studies, 1085
    clinical significance of, 1088–1092
        in adult ALL, 1090–1091
        in childhood ALL, 1088–1089
        risk classification using, 1091–1092
   role of, in prognosis of adult ALL, 1012–1013
   use in optimal selection for postremission therapy for ALL, 1100–1101
Molecular genetics, of acute lymphoblastic leukemia, 998–1003
    array-based comparative genomic hybridization, 999
    epigenetic changes associated with, 1003
    expression microarray analysis, 998–999
    perspectives for future, 1003
    resequencing of candidate genes, 1001–1003
    single nucleotide polymorphism array analysis, 999–1001
    timing of mutations associated with, 1003
Molecular pathogenesis, of ALL, novel treatment strategies based on,
   1099–1119
    current status, 1109–1111
    expansion of therapeutic armamentarium in older adults, 1103–1109
    improving on existing regimens, 1102–1103
    molecular insights to guide treatment, 1100–1102
Monoclonal antibodies, newer, for ALL, 1104–1105
    alemtuzumab, 1104–1105
    CD19-directed, 1105
    epratuzumab, 1105
    ofatumumab, 1105
   novel anti-CD20, 964–965
   rituximab for ALL, **949–971**
Mutations, genetic, success rates for detection in ALL, 994

   N

Nelarabine, for relapsed or refractory T-lineage ALL or lymphoblastic lymphoma,
   1121–1135
    before stem cell transplant, 1127–1128
    in indolent non-Hodgkin's lymphoma, 1132
    in pediatric patients, 1128–1132
    new treatment strategies, 1132
    phase I trials, 1123–1124
Neurocognitive outcomes, long-term, in survivors of childhood ALL, 1066–1068
Neuroendocrine outcomes, long-term, in survivors of childhood ALL, 1068–1069
Neurologic outcomes, long-term, in survivors of childhood ALL, 1068
Non-Hodgkin's lymphoma, indolent, use of nelarabine in, 1132
NOTCH1, targeting precursor T-cell ALL, 1108–1109
Nucleoside analogs, clofarabine, **1137–1144**

O

Obesity, long-term outcomes in survivors of childhood ALL, 1069–1071
Ofatumumab, 1105
Outcomes, long-term, in survivors of childhood ALL, **1065–1082**
    bone toxicities, 1071–1072
    neurocognitive, 1066–1068
    neuroendocrine, 1068–1069
    neurologic, 1068
    obesity and metabolic, 1069–1071
    other serious late effects of therapy, 1072–1073
    providing life-long risk-based care for, 1073–1074

P

Pediatric leukemia, acute lymphoblastic, risk-adapted treatment, **973–990**
    prognostic factors, age and leukocyte count at diagnosis, 974
        cytogenetics, 975–976
        early response to therapy, 976–977
        immunophenotype, 975
        treatment, 977–982
        CNS-directed therapy, 880–981
        continuation (maintenance), 979–880
        intensification (consolidation) and reinduction, 978–979
        remission induction, 977–978
        stem cell transplantation, 981–982
        targeted therapy, 982
    nelarabine for, 1128–1132
Pediatric-based treatments, replicating results of in young adults, 1102–1103
    vs. adult-based treatments for ALL in adolescents and young adults, 1034–1038
Pharmacogenomics, recognition of drug resistance in ALL, 1101–1102
Philadelphia chromosome-positive (Ph+) acute lymphoblastic leukemia, **1043–1063**
    allogeneic hematopoietic stem cell transplantation for, 1014–1018
    biology, 1043
    treatment in adults and children, 1044–1056
        central nervous system disease, 1055–1056
        future challenges in, 1056
        historical perspectives, 1044
        imatinib and imatinib-containing regimens, 1045–1049
        resistance to imatinib, 1052–1053
        role of allogeneic stem cell transplantation before and after imatinib era,
            1049–1052
        second-generation tyrosine kinase inhibitors, 1053–1055
Polymerase chain reaction (PCR) studies, monitoring minimal residual disease in adult and
    pediatric ALL with, 1085
Precursor B-cell acute lymphoblastic leukemia, rituximab therapy in, 958–960
    adult Ph-negative, 958–960
    pediatric, 960
Prognostic factors, cytogenetics, relevance in ALL, 994–998
    in adult ALL, 1012
    in pediatric ALL treatment, 974–977
        age and leukocyte count at diagnosis, 974

Prognostic (*continued*)
    cytogenetics, 975–976
    early response to therapy, 976–977
    immunophenotype, 975
  minimal residual disease in ALL, 1088–1092
  adult ALL, 1090–1091
  childhood ALL, 1088–1089
  use in risk classification, 1091–1092
 novel treatment strategies based on molecular pathogenesis of ALL, **1099–1119**
  current status, 1109–1111
    expansion of therapeutic armamentarium in older adults, 1103–1109
    improving on existing regimens, 1102–1103
    molecular insights to guide treatment, 1100–1102
Proteasome inhibition, 1108

R

Radioimmunoassay, transplant regimens for ALL based on, 1022–1023
Reduced intensity conditioning, for ALL, 1020–1021
Refractory acute lymphoblastic leukemia, allogeneic hematopoietic stem cell
  transplantation for primary, 1018
  nelarabine for, **1121–1135**
Reinduction, intensification and, in treatment of pediatric ALL, 978–979
Relapse, of acute lymphoblastic leukemia, allogeneic hematopoietic stem cell
  transplantation for, 1018
  management of, after allogeneic transplant for, 1023–1024
  nelarabine for, **1121–1135**
Remission induction, in treatment of pediatric ALL, 977–978
Resequencing, of candidate genes, in ALL, 1001–1003
Resistance, drug, mechanisms of, for rituximab, 963–964
  recognition of, in development of novel strategies for ALL, 1101–1102
  to imatinib in Ph+ ALL, 1052–1053
  to imatinib, strategies to overcome, 1106
Response, early, to therapy, in prognosis of pediatric ALL, 976–977
Risk-adapted treatment, novel strategies based on molecular pathogenesis of ALL,
  1099–1119
    current status, 1109–1111
    expansion of therapeutic armamentarium in older adults, 1103–1109
    improving on existing regimens, 1102–1103
    molecular insights to guide treatment, 1100–1102
  of pediatric ALL, **973–990**
    prognostic factors, age and leukocyte count at diagnosis, 974
      cytogenetics, 975–976
      early response to therapy, 976–977
      immunophenotype, 975
    treatment, 977–982
      CNS-directed therapy, 880–981
      continuation (maintenance), 979–880
      intensification (consolidation) and reinduction, 978–979
      remission induction, 977–978
      stem cell transplantation, 981–982
      targeted therapy, 982

Rituximab, for ALL, **949–971**
    effects on detection of minimal residual disease, 962–963
    for adult Burkitt-type leukemia/lymphoma, 954–958
    for adult Ph-negative precursor B-cell ALL, 958–960
    for CNS disease in ALL, 962
    for pediatric Burkitt-type leukemia/lymphoma and precursor B-cell ALL, 960
    future directions, 965
    immunophenotypic classification of ALL, 949–950
    mechanisms of resistance to, 963–964
    novel anti-CD20 monoclonal antibodies, 964–965
    principles of monoclonal antibody therapy with, 953–954
    prognostic significance of CD20 expression in precursor B-cell ALL, 950–951
    toxicity of, 963
    upregulation if CD20 expression in precursor B-cell ALL, 951–953
    with allogeneic stem cell transplant, 961

S

Second malignancies, in survivors of childhood ALL, 1073
Signaling pathways, aberrant, targeting for therapy of ALL, 1105–1108
Single nucleotide polymorphism array analysis, in ALL, 999–1001
Stem cell transplantation, allogeneic hematopoietic, for ALL in adults, **1011–1032**
    autologous, 1024–1025
    cell sources for, 1025
    for Ph+ ALL, 1014–1018
    for relapsed or primary refractory ALL, 1018
    future considerations, 1026–1027
    in first complete remission, 1013–1014
    management of relapse after, 1023–1024
    prognostic factors, 1012
    reduced intensity conditioning, 1020–1021
    regimen development for, 1021–1023
        radioimmunoassay-based, 1022–1023
    role of graft *versus* leukemia effect in, 1019–1020
    role of minimal residual disease, 1012–1013
    treatment strategy for, 1026
    umbilical cord transplantation, 1025–1026
    unrelated, 1019
    with rituximab-based chemoimmunotherapy, 961
  in pediatric ALL, 981–982
  nelarabine before, 1127–1128
  role in ALL in adolescents and young adults, 1038–1039
  role in Ph+ ALL before and after imatinib era, 1049–1052
Survivors, cancer, of childhood ALL, long-term outcomes in, **1065–1082**
    bone toxicities, 1071–1072
    neurocognitive, 1066–1068
    neuroendocrine, 1068–1069
    neurologic, 1068
    obesity and metabolic, 1069–1071
    other serious late effects of therapy, 1072–1073
    providing life-long risk-based care for, 1073–1074

T

T-lineage acute lymphoblastic leukemia, nelarabine for relapsed or refractory,
    1121–1135
Targeted therapy, in pediatric ALL, 982
Toxicity, bone, long-term outcomes in survivors of childhood ALL, 1071–1072
    of rituximab, 963
Tyrosine kinase inhibitors, second-generation, for Ph+ ALL, 1053–1055

U

Umbilical cord transplantation, for adult ALL, 1025–1026
Unrelated donors, for hematopoietic stem cell transplantation for ALL, 1019

Y

Young adults, ALL in adolescents and, **1033–1042**
        clinical and biological characteristics in, 1033–1034
        pediatric-based *vs.* adult-based treatments, 1034–1038
        role of hematopoietic stem cell transplantation in, 1038–1039
        when should adolescents be treated, 1039–1040

United States Postal Service

Statement of Ownership, Management, and Circulation
(All Periodicals Publications Except Requestor Publications)

1. Publication Title	2. Publication Number	3. Filing Date
Hematology/Oncology Clinics of North America	0 0 2 - 4 7 3	9/15/09

4. Issue Frequency	5. Number of Issues Published Annually	6. Annual Subscription Price
Feb, Apr, Jun, Aug, Oct, Dec	6	$283.00

7. Complete Mailing Address of Known Office of Publication (Not printer) (Street, city, county, state, and ZIP+4®)

Elsevier Inc.
360 Park Avenue South
New York, NY 10010-1710

Contact Person
Stephen Bushing
Telephone (Include area code)
215-239-3688

8. Complete Mailing Address of Headquarters or General Business Office of Publisher (Not printer)

Elsevier Inc., 360 Park Avenue South, New York, NY 10010-1710

9. Full Names and Complete Mailing Addresses of Publisher, Editor, and Managing Editor (Do not leave blank)

Publisher (Name and complete mailing address)

John Schrefer, Elsevier, Inc., 1600 John F. Kennedy Blvd. Suite 1800, Philadelphia, PA 19103-2899

Editor (Name and complete mailing address)

Kerry Holland, Elsevier, Inc., 1600 John F. Kennedy Blvd. Suite 1800, Philadelphia, PA 19103-2899

Managing Editor (Name and complete mailing address)

Catherine Bewick, Elsevier, Inc., 1600 John F. Kennedy Blvd. Suite 1800, Philadelphia, PA 19103-2899

10. Owner (Do not leave blank. If the publication is owned by a corporation, give the name and address of the corporation immediately followed by the names and addresses of all stockholders owning or holding 1 percent or more of the total amount of stock. If not owned by a corporation, give the names and addresses of the individual owners. If owned by a partnership or other unincorporated firm, give its name and address as well as those of each individual owner. If the publication is published by a nonprofit organization, give its name and address.)

Full Name	Complete Mailing Address
Wholly owned subsidiary of	4520 East-West Highway
Reed/Elsevier, US holdings	Bethesda, MD 20814

11. Known Bondholders, Mortgagees, and Other Security Holders Owning or Holding 1 Percent or More of Total Amount of Bonds, Mortgages, or Other Securities. If none, check box ☐ None

Full Name	Complete Mailing Address
N/A	

12. Tax Status (For completion by nonprofit organizations authorized to mail at nonprofit rates) (Check one)
The purpose, function, and nonprofit status of this organization and the exempt status for federal income tax purposes:
☐ Has Not Changed During Preceding 12 Months
☐ Has Changed During Preceding 12 Months (Publisher must submit explanation of change with this statement)

PS Form 3526, September 2007 (Page 1 of 3 (Instructions Page 3)) PSN 7530-01-000-9931 PRIVACY NOTICE: See our Privacy policy in www.usps.com

13. Publication Title	14. Issue Date for Circulation Data Below
Hematology/Oncology Clinics of North America	August 2009

15.	Extent and Nature of Circulation		Average No. Copies Each Issue During Preceding 12 Months	No. Copies of Single Issue Published Nearest to Filing Date
a.	Total Number of Copies (Net press run)		1981	1700
b. Paid Circulation (By Mail and Outside the Mail)	(1)	Mailed Outside-County Paid Subscriptions Stated on PS Form 3541. (Include paid distribution above nominal rate, advertiser's proof copies, and exchange copies)	701	628
	(2)	Mailed In-County Paid Subscriptions Stated on PS Form 3541 (Include paid distribution above nominal rate, advertiser's proof copies, and exchange copies)		
	(3)	Paid Distribution Outside the Mails Including Sales Through Dealers and Carriers, Street Vendors, Counter Sales, and Other Paid Distribution Outside USPS®	479	466
	(4)	Paid Distribution by Other Classes Mailed Through the USPS (e.g. First-Class Mail®)		
c.	Total Paid Distribution (Sum of 15b (1), (2), (3), and (4))	▶	1180	1094
d. Free or Nominal Rate Distribution (By Mail and Outside the Mail)	(1)	Free or Nominal Rate Outside-County Copies Included on PS Form 3541	137	137
	(2)	Free or Nominal Rate In-County Copies Included on PS Form 3541		
	(3)	Free or Nominal Rate Copies Mailed at Other Classes Through the USPS (e.g. First-Class Mail)		
	(4)	Free or Nominal Rate Distribution Outside the Mail (Carriers or other means)		
e.	Total Free or Nominal Rate Distribution (Sum of 15d (1), (2), (3) and (4)	▶	137	137
f.	Total Distribution (Sum of 15c and 15e)	▶	1317	1231
g.	Copies not Distributed (See instructions to publishers #4 (page 43))	▶	664	469
h.	Total (Sum of 15f and g)	▶	1981	1700
i.	Percent Paid (15c divided by 15f times 100)	▶	89.60%	88.87%

16. Publication of Statement of Ownership

☐ If the publication is a general publication, publication of this statement is required. Will be printed in the October 2009 issue of this publication.   ☐ Publication not required

17. Signature and Title of Editor, Publisher, Business Manager, or Owner	Date:
[signature]	September 15, 2009
Stephen R. Bushing – Subscription Service Coordinator	

I certify that all information furnished on this form is true and complete. I understand that anyone who furnishes false or misleading information on this form or who omits material or information requested on the form may be subject to criminal sanctions (including fines and imprisonment) and/or civil sanctions (including civil penalties).

PS Form 3526, September 2007 (Page 2 of 3)

Finish Strong.

Get a Superior USMLE Step 3 Score to Strengthen your Fellowship Applications

Step 3 CCS Bank + Question Bank:

- Be the best of the best with a superior CCS prep tool online!

- Use more than 1500 questions and 100 case simulations to get as close to the real test as possible

- Select cases by specialty, setting or topic to customize your experience

- Review question bank results by setting, problem/disease, clinical encounter, physician task, patient age

SUBSCRIBE TODAY TO SAVE 30%*

+ BONUS!

FREE Step 3 Scorrelator™ with purch of any Question Bank to see how your scores compare to others' USMLE Step and COMLEX Level III performance

NEW FRED V2 test interface for a more accurate simulation experier

Simple instructions to start boosting your scores:
1. Visit www.usmleconsult.com
2. Choose your Step, product and subscription length
3. Register or log in with your personal details
4. Activate discount code **CLINICS30** to calculate savings

DON'T FORGET!
USMLE Consult is MAC-compatible!!

Turn to USMLE Consult for the best remediation in the business!

Elsevier is the proud publisher of USMLE Consult, Adam Brochert's Crush Step 3, and The Clinics of North America.

* Activate discount code **CLINICS30** in the shopping cart to redeem savings. Offer includes all Step 3 products and all subscription lengths. Expires 12-31-2010.

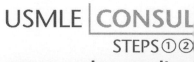

USMLE | CONSUL
STEPS ① ②
www.usmleconsult.co

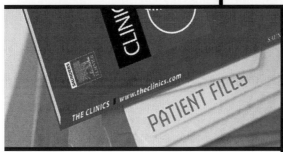

Moving?

Make sure your subscription moves with you!

To notify us of your new address, find your **Clinics Account Number** (located on your mailing label above your name), and contact customer service at:

Email: journalscustomerservice-usa@elsevier.com

800-654-2452 (subscribers in the U.S. & Canada)
314-447-8871 (subscribers outside of the U.S. & Canada)

Fax number: 314-447-8029

Elsevier Health Sciences Division
Subscription Customer Service
3251 Riverport Lane
Maryland Heights, MO 63043

*To ensure uninterrupted delivery of your subscription, please notify us at least 4 weeks in advance of move.

Printed and bound by CPI Group (UK) Ltd, Croydon, CR0 4YY

17/10/2024

01775303-0001